The Social Dimensions of Health and Health Care in Canada

Terrance J. Wade
Brock University

Ivy Lynn Bourgeault
University of Ottawa

Elena Neiterman
University of Toronto

PEARSON

Toronto

To my mother and father who were both far too young to be taken by cancer
TJW

To Lauren, Tyra and Adam Jutai for their inspiration and eternal patience.
ILB

To my family
EN

Acquisitions Editor: Matthew Christian
Marketing Manager: Christine Cozens
Program Manager: Madhu Ranadive
Project Managers: Madhu Ranadive and Marissa Lok
Development Editor: Cheryl Finch
Production Services: Rashmi Tickyani, Aptara®, Inc.

Permissions Project Manager: Kathryn O'Handley
Text Permissions Research: Varoon Deo-Singh, EPS
Photo Permissions Research: Dimple Bhorwal, Aptara®, Inc.
Cover Designer: Anthony Leung
Cover Image: Shutterstock

Credits and acknowledgments for material borrowed from other sources and reproduced, with permission, in this textbook appear on the appropriate page within the text.

If you purchased this book outside the United States or Canada, you should be aware that it has been imported without the approval of the publisher or the author.

Library and Archives Canada Cataloguing in Publication

Wade, Terrance J., author
The social dimensions of health and health care in Canada / Terrance J. Wade
(Dept. of Health Sciences, Brock University), Ivy Lynn
Bourgeault (University of Ottawa), Elena Neiterman (Department of Sociology, University of Totonto).

Includes bibliographical references and index.
ISBN 978-0-13-208811-4 (pbk.)

1. Social medicine—Canada.   2. Health—Social aspects—Canada.
I. Bourgeault, Ivy Lynn, -author   II. Neiterman, Elena, -author
III. Title.

RA418.3.C3W23 2014   306.4'610971   C2014-905809-8

10 9 8 7 6 5 4 3 2 1 [WC]

PEARSON

ISBN-13:   978-0-13-208811-4

Contents

8   Social Dimensions of Mental Illness   164

9   Social Dimensions of Aging, Health, and Care   190

10   Self Care and Health Care Behaviour   215

11   Health and Illness Experiences   235

Preface

Health is a central aspect of contemporary Canadian society. Health as a concept, however, has been very difficult to define, to conceptualize, and to measure. What does it mean to be "healthy"? Health can mean different things to different people at different times based on their culture, their age, their gender, and a multitude of other factors. Health to some could mean not being sick (i.e., a negative definition) while to others it may mean being able to do certain activities (i.e., a positive definition). People interpret health very differently depending on the context of their lives, which illustrates the social nature of health. Even people who have chronic diseases such as cancer or heart disease may see themselves as healthy, apart from their disease. So how do we begin to understand health? While the concept of health is discussed in detail in Chapter 1, it is informative to examine health more generally here.

The most common way to look at health and health research has been through the prevailing biomedical perspective. What do we mean by a biomedical perspective? First, a perspective is a way of looking at, interpreting, and evaluating the things around us. Each perspective makes certain assumptions about the world, and these assumptions filter observations in light of preconceived notions. As such, a person's perspective will influence his or her view of the world and the activities undertaken within it. The **biomedical perspective** of health and illness is rooted within the medical science enterprise, applying the tenets of science, including objectivity, logic, rationality, and cause and effect in a mechanistic fashion. This mechanistic-based perspective objectifies illness and disease, separating it from the person as well as the larger cultural, political, and social context. In this sense, an illness or disease is a physiological or biological deviation from what is defined as normal (Mishler et al., 1981). The deviation can be identified by the physician, assessed as to the cause, and then cured just as a mechanic fixes a car. The physician need not be concerned with the person, just the disease.

The biomedical perspective has been the dominant perspective in health and health research. This dominance is understandable because it has historically demonstrated a great deal of success in dealing with some diseases. It is limited, however, by its underlying assumptions and in its inability to fully understand some dimensions of health. Moving outside the biomedical perspective permits us to examine health and health care using different lenses to assess and challenge commonly held beliefs. To this end, this text largely employs a broader sociological perspective of health.

Sociology, as a scientific discipline, was defined in 1830 by Comte as being "[T]he science of society, social institutions, and social relationships; specifically: the systematic study of the development, structure, interaction, and collective behavior of organized groups of human beings".[†]

[†]By Permission. From Merriam-Webster's Collegiate® Dictionary, Eleventh Edition © 2014 by Merriam-Webster, Inc. (www.Merriam-Webster.com).

A **sociological perspective** (or a *sociological imagination*, as C. Wright Mills, 1959 coined) permits us to see how personal issues are connected to larger social and structural entities. Mills argues that a sociological imagination allows us to understand how personal troubles affecting people and those close to them, such as family (biography), are rooted in the past development (history) of the current arrangement of society (structure). For example, the death rate among younger cohorts is significantly higher among those who earn less income. Is this a personal trouble? Or are there some common factors among people in lower income brackets that sentence them to a shorter life expectancy? It is this ability to look past the *individualist* approach (personal troubles) where everyone is responsible for his or her own fate, to examine how the historical and structural organization of society may be a source of the problem.

The **sociology of health**, or medical sociology, is a subdiscipline of sociology that focuses on the systematic study of human society in relation to health, illness, and health care. It examines the social aspects of health and health care taking a broad perspective from society at large (the *macro* level) and institutions (the *meso* level) to individuals and relationships (the *micro* level). Although disease and death occur at the individual level, a sociological perspective allows us to identify associated social patterns at higher meso and macro levels; that is, how disease and death are differentially distributed across groups and what the reasons are for these differences.

Sociologists differ among themselves in their approach to health issues—they choose different theories, different areas of inquiry, and different methods of study. Looking at social structures and social conditions at the *macro* level, sociologists are interested in understanding the relationship between social conditions and health. Why, they may ask, are some countries healthier than others? What creates these health inequalities? At the *meso* level, sociologists study health and illness at the level of institutions. They might be interested in understanding the dynamics of the relationships in hospitals or explore how and why the health professions are gendered. At the *micro* level, sociologists examine how social interactions among individuals shape the experiences of health and illness. What meaning do people attach to the concepts of health and illness and how is this meaning created in communications with others? Although sociologists employ a number of different theoretical perspectives (or lenses) and methodologies to view and interpret the existence, prevalence, and lived experience of health and illness as well as the social organization of how health care is delivered and distributed across groups, the goal remains the same—to understand health and illness as social phenomena that are experienced and situated in society.

MEDICAL SOCIOLOGY AND THE SOCIOLOGY OF HEALTH

The origins of medical sociology are found in public health and social medicine initiatives in the nineteenth century that grew into a specific subfield from its parent discipline of sociology in the late 1940s (Bloom, 2002). Just as sociology is the study of the social causes of consequences of behaviour, medical sociology is the study of the social causes of illness and disease. The sociology of health moves beyond medical sociology to focus not only on disease but also on the social causes and consequences of health, health behaviours, and health care. Behaviour, in this sense, is a broad term encompassing individual behaviours and social interaction as well as institutional and societal behaviours and actions. Medical sociology and its evolution into a sociology of health has carved out its own niche from its parent discipline by focusing on the social conditions that help to promote well-being and disease prevention as well as those that cause illness and disease. To facilitate research and the interaction among researchers in the sociology of health in Canada and other countries, various academic associations have been established. (See Box P.1 on the Canadian Society for the Sociology of Health.)

A historical distinction within medical sociology is between the **sociology of medicine** and the **sociology in medicine**. First articulated by Robert Straus (1957), the sociology *of* medicine is oriented toward a better understanding of society or sociological concepts through the lens of health problems, medical settings, or the organization of health care. For example, Elliot Freidson (1970a, 1970b) presents the case that the medical field has laid claim to expertise on a broad array of behaviours, far beyond its demonstrated capacity to treat and cure. Through political lobbying, legislation, and other means, the medical field has taken over many behaviours that used to be in the domain of other institutions, such as the legal system and religion. Determinations such as being "not guilty by reason of insanity" redefine behaviours that were previously considered immoral as a sickness, beyond the control of the individual. It also moves these behaviours from the domain of the legal system to the medical system. Even the difficult or overly rambunctious child whose behaviour used to be defined as unruly and controlled

Box P.1

The Canadian Society for the Sociology of Health

The Canadian Society for the Sociology of Health/Société Canadienne de Sociologie de la Santé (CSSH/SCSS) is dedicated to the promotion of the sociological study of health, illness, and health care issues in Canada in both our official languages. The Society began in 2008 with the hosting of the Interim Conference of the Research Committee on Medical Sociology of the International Sociology Association in Montreal. This served as an important crystallizing event for Canadian medical sociology. The primary objectives of the CSSH/SCSS are to provide a bilingual venue to bring together Anglophone and Francophone medical sociologists to present cutting-edge research on a variety of critical topics, to advance the discipline and our understanding of health and health care issues in Canada, and to foster greater translation of the knowledge we create to key users to better address health issues in Canada and abroad.

For more information on the CSSC/SCSS, go to www.cssh-scss.ca

through behaviour adjustments and physical restraint is defined now as attention deficit hyperactivity disorder (ADHD) and is controlled through pharmacological restraint.

Alternatively, sociology *in* medicine is generally oriented toward a better understanding of health-related problems or the development of health policy and programs. Much of the work centred within a sociology-*in*-health perspective occurs in the health field where researchers examine the social causes of illness and disease. For example, children manifesting high levels of problem behaviour or diagnosed with ADHD are examined to attempt to understand the social factors associated with their behaviour. Such researchers reveal that various social institutions encountered across the lifecourse, including the family, school, and marriage, may explain why some people are hyperactive as children, become risk-takers as adolescents, and in some cases, criminals as adults (Sampson & Laub, 1993). This perspective also describes how the social environment of various groups leads to higher rates of depression and other mental health problems. Researchers have shown that persons in social positions that are associated with higher levels of social stress, be it at home or at work, are more likely to manifest depression and other mental health problems (Avison & Gotlib, 1994).

Although the distinction between a sociology *in* medicine and a sociology *of* medicine is important to make, it is not a clear dichotomy. Many sociologists examining health are engaged in both. Initially the work of some sociologists and social psychologists such as Erving Goffman (1963), David Rosenhan (1973), and Talcott Parsons (1951) took more of a sociology *of* medicine approach. Goffman examined how the label of mental illness was stigmatizing to persons, spoiling their identity and making them less worthy than *normal* people. Rosenhan examined how people can easily be involuntarily hospitalized and kept confined against their will in psychiatric hospitals by merely pretending to report symptoms that would be consistent with schizophrenia. Parsons examined how society relates to people who are sick by identifying a specific, agreed-upon role that these people play. However, the overwhelming majority of the work on the social aspects of illness and disease was done within the health system using a medically defined approach to examine how these diseases manifested and who was more likely to become sick.

Sociology is not the only social science to focus on health and health care, to understand health and illness as social phenomena. Other social scientific disciplines can help to inform various health and health care issues. Throughout the text, we will complement the sociological perspective with other disciplines such as psychology, demography, epidemiology, geography, political science, economics, and anthropology. For example, when we examine health care seeking behaviour (in Chapter 10) and aging and development (in Chapter 9), we discuss various psychological theories and models. In Chapter 10, we also examine some of the economic arguments for medical tourism, seeking medical care and procedures in other countries. Comparing these explanations with various sociological explanations provides a more thorough understanding of how our social world both influences and is influenced by health and health care. Even various medical subdisciplines can help to inform some of these debates. As such, we intentionally titled the book,

The Social Dimensions of Health and Health Care to embrace this larger "social" framework to complement the sociological perspective to examine various health and health care issues.

OBJECTIVES OF THIS TEXTBOOK

This preface presents a introduction to the importance of taking a *social dimensions* approach to health and health care. Since the social examination of health is such a large area, this text is structured in a way to provide the broad array of content in a coherent and comprehensible manner. The oversight and writing of the text as a whole was done by the three primary authors. However, since no one can be an expert in all things, various chapters are co-authored with experts in specific areas relevant to those topics. This ensures that a comprehensive coverage of topics is presented while the overall text maintains a consistently clear and fluid presentation.

The text is organized into 13 chapters. The first two chapters provide an overview of theoretical and methodological tools that cut across the thematic content areas presented in three overarching sections. Chapter 1 defines health and presents the theoretical perspectives commonly used in examining the social aspects of health. Chapter 2 presents methodological tools that provide us with a systematic manner in which to collect and evaluate information to help confirm or reject arguments consistent with various theoretical perspectives. These two introductory chapters will be most useful for those who may not be familiar with sociological theory or social research methods but will also provide a good review for others. With these tools, readers are prepared to begin the task of working through the thematic content areas.

We then shift our focus to the health care system in Canada. In Chapter 3, we examine the historical development of the Canadian health care system with a focus on policy and legislation. This provides a foundation for better understanding the current organization of the system. In Chapter 4, we explore professions within the health care system, its division of labour, and how various factors, such as training, professionalization, licensing, and credentialing, influence this division. Moving from professions, Chapter 5 focuses on the various institutions such as hospitals, nursing homes, and facilities for long-term care; their organization within the medical system; and how they influence the delivery of health care. We also examine the process of government decentralization and institution centralization through the regionalization of local health systems.

Next, we focus on population health and the social determinants of health. As discussed, health is generally thought of as an individual issue. In Chapter 6, we move from an individual perspective to a population perspective to discuss health. In doing so, we introduce the discipline of epidemiology and provide a look at the changing demographics of the Canadian population and examine patterns of mortality and life expectancy. Moving from this, in Chapter 7, we employ this population perspective to explore how social factors are associated with health disparities and examine how health and health care is disproportionately distributed across advantaged and disadvantaged groups. This perspective allows us to see past individual-level troubles to look at how health and illness are distributed across populations. In Chapters 8 and 9, we examine both mental health and aging as two key population health issues because of the important implications they have for Canada now and in the future.

Next, we examine how people experience health and illness and how they encounter the health care system. In Chapter 10, we examine health care seeking behaviour and why some people are more likely to seek care than others. From here, in Chapter 11 we attempt to understand the experience of health and illness. While having an illness can be a physiological experience, how people personally experience illness and how others treat people with various illnesses is very much influenced by social factors. Moreover, the definitions of what constitute illness and disease itself are open to much debate, which we will also describe here. In Chapter 12, we discuss the social factors that may play a role in the identification, definition, and treatment of what we label illness and disease. We also examine the role that institutions such as medicine and industries such as the pharmaceutical industry play in medicalization.

Finally, in Chapter 13, we discuss the social aspects of food and agriculture, an area of critical importance to health but relatively new to our discipline. Examining a variety of issues such as historical changes in food production and food consumption, and current health trends such as obesity and diabetes, we explore the connections between government, industry, and populations, and how these connections influence our consumption habits and, ultimately, our health.

Chapter Features

Each chapter begins with an outline to identify the topic of discussion. We present a list of objectives to orient readers as to the general themes and ideas that you should be able to take away from a specific chapter. It is helpful to keep these in mind as you work through the content. At the end of each chapter, these learning objectives are complemented by a series of critical thinking questions, a list of key terms, and suggestions for additional readings and resources, including reports, websites, and other media for further learning. The key terms are important in any research discipline since engaging in any new area of research is partly the ability to learn some of the jargon and key concepts. Finally, to complement each chapter, we include a series of information boxes and researcher profiles to add to and expand on specific content and to highlight some of the key historical and contemporary Canadian health researchers and their research programs. Although certainly not exhaustive, these information boxes and researcher profiles provide readers with a country-wide view of some of the important work that is being pursued by Canadian researchers and educates them as to the array of potential research opportunities across Canada.

To conclude, it is our intent to challenge readers to move past commonly held beliefs about health and health care to broaden their understanding of how our social world influences health and illness. In doing this, we introduce readers to a broad array of health and health care issues from different perspectives. We hope that students reading this book will walk away with a better understanding of the social influences on health and health care with a particular focus on the Canadian context.

KEY TERMS

Biomedical perspective—a mechanistic-based view that objectifies illness and disease based solely on physiological factors, separating it from the individual as well as from the larger cultural, political, and social context in which it occurs.

Sociological perspective—a perspective that examines how personal issues are patterned across groups and are connected to the larger social and structural organization of society.

Sociology in medicine—sociological inquiry that is generally oriented toward a better understanding of health-related problems or the development of health policy and programs.

Sociology of health—a subdiscipline of sociology that focuses on the systematic study of human society in relation to health and health care.

Sociology of medicine—sociological inquiry oriented toward understanding medical settings, the organization of health care, or the construction and definitions of disease through the lens of health problems.

FURTHER READINGS AND RESOURCES
Relevant Academic Journals

The following are useful journals where key articles in sociology of health, illness, and health care are published:

Health and Canadian Society—includes key social science and health articles with a Canadian context

International Journal of Health Services—particularly for studies from a materialist perspective

Journal of Health and Social Behavior—the American Sociological Association's flagship health journal, a general health journal focusing on all sociology of health areas

Research in the Sociology of Health Care—published once a year on key themes of sociology pertaining to health care

Social Science & Medicine—an international journal incorporating a variety of social scientific perspectives on health, illness, and health care

Sociology of Health and Illness—the journal of the British Medical Sociology group, leans more toward theoretical articles and those from a critical interactionist or constructionist perspective

Women & Health—focuses on studies of health, illness, and health care organization and provision from a feminist perspective, broadly defined

Relevant Websites

Canadian Society for the Sociology of Health (CSSH)
www.cssh-scss.ca/

American Sociological Association (ASA) – Medical Sociology Section
www2.asanet.org/medicalsociology/

Health Sociology group of The Australian Sociological Association
www.tasa.org.au/thematic-groups/groups/health/

Medical Sociology Group of the British Sociological Association
www.britsoc.co.uk/medical-sociology.aspx

Sociology of Health website
www.sociosite.net/topics/health.php

Society for the Study of Social Problems (SSSP)
www.sssp1.org/

SUPPLEMENTS

CourseSmart for Instructors

CourseSmart goes beyond traditional expectations—providing instant, online access to the textbooks and course materials you need at a lower cost for students. And even as students save money, you can save time and hassle with a digital eTextbook that allows you to search for the most relevant content at the very moment you need it. Whether it's evaluating textbooks or creating lecture notes to help students with difficult concepts, CourseSmart can make life a little easier. See how when you visit **www.coursesmart.com/instructors**.

CourseSmart for Students

CourseSmart goes beyond traditional expectations—providing instant, online access to the textbooks and course materials you need at an average savings of 60%. With instant access from any computer and the ability to search your text, you'll find the content you need quickly, no matter where you are. And with online tools such as highlighting and note-taking, you can save time and study efficiently. See all the benefits at **www.coursesmart.com/students**.

Learning Solutions Managers

Pearson's Learning Solutions Managers work with faculty and campus course designers to ensure that Pearson technology products, assessment tools, and online course materials are tailored to meet your specific needs. This highly qualified team is dedicated to helping schools take full advantage of a wide range of educational resources, by assisting in the integration of a variety of instructional materials and media formats. Your local Pearson Education sales representative can provide you with more details on this service program.

Pearson Custom Library

For enrollments of at least 25 students, you can create your own textbook by choosing the chapters that best suit your own course needs. To begin building your custom text, visit **www.pearsoncustomlibrary.com**. You may also work with a dedicated Pearson Custom editor to create your ideal text—publishing your own original content or mixing and matching Pearson content. Contact your local Pearson Representative to get started.

peerScholar

Firmly grounded in published research, peerScholar is a powerful online pedagogical tool that helps develop your students' critical and creative thinking skills. peerScholar facilitates this through the process of creation, evaluation and reflection. Working in stages, students begin by submitting a written assignment. peerScholar then circulates their work for others to review, a process that can be anonymous or not depending on your preference. Students receive peer feedback and evaluations immediately, reinforcing their learning and driving the development of higher-order thinking skills. Students can then re-submit revised work, again depending on your preference. Contact your Pearson Representative to learn more about peerScholar and the research behind it.

ACKNOWLEDGEMENTS

Health and health care is one subject about which every Canadian has strongly held opinions and beliefs. Oftentimes, if Canadians aren't talking about the weather, they are talking about their own health and health care experiences or those of their family and friends. People are eager to share these experiences and stories (especially their bad experiences and stories) and do so with a great deal of passion and emotion with anyone willing to listen. It is through these personal experiences and the stories from others that people form the basis of their opinions and beliefs about Canadian health care. While everyone is certainly entitled to their own views, in this text, it was our intent to make students challenge these personal opinions and beliefs in light of evidence to give them an opportunity to develop a better understanding of the issues surrounding health and health care in Canada.

The building of any textbook is a long journey. And with any journey, there are many people along the way who have had an influence on this project. This project originally stemmed from a textbook previously published by Gail Parry (nee Frankel), Mark Speechley, and Terrance Wade in 1996. We thank both Gail and Mark for allowing us to use some of that material in this textbook. The oversight and writing of the text as a whole was done by the three primary authors. Since no one can be an expert in all things, we enlisted co-authors with expertise in specific areas to assist as required. As such, we thank John Cairney (Chapter 8), Margaret Denton (Chapter 9), and Paul Millar (Chapter 13) for their valuable contributions to improve the overall quality and breadth of the material.

Thank you also to the following instructors who reviewed early versions of the manuscript: Seema Ahluwalia, Kwantlen Polytechnic University; Heather Bromberg, Carleton University; Weizhen Dong, University of Waterloo; Daniel S. Popowich, Mohawk College; Steven Prus, Carleton University; and Angela Aujla, Humber College.

We thank the editorial team at Pearson. There have been a number of people involved in the development of this project as we progressed, including Madhu Ranadive, Cheryl Finch, Joel Gladstone, Matthew Christian, Rashmi Tickyani, Ruth Chernia, and Susan Bindernagel.

Finally, we thank our students who, over the years, continue to show an intense enthusiasm, dedication, and passion toward the social dimensions of health and health care. It is both humbling and inspiring to witness their critical engagement with the material as they learn about how our social world is intimately tied to health. It is our sincere hope that we inspire future students who read this book to think more critically about health and health care as they reach out into the world in their future roles.

About the Authors

Terrance J. Wade, PhD, is a Professor in the Department of Health Sciences and the Department of Child and Youth Studies at Brock University. He is the past Canada Research Chair in Youth and Wellness as well as the past Chair of the Department of Health Sciences.

Ivy Lynn Bourgeault, PhD, is a Professor in the Institute of Population Health and the Telfer School of Management at the University of Ottawa and the Canadian Institutes of Health Research Chair in Gender, Work and Health Human Resources. She is also the Scientific Director of the Pan-Ontario Population Health Improvement Research Network, the Ontario Health Human Resource Research Network and the Pan Canadian Health Human Resources Network. She has garnered an international reputation for her research on health professions, health policy and women's health.

Elena Neiterman is a postdoctoral fellow in the Department of Sociology at the University of Toronto. Her research interests concern health and health care systems, aging, health care professions, and women's experiences of pregnancy and postpartum, and the interdisciplinary study of the body.

Chapter 1

Theoretical Tools for a Sociological Analysis of Health and Health Care

Chapter Outline

- **Learning Objectives**
- **Understanding Health as a Concept**
- **Multiple Perspectives in Health Research**
- **Structural Functionalism**
- **Materialism**

- **Feminism**
- **Antiracism and Postcolonialism**
- **Symbolic Interactionism and Social Constructionism**
- **Postmodernism**
- **Theoretical Interpretations of Health and Sickness**

Learning Objectives

After studying this chapter, you will be able to:

1. Define health, and differentiate between it and the related concepts of disease, illness, sickness, and wellness;

2. Identify, explain, and compare various sociological theories that have been used to examine health, illness, and health care;

3. Identify how various theories use a variety of levels of analysis, differentiating between macro-levels and micro-levels;

4. Use these theoretical tools to critically evaluate the different aspects of health and health care presented throughout the text.

In this chapter, we introduce how issues of health, illness, and health care are understood and conceptualized from a sociological perspective. We differentiate this perspective from the more traditional biomedical model for understanding health, and examine health as both a negative (less health/poor health) and positive (good health) phenomenon. We accomplish this by first defining *health* and differentiating it from some terms often used interchangeably with health, including *illness, disease, sickness,* and *wellness*. Next, we discuss various sociological theories that react to the biomedical perspective (as much as they react to each other) and how they are used in examining the broader social dimensions of health and health care. Although numerous books have been written on social theory, our discussion will include a brief overview to prepare readers to better understand and critically evaluate the ways in which health and health care are products of our social world. At the end of the chapter, we employ some of these theoretical tools to examine the social aspects of health and sickness and to illustrate how taking different perspectives informs our understanding.

UNDERSTANDING HEALTH AS A CONCEPT

When people talk about health, they usually couch it within the legacy of the mechanistic, biomedical perspective: health is based on the presence or absence of a disease or sickness. Individuals who have a disease cannot be defined as healthy, nor can they perceive themselves as healthy. But it is not quite so clear. There are many factors at both the individual and societal levels that affect health and your self-perception of being healthy. It depends on the comparison of your condition to others in similar circumstances (e.g., age), to yourself over time, and to your overall perceptions, given the presence of a health condition or disease. As such, health is very much based on the context of your life. When asked, many people with chronic health conditions rate themselves as being in good, very good, or excellent health. Similarly, people with a disability may rate their health as just as good as someone without a disability.

Perhaps the most recognized definition of health comes from the World Health Organization (WHO). The 1986 Ottawa Charter for Health Promotion reiterated the original WHO definition of health as a "state of complete physical, mental and social well-being, and not merely the absence of disease and infirmity" (WHO, 1986/1948, preamble). While this definition challenges the prevailing biomedical perspective, it presents an idealistic, and, some would argue, unattainable goal of health (Rootman & Raeburn, 1994). Rootman and Raeburn provide an alternative definition that is less idealistic and addresses some of the structural and environmental factors that influence our health status:

> Health . . . has to do with the bodily, mental, and social quality of life of people as determined in particular by psychological, societal, cultural, and policy dimensions. Health is . . . to be enhanced by sensible lifestyles and the equitable use of public and private resources to permit people to use their initiative individually and collectively to maintain and improve their own well-being, however they may define it. (p. 69)

Health, or being healthy, can also be seen as a state of obliviousness to one's body. We usually do not notice our bodies until we get sick. Only then, when we have difficulty performing routine activities, do we begin to regard ourselves as being unhealthy. This could be something as simple as a cold or flu or it could be something as serious as a diagnosis of cancer or heart disease. In the case of chronic health conditions, over time we recalibrate our self-perception of health, taking into account the new status of having a chronic illness (Charmaz, 1995). Finally, health and our perception of health are also influenced by external factors, such as the availability of health care or advertisements by pharmaceutical companies. For example, the pharmaceutical industry makes its money by convincing us that we need drugs to maintain and improve our health and to correct our deficits. Many of these external factors are discussed in depth in subsequent chapters.

To further complicate matters, any definition of health often overlaps with the concepts of sickness, disease, illness, and wellness. In fact, there are often tautologies in defining these various concepts. For example, health is thought of as not being ill, whereas illness is thought of as not being healthy. While it is difficult to differentiate between them, there are distinct nuances and differences that make it useful to make the attempt. **Health**, previously defined, is usually thought of as soundness in mind and body. **Illness**, often defined as the opposite of health, is a *feeling* of unsoundness, or that some problem exists. This is different from having a disease because the feeling may have no objective or scientific basis. **Disease** entails the *objective presence* and possible identification or validation of some deficit or mechanical issue that is usually biologically based (but not necessarily). Validation can take many forms, including medical tests to identify biological abnormalities or through a clinical assessment to identify a mental illness. You can have a disease but not feel ill, such as when someone has a cancer that has yet to be identified. But you can also feel ill with no objective basis. A visit to the physician may or may not validate your perception of illness as a clinical issue or a disease. The validation of an illness or the awareness of a disease would lead the person to being labelled "sick." As such, **sickness** is the combination of both the presence of an objective (validated) disease and the perception of being ill. A sickness, discussed in depth in Chapter 11, is where one legitimately assumes the role of a sick person with all of the benefits and responsibilities that come with that role.

Another related concept, **wellness** (and well-being), is considered more than just being of good health. Good health should be a necessary component for wellness, but wellness also infers a high quality of life and a satisfaction with living conditions (Bruhn et al., 1977; Rootman & Raeburn, 1994). Wellness implies an ability to thrive in life, to reach our desired goals, and to achieve a high level of life satisfaction and a sense of contentment. The concepts of health and wellness, and illness, disease, and sickness will be revisited several times as we proceed. Although in daily life we often use these concepts interchangeably when we discuss health and illness as the products of social life, it is important to understand the different meaning attached to each of these concepts. In the next section, we examine some of the various sociological theories that examine health and related concepts.

MULTIPLE PERSPECTIVES IN HEALTH RESEARCH

Before we proceed, here is some context. The ability to observe anything is conditioned and constrained by your perspective. It is akin to the parable of the blind men and the elephant. Some blind men were asked to describe an elephant. The blind man who felt its tail said an elephant is like a rope. The blind man who examined the leg said the elephant was like the trunk of a tree. A blind man examined the elephant's trunk and said it was like a snake. The blind man who felt the middle of the elephant described it as like a wall. The final blind man felt the ear and said it was like a fan. All described different features of an elephant and all were equally correct but by themselves only provided an incomplete piece of the picture. Taken together, the blind men provided a more complete description of what an elephant looks like.

In the same way, different theoretical perspectives make certain assumptions about the world—including the biomedical perspective—and these assumptions affect subsequent observations (Figure 1.1). Therefore you should be open to examining individual and organizational activities and behaviour from different points of view. None are necessarily right or wrong, nor are any better or worse. They simply present different perspectives by highlighting different aspects of the medical and social worlds. For example, some theories present a more societal view (macro-level) while others are focused more on the individual (micro-level). It is unimportant to debate which level of analysis—macro- or micro-—is most correct. What is relevant is that they are connected and complementary in our understanding. The tension between individual human action and self-determination (agency) versus the social structural constraints and opportunities placed upon individuals (structure) is very much a central debate in sociology (Giddens, 1984). It is useful to see how each permits different interpretations of the same social phenomena. It is the multi-layered perspectives that add strength to our ability as scholars to better understand health and health care. The key feature of each of these perspectives—to a greater or lesser extent—is how they each enable a critical analysis of common and often unquestioned assumptions of how society *is* and how society *ought to be*.

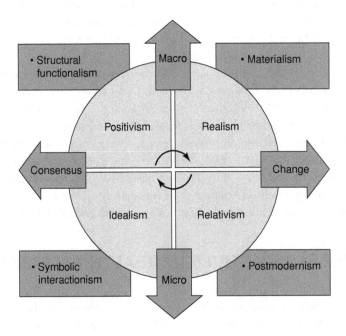

Figure 1.1 Assumptions of Different Theoretical Frameworks

STRUCTURAL FUNCTIONALISM

As a theoretical perspective, structural functionalism is based on the works of Emile Durkheim (1858–1917), highlighting the importance of social systems on individual behaviours. His classic work on suicide (Durkheim, 1897/1951) identified how social institutions such as religion and marriage explain variations in the rates of suicide among groups. His term **anomie** was used to identify those who are more likely to commit suicide because they felt alienated and less attached to their community. Similarly, Ratcliffe-Brown (1940) argued that the social structures in any society have essential functions for one another such that the continued existence of the one element is dependent on that of the others and for society as a whole.

If you think of the human body as a metaphor, all organs (structures) contribute specific roles (functions) for the survival of the body as a whole. Moreover, the body itself is defined as more than just the mere sum of the individual parts (organs, skeleton, and so on). It takes on a life of its own that strives at maintaining equilibrium or homeostasis. Without all organs working together, the body ceases to exist. Society then, as a body, has various parts (structures) that provide specific complementary functions that contribute to the overall survival and equilibrium of the whole. If something threatens the equilibrium of the body, it works to re-establish balance to ensure its overall survival. Just as the organs of the body work together fulfilling defined roles, so too in society people and institutions work together fulfilling specific social roles for the survival of the whole. The relationships among these various social roles and groups are necessary for the balance and overall survival of society (Lachmann, 1991). In this sense, the individual person *per se* does not matter; it is the social role that the person occupies that is important. Be it a doctor or a patient, a mother or a child, a pastor or a sinner, each social role provides a specific function for society. Each social role has commonly agreed-upon responsibilities and privileges. Each position has a certain value attached to it that provides it with more or less social worth and power.

Talcott Parsons (1902–1979) was instrumental in relating this particular theory to the social study of health. His work, *The Social System* (Parsons, 1951), theorized how the medical profession functions with a particular focus on the complementary roles of physicians and patients. He conceptualized the *sick role* as a deviation from people's functional normal social roles that threatened the status quo. To alleviate this threat to society, occupying the sick role came with an agreed-upon set of rights but also responsibilities for the individual. In order to re-establish equilibrium for the body (society), occupancy of this role permitted a temporary exemption, such as time off work, from the responsibilities of the other social roles an individual occupied. This exemption came with an obligation to do all a person could, including seeking and following medical advice, to try to get better so the sick person could return to his or her previous social roles. Necessarily, the counterpart to the sick role was the role of the physician who validates and legitimizes the sick condition and works at making the person healthy again to go back to his or her normal social roles. Discussed in depth in Chapter 11, the sick role has had a large impact on our understanding of the social dimensions of health and illness and has been the target of much criticism.

Although there are many critiques of the structural-functionalist paradigm, for our purposes, we focus on the distribution of power underlying the theoretical suppositions of the sick role and the overarching functionalist paradigm. For some, differential power across social roles is not functional because the organization of society is not based on consensus and equilibrium but rather on conflict over the distribution of scarce societal resources. In this sense, there are winners and losers in any competition, and to the victor go the spoils. This critique has come from two different theoretical perspectives: materialism and interactionism.

MATERIALISM

Referred to by some as *conflict theory*, *materialism* takes on a societal, macro-level of analysis consistent with structural functionalism. However, instead of assuming consensus and equilibrium, it argues that society is based on conflict and the differential distribution of power resulting in an inequitable allocation of scarce resources. The materialist perspective is based originally on the works of Karl Marx (1818–1883) and Friedrich Engels (1820–1895). Marx and Engels argued that modern industrial society is organized into two strata: the *capitalist class*, who own the means of production (land, labour, and **capital**) and the **proletariat**, who sell their labour. The capitalist class derives profit, or capital accumulation, from exploiting and separating labour from the value of the goods they produce. By paying labourers less than the value of what they produce, residual capital is siphoned off as profit for the capitalist. It is in the best interest of the capitalist to maximize profit by raising productivity levels and keeping wages as low as possible. This provides those owning the means of production and the wealth associated with that power with the ability to successfully lobby to form laws, policies, and regulations to maintain their privileged position at the expense of others. Class differences in health result from these social structural differences based on the competitive character of capitalism. Differences in health between the capitalist and proletariat classes are related to poverty, poor housing, and differential educational attainment. As Engels wrote,

> All conceivable evils are heaped upon the poor . . . They are given damp dwellings, cellar dens that are not waterproof from below or garrets that leak from above. . . . They are supplied bad, tattered, or rotten clothing, adulterated and indigestible food. They are exposed to the most exciting changes of mental condition, the most violent vibrations between hope and fear. . . . They are deprived of all enjoyments except sexual indulgence and drunkenness and are worked every day to the point of complete exhaustion of their mental and physical energies. (Engels, 1845/1987, p. 83)

Obviously the concepts of inequality, power, and control have consequences for both health and health care. The capitalist mode of production is a production mode for disease. Workers have less connection to their personal labour, have less say in the process, are exposed to more hazards and risks on the job, and benefit less from their participation. For example, black lung disease prevalent in coal miners (Smith, 1981), brown lung disease (*asbestosis*) prevalent among asbestos workers (Greenberg et al., 2005), and cuts and severed extremities prevalent with meat-packaging workers (Novek, Yassi, & Spiegel, 1990) are all hazards for labourers. Increasing the pace of work, demanding higher levels of productivity, and cutting expenses to maximize profit threaten safety and put workers at greater risk for accidents and disease. Vicente Navarro (1976, 1986), a contemporary Marxist theorist, argues that this capitalist mode of production also applies to the health care industry. Health care workers, especially those at lower levels of the hierarchy of professions, have an increased risk similar to workers in other industries. Pat and Hugh Armstrong (2002) argue that health care management strategies, in part a consequence of the private, for-profit sector, work to control costs through intensifying work, deskilling labour, and reducing safety standards. In addition to the adverse health impacts on the labour process of capitalist society, the driving down of wages and general economic inequality has also been shown to directly influence health.

While viewed by some as an overly simplistic portrayal of society, one of the outcomes of the historic materialist perspective is its elemental basis for the development of other theoretical perspectives such as *feminism* and *antiracism* that usurp its general framework but critically appraise its premise. That is, materialism provides the foundation for these theories to examine social cleavages but is also a target for the critiques levelled by these theoretical positions.

FEMINISM

For feminism, the primary social cleavage rests with the current system of **patriarchy**, the system of male domination in society, and the resulting gender inequality. Seen as both a theoretical perspective and a political movement, there are many variants of feminism with a diversity of viewpoints from micro- to macro-level analyses. However, all are based on the **lived experiences** of women and the institutionalization of their disadvantaged access to resources that other theoretical perspectives do not acknowledge. Dorothy Smith (1993), a Canadian feminist scholar, employs an institutional ethnographic approach to examine the link between the lived experience of women and what she refers to as the "relations of ruling" not afforded in theoretical perspectives previously discussed (see Researcher Profile 1.1).

Feminism has had important implications for the study of health and health care. One dominant focus of feminism has been on how so many aspects of women's lives and bodies have been *medicalized* and how this reflects the purported role of women within society. Feminist analyses have revealed how natural life events from pregnancy and childbirth (Katz Rothman, 1993; Oakley, 1980) to menopause (McCrea, 1983) have increasingly come under medical control, and they question the necessity of many biomedical interventions. Another key focus of feminist studies is the predicament of females in providing health care both formally (paid) and informally (unpaid)

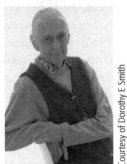

Courtesy of Dorothy E Smith

Dorothy Smith, born in England in 1926, completed her schooling at the London School of Economics and the University of California, Berkeley, receiving her PhD in 1963. She came to Canada in 1967 to the University of British Columbia (UBC), Vancouver. She has taught at UBC until 1977 when she moved to the Ontario Institute for Studies in Education (OISE). Upon retirement in 1994, Smith went to the University of Victoria.

During her undergraduate studies at the London School of Economics, she became fascinated with sociology. She has made many contributions to Canadian sociology and feminist scholarship publishing a number of books, including *The Everyday World as Problematic: A Feminist Sociology* in 1987, for which she received the 1990 Canadian Sociology and Anthropology Association (CSAA) Outstanding Contribution Award and the John Porter Book Award. Smith is best known for her work on standpoint feminist theory as well as the methodology of institutional ethnography.

(e.g., Reverby, 1987). Among the paid health care workforce, women are more prevalent in the lower paid and lower valued occupations. Even among medical doctors who are at the top of the health care hierarchy, females are more likely to be in lower-paid and lower-valued specializations such as primary health and obstetrics instead of orthopedics and surgery.

Feminist medical sociology links social structural aspects of patriarchy to the lived experience of women as both providers and recipients of care more explicitly than other sociological perspectives that examine health, illness, and health care. Some feminist scholars argue, however, that by treating all women as a universal group, it has neglected the differences among the subgroups of women, in particular working-class women and women of colour (Collins, 1990). This critique has also spurred the development of other cleavage-based social perspectives, including *antiracism* and *postcolonialism*.

ANTIRACISM AND POSTCOLONIALISM

As with feminism, antiracism is based on the belief that power and resources are unequally distributed in society through an institutionalized expression of prejudice and discrimination. The unequal distribution across racial lines is based on the historical organization of society (Dei, 1996). Consistent with this is the postcolonial perspective based on the historical relations between imperialist and colonized countries. It is connected to antiracism in that race is a principal differentiating characteristic between these groups of nations that results in the treatment of colonized populations as less worthy or less human (Castagna & Dei, 2000). Antiracism and postcolonialism perspectives are both relative newcomers to medical sociology, so their impact in the area of health and health care is still developing; however, they hold significant promise. For example, the destruction of traditional cultures and health practices among Aboriginal groups following European contact (Frideres, 1994; Ponting, 1997; Wotherspoon, 1994) has been linked to their poorer health and higher mortality rates. The systemic poverty and inadequate living standards of Aboriginal peoples is rooted in the historical context of colonization. An antiracist perspective also enables a better elucidation of the systematic racism experienced by internationally educated health professionals who come to Canada as immigrants (Nestel, 1996/1997).

SYMBOLIC INTERACTIONISM AND SOCIAL CONSTRUCTIONISM

Symbolic interactionism and social constructionism derive their theoretical roots from German **idealism**, American pragmatism, the interpretivist tradition that is evident in the works of Max Weber (1864–1920), and in the works of various scholars such as George Herbert Mead (1863–1931) and Charles Cooley (1864–1929) (Meltzer, Petras, & Reynolds, 1975). Max Weber, expanding on the historical materialist framework of Marx and Engels, added the importance of individuals and their active interactions within the structured organization of society. Weber, in his term **Verstehen**, referred to the importance of individuals in their interpretation and meaning of the social situation. The concept of the **definition of the situation** by W. I. Thomas (1863–1947) is perhaps most illustrative of symbolic interactionism as a perspective, that is, *if one defines a situation as real, then it is real in its consequences.* In this sense, the meaning of objects, events, and situations are subjective and actively defined by people through interaction and interpretation (Blumer, 1969). Contrary to materialism, interactionism suggests that actions taken by individuals are purposive and meaningful and not just dictated by the macro-structural forces within society. Employing this perspective, Becker and colleagues (1961) examined the process of medical socialization among doctors. Far from the more structural-functionalist account by Merton, Reader, and Kendall (1957), who saw medical training as mastering the skills and knowledge necessary to become a physician, Becker et al. (1961) saw medical socialization as a process of "getting through" the program, causing medical students to be cynical about their ability to cope with the vast knowledge and skills.

Erving Goffman (1922–1982), a Canadian-born sociologist, contributed to medical sociology by studying identity development of patients in mental asylums (Goffman, 1961). Such patients are removed from society, and much of their daily lives are controlled in a formal and regimented existence. Their self-identities become that of patients—they see themselves and are seen by others through the lens of their mental illnesses (Weitz, 1996). Analyzing how individuals deal with the identity that does not conform to social norms and regulations, Goffman advanced the concept of a spoiled identity and the stigma associated with it (Goffman, 1963). *Stigma*, Goffman described, is a discrediting of one's social identity based on our stereotypes of what individuals should be, with society labelling them as unworthy, different, evil, or less than human. Labelling can be based on physical characteristics, moral behaviour and character, or group membership. While these attributes in and of themselves may not be negative, such as having a physical disability, a mental illness, or malformation, it is in the relationship to others that label them as bad or deviant based on being different. In fact, among other groups or cultures, these same attributes may be defined as positive, indicating that labelling and stigma are socially localized, rooted in both time and place (see Researcher Profile 1.2).

If we recognize that the same condition or feature can be perceived as good or bad in different cultures and that the definition is actually dependent on cultural beliefs and social norms, then the objective nature of any condition or feature can be challenged. This is a major assumption for the social constuctionist theory that moved symbolic interactionism even further by questioning supposedly self-evident truths

Researcher Profile 1.2

Erving Goffman

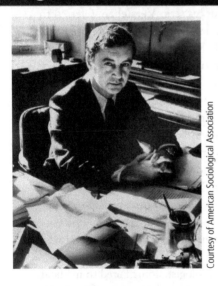

Courtesy of American Sociological Association

Erving Goffman (1922–1982) was born in Mannville, Alberta (half way between Edmonton and Lloydminster). He studied sociology and anthropology at the University of Toronto, graduating with a Bachelor degree. From there, he continued his studies at the University of Chicago, completing his PhD in Sociology in 1953. Aside from working at the National Institute of Mental Health in Bethesda, Maryland, he held academic appointments at the University of California, Berkeley, and the University of Pennsylvania.

He developed the dramaturgical approach that analyzes social interactions as a staged play in his book, *The Presentation of Self in Everyday Life* (1959). While his sociological accomplishments are many, he is probably best remembered for his work on mental illness, where he created the concept of the *spoiled identity*, which was instrumental for labelling theory, in his publications *Asylums* (1961) and *Stigma: Notes on the Management of Spoiled Identity* (1963).

and facts that people commonly take for granted. Berger and Luckmann (1966), pioneers in this perspective, argued that facts are created through social interaction and the interpretation of these interactions. According to this perspective, illness does not exist in any objective sense but only in so far as it serves a purpose for those defining it. That is, illnesses—and psychiatric illnesses are particularly prone to this criticism—are socially created political successes that are advantageous for the group creating the illness category. The group creating the illness category benefits by claiming ownership over certain behaviours because it creates both a domain of practice and their control over it.

Working under the social constructionist perspective, researchers examined the emergence of many sicknesses, including ADHD, erectile dysfunction, mental illness, alcoholism, and various other conditions (Conrad, 2007). The goal of their analyses is not to dispute the existence of these conditions but to understand how and under what social circumstances they have come to be defined as sicknesses that can be diagnosed and treated by medical doctors (Conrad, 2007).

POSTMODERNISM

Often associated with Michel Foucault, Jacques Derrida, and Jean Baudrillard, postmodernism, or poststructuralism, critiques any attempt to explain the organization of society in macro-level terms. Instead, subjectivism, **relativism**, and pluralism are principal tenets; truth and knowledge cannot be absolute across time or space. Foucault's work, and Turner's presentation of it, is perhaps most relevant for a sociological analysis of health. Turner argues that changes in language and discourse over time toward things like mental illness and sexuality have been the primary manner in which the medical profession has been able to exert more and more control over the body (Cockerham & Ritchey, 1997), or what Turner (1992) coined *the government of the body*. Disease is not a natural event but exists only within medical discourse (Turner, 1995). Expanding medical discourse into broad areas of everyday life results in extending the control of medicine over behaviours that become redefined within a health and illness framework. Health, wellness, illness, and sickness become the new morality in which to evaluate others (Turner, 1995). For example, for most religions and cultures, homosexuality is a sin. But in the United States and Canada as well as most Western, secular societies, it was redefined as a psychiatric disorder in the 1968 edition of the *Diagnostic and Statistical Manual of Mental Disorders* (DSM-II, American Psychiatric Association, 1968), the principal psychiatric clinical guide for the American Psychiatric Association. In subsequent editions of the DSM (DSM-III onward), homosexuality was delisted and is now defined as a sexual preference or lifestyle by the medical community. Another example is obesity. Historically perceived as a display of wealth and affluence, it is now thought of as a medical condition that requires interventions ranging from physical activity and dieting to medical procedures such as gastric banding or stomach stapling. And now people evaluate the worth and morality of others negatively based solely on excessive body weight. Postmodernism, then, can help to bring a different focus on the consequences of how the body is defined and analyzed complementing other disciplines such as feminism in further understanding the **medicalization** of women's bodies.

THEORETICAL INTERPRETATIONS OF HEALTH AND SICKNESS

We have provided a thorough description of some sociological theories used in health research. As tools, these perspectives are used throughout the text to assist in interpreting various social aspects of health and health care differently depending on your perspective. In this section, we examine the related social components of health and sickness in relation to various theories as a primer.

From a structural-functional perspective, health and sickness are measured by the ability to fulfill one's regular social roles. Being labelled as sick would necessitate the person to move into the sick role. But in order to move into this role, there must be some legitimate validation to exempt the sick person from his or her usual roles and responsibilities. Traditionally, a physician authorizes this validation. Once the patient has improved, he or she would be expected to resume his or her regular social roles.

Within an historical conflict or materialist perspective, being healthy would mean the ability to continue to work and produce value. Once a worker is unhealthy or unable to perform the work due to illness or injury, he or she is discarded and replaced by someone who can perform the tasks. There is no value in an unproductive worker as he or she reduces both productivity and profit. Moreover, the more an owner has to spend on the health and safety of workers, the lower the profits. Conflict arises because of the continual struggle between labourers and employers to improve health, safety, and standard of living for workers versus maximizing profits for employers. Another issue for health and sickness within the materialist perspective is the authority and power to validate sickness. To control the right to identify, validate, and treat disease and sickness both creates and maintains the inequitable societal distribution of power and resources.

From other theoretical perspectives such as social constructionism and symbolic interactionism, health depends on individual perceptions. Health will depend upon the subjective interpretation of one's body. In this case, the body is much greater than its mere physical components, incorporating other dimensions such as those included in the WHO definition of health stated earlier in this chapter. Moreover, lifestyle behaviours that are deemed to be unhealthy, such as smoking, will lead others to define and stigmatize people who engage in these acts. As such, a status of good versus poor health may be thrust upon individuals through stigmatizing of behaviours. This may facilitate efforts to control behaviours of others who are deemed to be unhealthy. Going even further, unhealthy behaviours such as smoking are redefined to be bad or even immoral, and those engaging in them become stigmatized and perceived as less worthy.

SUMMARY

Theoretical tools provide a means to view issues from a variety of angles (theoretical perspectives) to gain a more thorough understanding of them. Although health issues are broad and diffuse, and social researchers employ a wide variety of theoretical perspectives, they are united in their attempt to understand the studied phenomena, and to locate them within the social conditions, structure, meanings, context, and processes of society. There are multiple ways in which to interpret medical, health, and social phenomena. No one theory is correct or incorrect; rather they are tools to allow us to better contextualize health within contemporary society. Throughout the text, these perspectives will be juxtaposed against one another and against other prevailing perspectives, most notably the otherwise dominant biomedical perspective. Using this broad array of theoretical tools will enable a deeper level of understanding of the many social relations that are relevant to the study of health and illness. In the next chapter, we explore various methodological tools to provide us with a systematic manner in which to collect and evaluate information (evidence) to help support or challenge various theoretical perspectives used to understand and interpret social phenomena.

Key Terms

Anomie—the term used by Emile Durkheim to identify the feeling of social isolation, alienation, and detachment from society

Capital—financial, social, and cultural wealth that is predominantly accumulated by and concentrated within the higher social class in our society

Definition of the situation—also known as a W. I. Thomas (1863–1947) theorem. It suggests that if people define the situation as real, then it is real in its consequences.

Disease—the objective identification or medical validation of some deficit or mechanical issue that is usually biologically based (but not necessarily)

Health—usually thought of as soundness in mind and body

Idealism—school of thought that sees social life as only comprehensible through understanding the meaning that people attach to it

Illness—feeling of unsoundness, or the perception by someone that some problem exists

Lived experiences—an attempt to capture the day-to-day experiences of the participants in social (mostly qualitative) research

Medicalization—a process by which non-medical conditions become redefined and treated as medical

Patriarchy—domination of men over women that is embedded in social relations and social structures

Proletariat—individuals who have to sell their labour for money, also referred to as working class

Relativism—a school of thought that believes that it is impossible to grasp the existence of social reality independently of subjective influence of the observant and/or researcher

Sickness—the combination of both the presence of an objective (validated) disease and the perception of being ill

Verstehen—the term used by Max Weber to refer to the importance of meaning and interpretation that people attach to social phenomena

Wellness (well-being)—a high level of satisfaction and contentment with one's life and one's living conditions of which health would likely be an important component

Critical Thinking Questions

1. What is the utility of differentiating among health, disease, illness, sickness, and wellness from a "social dimensions of health" perspective?
2. Compare and contrast the underlying assumptions that guide macro-level theories and micro-level theories.
3. Discuss how a lifestyle behaviour such as smoking might be interpreted using different theoretical perspectives.

Further Readings and Resources

Albrecht, G. L., Fitzpatrick, R., & Scrimshaw, S. (Eds.) (2000). *Handbook of social studies in health and medicine.* Thousand Oaks, CA: Sage.

Canadian Institutes for Health Information (CIHI) (1999). *Health information roadmap: Beginning the journey.* Retrieved from www.cihi.ca

Scambler, G. (Ed.) (1987). *Sociological theory and medical sociology.* New York, NY: Tavistock.

Turner, B. (2004). *The new medical sociology: Social forms of health and illness.* New York, NY: Norton.

Chapter 2

Methodological Tools for a Sociological Analysis of Health, Illness, and Health Care

Chapter Outline

Learning Objectives

After studying this chapter, you will be able to:

1. Identify, describe, and compare the key components of quantitative and qualitative methodologies;

2. Connect these methodologies with theoretical perspectives presented previously to determine the appropriate study designs for research questions and to critically evaluate existing health research;

3. Explore the various health data collection initiatives by Statistics Canada and other agencies to see how they are being used to inform the national health and health care policy debate;

4. Advance a mixed-methods approach that attempts to bridge and combine quantitative and qualitative methodologies into a unifying methodological framework.

In this chapter, we move from a discussion of the various theoretical perspectives to discuss methodological tools used to examine the broader social dimensions of health and health care. Our discussion of these methodological techniques and issues deals with the basic tenets of both quantitative and qualitative approaches. Methodological tools complement our previous discussion on theoretical perspectives by equipping readers with an appreciation of the broader landscape of what is knowable about health, illness, and health care that a sociological lens affords. The methodological tools provide an understanding of the ways in which we can explore the extent of our knowledge using appropriate methods of inquiry to gather supporting and refuting evidence. In addition, we present a discussion of some recent government data used to evaluate population health, its distribution across groups, and the Canadian health care system. At the end of the chapter, we briefly discuss the use of a mixed methods strategy that integrates qualitative and quantitative methodologies in a complementary fashion.

METHODOLOGICAL TOOLS IN HEALTH RESEARCH

In this section, we provide an introduction to some pertinent methods of inquiry and methodological concepts that are employed in both health research and a critical sociological analysis of health research and health data. Principally, a **methodology** is a systematic approach of inquiry, or a structured process, to gather information and evidence to better understand a particular phenomenon. It is important, first, to be familiar with several key terms and approaches. A distinction is often made between *quantitative* and *qualitative* methods. Quantitative methods are based on numbers, statistics, and inference; qualitative methods are based on understanding, meaning, and interpretation. More often than not, qualitative methods are framed within symbolic interactionist, feminist, and antiracist approaches. Quantitative methods, by contrast, are more consistently framed within normative and realist approaches, including structural functionalism and some perspectives within contemporary materialism. Table 2.1 provides a comparison of quantitative and qualitative methods on some key criteria.

QUANTITATIVE RESEARCH METHODS

In general, quantitative methods investigate the differences or variation in something, or a **variable**, associated with or predicting variation in something else. Thus, the primary goal of these methods is to explain relationships among variables, ideally causal relationships that can be measured and counted. Some of the key assumptions of researchers who employ quantitative methodological approaches include that this is a reality (i.e., realism) that is largely agreed upon by societal members (normative), and that it can be analyzed (measured)—that is, separated into its constitutive components (i.e., reductionism). The objectivity of the research is critical and all aspects of the approach to research are usually determined beforehand and applied deductively. At times, however, ideas are generated from the data that lead to new and innovative avenues of research.

Table 2.1 A Comparison of Quantitative and Qualitative Research Methods

	Quantitative Methods	Qualitative Methods
Overall goal	To explain relationships, ideally causal, among variables that can be measured, counted, and controlled.	To provide insight into social phenomena and their context and meaning for various participants.
Data	Quantitative, in the form of numbers, categories, and statistics	Qualitative, in the form of words, such as descriptions of actions, pictures, and context
Theoretical assumptions	Realism, reductionism, and normative	Relativism, holism, and interpretive
Position of researcher	Objective: Researchers remain detached, measure variables precisely, and make careful observations using standardized techniques	Subjective: Researchers are the primary data gathering "instrument" and develop and maintain close personal interactions with participants
Process of inquiry	Usually deductive: Begin with theory, develop hypothesis, collect then analyze data, and confirm or disconfirm hypothesis and theory	Usually inductive: Begin with observation, data collection, and analysis concurrent; detect patterns and develop theory or hypothesis
Study Designs	All aspects of the study design are controlled and determined before data are collected. Key examples include experimental, quasi-experimental, and survey designs	Many aspects of the study design emerge during the data collection process; analysis occurs concurrently. Key examples include participant observation, in-depth interviews, and documentary analysis
Evaluation of Quality	Validity and reliability	Transferability and trustworthiness

Variables and Measurement

The predictor variable is referred to as the *independent* variable while the consequence or outcome is referred to as the *dependent* variable. As its root *vary* infers, a variable must have variation. For example, income can be an independent variable with the variation being lower and higher levels of income. This might be used to predict variation in another phenomenon such as age at death. Income and death are fairly clear examples of phenomena that are not difficult to define, measure, and interpret. Many other phenomena of interest in health research are more vague, abstract, and difficult to measure and conceptualize.

In the sociological study of health, we often look at various societal (macro-level), community (meso-level), and family and individual (micro-level) characteristics or concepts. Many of these concepts are difficult to define and measure. For example, we might look at societal cohesion, community connectedness, family functioning, or individual health-related quality of life (HRQL). What do we mean by these concepts? How would we go about defining them? How would we go about measuring them in order to examine relationships? This is a process that involves both theory and measurement. First, we need to conceptualize and define a concept or what we label a **theoretical construct**, such as Durkheim's construct of *anomie*, a person's connection to his or her community (discussed in the previous chapter). Second, we need to be able to decide what we could use to identify this abstract construct or operationalize it so we can actually observe it and measure it. **Operationalization** is the process of taking an abstract theoretical construct and defining it as an observable phenomenon in such a way that you can measure its presence or degree. Durkheim, for example, operationalized anomie through two measureable phenomena or variables, religion (being Catholic or Protestant) and marriage (being married or not). He found that Protestants were more likely to commit suicide than Catholics and that unmarried people were more likely to commit suicide than married people. From this, he concluded that people with a weaker connection or tie to their community (anomie, his theoretical construct), were more likely to commit suicide. Interestingly, he did this using previously collected data from secondary and administrative sources to identify patterns.

Box 2.1

Sources of Data

Data—both qualitative and quantitative—come from a variety of sources and can be grouped into three main categories, *primary*, *secondary*, and *tertiary*. In primary data, the researcher collects the data necessary for the study at that time. It can be exploratory—to further assist in understanding a topic—or it can be confirmatory—to test a given hypothesis. Secondary data is data that have been collected previously for another purpose. They can be anything that has been previously collected, such as but not limited to historical records (e.g., birth and death statistics, enactment of new laws), institutional administrative records (e.g., medical records), or surveys that were previously administered. Since these data were collected for another purpose, you must appraise them critically to ensure they will meet the current needs and are not biased based on the original intent of collection (Wade & Brannigan, 2010). In tertiary data, published research studies are examined to provide a synthesis of previous work either through a critical review or through a statistical analysis that pools the various correlations of studies together to assess an overall pattern of relationships. It is sometimes called a meta-analysis, or an *analysis of analyses* (Glass, 1976).

Validity and Reliability

The process of linking theoretical constructs to measureable observations is based on two related concepts: validity and reliability. While there are many ways in which the term validity is used in research, **validity**, simply, is how we know that we are actually measuring what it is we purport to measure. How valid or accurate is our measure or instrument? How valid was Durkheim's measure of anomie? That is, were religious affiliation and marriage an accurate way to concretely identify anomie? This type of validity is *construct* validity, that is, how well a measure links to the theoretical construct it purports to measure. Construct validity has been further broken down into *concurrent* validity and *predictive* validity. For example, an exam is routinely used to measure your grasp of the content in a course. How well the exam accurately measures your knowledge of the course material is an assessment of the exam's concurrent validity. Predictive validity could be thought of as how well a present measure predicts a person's success at something in the future. A common example is the Medical College Admissions Test (MCAT), used by many institutions as a way to select students for entry into medical school because it is thought to accurately predict future success in the program and as a physician.

Two other types of validity that are important in health research are *internal validity* and *external validity*. Internal validity, sometimes called experimental validity, refers to the ability to draw inferences from a difference or change in something that caused a difference or change in something else. This is framed as a **hypothesis**, a proposed relationship between an independent variable and a dependent variable. A hypothesis is usually informed by a theoretical perspective and is an educated guess of what is expected to happen to something if something else occurs. Internal validity is the level of certainty that we can discount that other things occurring may have caused the outcome instead of our predicted independent variable.

External validity is an assessment of how well an identified relationship between two variables would be applicable or generalizable to the larger group, population, or other populations and settings. It is based, in part, on how representative the people who participated in the study are of the target population of interest. One way that researchers achieve greater representativeness is to select a random sample from the population. A **sample** is simply a collection of individuals from a defined population that is used to gather research data that is then used to make inferences about that population. A **random sample** would be systematic selection of individuals from the population where everyone has a chance to be selected. Then, within a certain statistical margin of error, the results would be an accurate reflection of that population. For example, we are inundated by polls published in the media indicating that significantly more people are for or are against physician-assisted suicide, accompanied by the caveat that the results are accurate to within plus or minus some percentage, 19 times out of 20. This caveat is the statistical margin of error that makes the results more or less accurate of the expected views of the population.

Reliability is the ability to consistently measure the same construct across time, space, or persons. There are three different types of reliability that are commonly presented in health research. *Inter-rater reliability* refers to the consistency of measurement with different people doing the measuring. For example, the capability of different radiographers to diagnose a tumour from the same image would be inter-rater reliability. *Test-retest* is another type of reliability. This refers to the consistency of someone or something to measure the same construct over two or more points in time. Using the same example, it would be the likelihood that the same radiographer would come up with the same diagnosis using a subsequent image. Test-retest reliability does assume that nothing has happened in between time points that may affect the specific construct being measured, so it usually occurs in a short time frame. The final type of reliability is *inter-item reliability* (or internal consistency). One popular way to measure theoretical constructs is to develop a set of questions or items that accurately measure it. This set of items is commonly referred to as a measurement **instrument**. Since many theoretical constructs are nebulous, an instrument is the collection of items that cumulatively would provide an operational measure of the construct. Inter-item reliability refers to the consistency of single items in relation to the total scale. We will discuss measurement instruments more in subsequent chapters.

Study Designs

Experimental Study Design   The experiment is considered the strongest quantitative study design as it ensures the highest level of internal validity and provides the most stringent test of a hypothesis. The two inter-related components that make the experiment the "gold standard" of methods are randomization and experimental control. **Randomization** is a process of randomly assigning subjects into either the experimental group (those who receive the intervention) or the control group (those who do not). This process assumes that distributing people across the experimental group and control group at random will cancel out any differences that exist between individuals and groups. **Experimental control** keeps constant all other things that might influence the dependent variable across both the experimental group and the control group. This ensures that some extraneous factor cannot be identified as a competing cause of any effect as it would have been assumed to have happened equally across both groups. External validity, however, is often a challenge in an experimental design because experiments usually occur in very sterile, artificial environments where the researcher can control or keep constant everything except the predictor variable of interest. The real world is much more complex.

Quasi-Experimental Study Design   The **quasi-experiment** is an alternative study design that attempts to increase external validity while minimizing threats to internal validity. This design is often used to test the implementation of a program or policy in the "real world" that, by its nature, would be unable to ensure the same level of experimental control as an experiment. In this case, full randomization across groups is not always possible so a matched-group design is employed. A **matched-group design** would match individuals or groups across as many characteristics as needed and then randomly assign them into the intervention or comparison group. Evaluation of the consequence of the presence or absence of the intervention (independent variable) on a change in some observable outcome (dependent variable) would provide evidence for its effectiveness. Instead of experimental control, **statistical control** is used as a way to adjust for, or keep constant, the effect of other factors when examining the relationship between an independent variable and a dependent variable. Because this design can be more easily implemented in the community, its results can be more readily transferable back to the community. However, as a cost, one can never be certain that there is not some extraneous, yet unidentified factor responsible for any identified change in the dependent variable. As such, with any increase in external validity, there is always some decrease in internal validity.

Survey Study Design   One of the most prevalent quantitative methods used in health research is the survey. A **survey** is a compilation of a list of questions and instruments distributed to a population or sample of a population. While the survey is a study design separate and apart from others, it can also be used as a component of the experiment and quasi-experiment to measure various constructs. Surveys are a collection of questions that tap the phenomena of interest. Usually additional information is collected in surveys on other factors identified in previous research that may be important to be able to account for them.

Most surveys are **cross-sectional**, that is, they gather information on all variables at the same time. Analyses of cross-sectional survey data examine relationships as statistical associations instead of causal effects because the temporal ordering of variables is often uncertain. It may be obvious for some relationships as to which variable comes first, for example, the relationship between gender and depression. Overall females have rates of depression about twice that as males (see Chapter 8). It would make no sense to talk about depression causing a person's gender. For other statistical associations, however, the causal ordering is not so clear, which results in ranking surveys lower in internal validity. To assist with this, however, the surveyor's theoretical perspective can assist in interpreting the presumed direction of a statistical association.

With respect to external validity, depending upon how the sample was selected, surveys are representative of the population from which participants were selected. Sometimes, surveys are administered to the same people at multiple time points to be able to examine how a change in one factor over time may be associated with a change in another variable. These are called **longitudinal surveys**. This is often done in quasi-experimental studies where the researcher is interested in the effect of some intervention introduced to the experimental group. Longitudinal surveys provide a better ability to assess a temporal ordering between factors; however, most often the data on both variables are still collected at the same points in time. We will discuss this further in the section that introduces current health data collection initiatives by Statistics Canada.

Statistics Canada and Current National Health Surveys

Throughout the text, we will refer to results (usually done through secondary analyses) across existing Canadian national, regional, and provincial surveys as well as surveys from other countries. It is important to have an understanding of how the current Canadian population health surveillance surveys came into being and how they have informed debates regarding Canadian health and health care. Kendall and colleagues provide an excellent historical inventory of Canadian national and provincial health surveys from the first national community-level household survey in 1950 (Kendall, Lipskie, & MacEachern, 1997). The 1950 Canadian Sickness Survey was funded by the Department of National Health and Welfare and implemented by the Dominion Bureau of Statistics (now called Statistics Canada). Several surveys have been conducted since that time, including, but not limited to, several General Social Surveys (GSS), the 1976 Canada Health Survey (CHS), the 1981 Canada Fitness Survey, the 1988 Campbell Survey on Well-Being, and the 1992 Canadian Heart Health Survey. The provinces and territories have also implemented many health surveys starting in 1977. Most of these surveys are still available for analysis and provide the ability to track changing health and health utilization patterns of our nation.

In 1994, Statistics Canada initiated two national longitudinal surveys representative of all provinces, the National Longitudinal Survey of Children and Youth (NLSCY) and the National Population Health Survey (NPHS). The NLSCY examined the developmental trajectories of 25 000 children from birth to 11, redoing the survey every two years as these children move into adulthood. Every two-year cycle, the survey recruits an additional sample of newborns to one-year-olds to replenish the survey among the younger cohorts. Respondents who answered the survey questions includes the person most knowledgeable (PMK) about the child (in most cases the mother) and the children themselves when they are 10 years and older.

The NPHS originally surveyed 17 628 persons aged 12 and older in 1994 and continues to re-interview them every two years. When someone dies, information from the death record gets added to the NPHS survey information. However, as there is no strategy to replenish respondents in the NPHS, it becomes less and less representative of the overall Canadian population with every cycle.

In a coordinated effort to complement these two longitudinal surveys, in 2000, Statistics Canada along with other federal government departments and provincial counterparts implemented the cross-sectional Canadian Community Health Survey (CCHS) initiative. Prior to 2007, the CCHS consisted of four two-part surveys completed every two years to provide an overall picture of the population health and the health system at a set time. The first part of each survey randomly sampled about 130 000 people and was large enough to inform and evaluate health policy at national, provincial, and smaller health-region levels. The second part randomly sampled about 35 000 people and focused on specific health issues, such as mental health (2001) or diet and physical activity (2003). In 2007, the data collection format for the CCHS changed to collect data annually from about 65 000 Canadians. This sample size is presumed to be a large enough sample to ensure the ability of accurate population estimates at the sub-provincial health-region level.

Why are these national health surveys important? These data allow researchers to examine health and health care at a national level without incurring the enormous costs involved with collecting primary data. Moreover, national data sets such as the NPHS, CCHS, and NLSCY permit researchers to make generalizations about the whole population, a problematic endeavour when trying to generalize from a local survey to other regions in Canada. In addition, the large numbers of respondents enable researchers to examine small subpopulations that are generally absent from most research studies. Finally, the longitudinal NPHS and NLSCY allow researchers to examine changes in health among individuals as they transition through their life stages. The ongoing CCHS allows researchers to examine patterns and changes in health and health care at a population level over time. For example, the NPHS and CCHS have enabled researchers to map out a national profile of mental illness in Canada that was not previously possible (cf. Cairney & Streiner, 2010). This will be elaborated on in Chapter 8 on mental health.

Many of these surveys, and thousands of others, are available for searching and data exploration and analysis through the Ontario Data Documentation, Extraction Service and Infrastructure (<odesi>) (see Box 2.2). In fact, <odesi> is one of the first data services with the capacity to search across thousands of datasets by key words (e.g., concepts, variables, etc.) to identify potential data sources to address research questions. It also provides a description of each survey and the technical survey methodologies used for them. This is an extremely novel and powerful tool for researchers and students.

Box 2.2

<odesi>
(Ontario Data Documentation, Extraction Service and Infrastructure)

"A data portal for researchers, teachers and students; inspiring, developing and supporting research excellence"

www.odesi.ca

<odesi> is a web-based service that permits data exploration, data extraction, and preliminary data analysis. Its innovative exploration capability provides the user with an ability to move past looking for specific surveys to instead search for keywords (variables) across all of the surveys in the collection. The extensive and continually expanding collection contains over 11 300 health, social science, and polling surveys, including surveys from a variety of producers such as Statistics Canada public-use surveys, Canadian Gallop, Ipsos Reid, and the Canadian Opinion Research Archive (CORA). Once a survey is identified, <odesi> provides access to general information such as who collected it and when, the content

of the survey, the population from which the survey comes, and any necessary sampling information. Moreover, it enables the researcher to conduct simple online analyses, including frequencies (a distribution of a single variable) and cross-tabulations (pattern between two variables) for preliminary research into various health issues. (In fact, some of the data presented in the next section and throughout subsequent chapters were acquired through <odesi>).

It also provides for the downloading of some survey data into statistical software formats (e.g., SAS, SPSS) for more sophisticated analyses. For surveys in its archive with more restricted accessibility, it provides information on where to go to seek permission to use and access the data. The website has an online tutorial for those interested in learning more about <odesi> and using it in their research.

QUALITATIVE METHODS

Qualitative research is more than simply the collection and analysis of data that are not easily reduced to numbers. It involves a systematic approach to better understanding social phenomena within their context and the meaning they hold for various participants. Indeed, the parable of the blind men and the elephant highlighted in the previous chapter is apropos to the relativism and appreciation of multiple realities of most qualitative researchers. Thus there is an affinity to qualitative approaches among those who approach the study of social phenomena as framed within idealism and relativism approaches, usually from a *symbolic interactionist, social constructivist,* or *intepretivist* perspective.

Qualitative researchers take on a more active and interpretive role in the research, appreciating their own subjectivity and influence on the research process. Indeed, the qualitative approach identifies the researcher as the key data-gathering instrument, though she or he is usually steered by an interview guide and perhaps also a preliminary conceptual framework. The data gathered is in the form of spoken or written text or other forms of expression such as photos, video, art, or song. Many aspects of the study design emerge or are otherwise constructed during the data collection process. As such, the study design often develops concurrently with the analysis. Unlike quantitative methods that generally follow more of a linear research process, qualitative approaches are more *iterative*, particularly when the tasks of data collection and analysis are involved. The term *writing as analysis* also indicates how the process of writing up research results occurs in a parallel fashion with the analysis process.

Qualitative Study Designs

Study designs that typically use quantitative data, specifically experiments, quasi-experiments, and surveys, can also collect qualitative data. The term "qualitative" not only applies to the form of data collected, but also to the researcher's approach to the research process. Some of the most noteworthy examples of qualitative approaches to data collection involve *participant observation, in-depth interviews,* and *documentary analysis.*

Participant Observation   Participant observation involves the simultaneous participation in and observation of a community or social phenomena. Data are collected in a naturalistic setting that is not manipulated by the researcher, with the purpose of providing thick or detailed descriptions of behaviour and how it is linked to particular situations. It is most often used in ethnographic types of qualitative research. Ethnographic approaches are derived from anthropology and traditionally focused on cultural beliefs and practices. **Ethnography** involves the close observation of, and often participation in, the social life of the group being researched. The researcher often assumes a learning role, that is, as an acceptable incompetent, to better understand and appreciate the context of the lives of the participants of particular social phenomenon.

In-Depth Interview   An in-depth interview can be undertaken concurrently with participant observation, but it can also occur without any observation component. The organization of the interviews can range from very structured to unstructured, with *semi-structured* interviews being most typical. In structured interviews, all of the questions are determined beforehand; *unstructured interviews* tend to follow a more conversational style. This latter form necessitates that the interviewer be very focused on the participants' responses to identify critical questions for follow up. It is not unusual for the first few interviews at the beginning of a study to be more unstructured with more structured interviews occurring towards the end—as the identification and analysis of key issues progress. Questions within structured or unstructured interviews can be either *open ended*—where the range of responses is not determined by the researcher—or *closed ended*, where the range of responses are determined by the researcher or where a simple "yes" or "no" answer is required. In-depth interviews that attempt to capture the day-to-day experiences of a participant are a key form of data collection in phenomenological research that is interested in the lived experiences of research participants. The researcher, in this case, must set aside her or his own beliefs, perceptions, and predispositions so as to better understand a phenomenon through the eyes of the participant.

Documentary Analysis   The final approach discussed here is another data collection strategy that can involve the analysis of text but can also be thought of more broadly as the analysis of any found artifacts. This could include photographs, audio or video files, artwork, and the like. The approach to the analysis of artifacts is not structured around any particular research objectives or questions, as is the case for interviews conducted or photographs taken specifically for research purposes. It is up to the researcher to create that structure through an analytic framework. The analysis of documents and other artifacts is typical of historical methods and policy analyses and, where possible, can also involve **key informant** interviews with important representatives and stakeholders involved in the policy or historical phenomenon being studied. These interviews differ somewhat from experiential interviews already discussed because the interview guide must be tailored to the unique perspective and information each key informant is able to provide.

Themes and Meaning

Meaning and understanding are essential concerns of all forms of qualitative research regardless of the design. To understand the meaning that people attach to a social phenomenon is the goal of symbolic interactionists (Blumer, 1969) and many other qualitative researchers. Max Weber, the father of symbolic interactionism, used the German term *Verstehen* [to understand, to know] (see Chapter 1) to capture the notion of the interpretive understanding of human interaction. The qualitative researcher is tasked with closely examining participants' words and actions to identify patterns of meaning, or *themes*, that emerge inductively from the data. This pattern recognition, or *content analysis*, requires the multiple readings of notes, transcripts, or text in a variety of different ways. Other techniques include *constant comparison* between and within participants' responses to create a more accurate and robust depiction of the phenomenon by those who most closely experience it. The researcher then organizes these themes, or clusters them, into broader categories to aid in the presentation of an account of the phenomenon.

In writing up qualitative research, the researcher presents these categories through representative examples of the themes in the participants' own words. This is often referred to as "staying close to the data."

Trustworthiness and Transferability

Quantitative methods are fundamentally concerned with issues of validity, reliability, and generalizability. Some argue that qualitative methods lack these metrics of research quality. However, others argue that these metrics do not apply to qualitative research because of the theoretical assumptions and the beliefs about the nature of social reality (Becker, 1970; Blumer, 1969). Because the theoretical assumptions of qualitative research differ from those of quantitative research, the concepts of validity and reliability need to be redefined for qualitative approaches (Table 2.1). Lincoln and Guba (1985), for example, argue qualitative research should be geared toward the trustworthiness of the researcher and the transferability of the findings. **Trustworthiness** is based on the *truth value*, which is the credibility of a particular study; **transferability** is the dependable *applicability* and *consistency* of the results beyond the bounds of the phenomenon studied to similar phenomenon among different people and settings. Although many are reluctant to accept trustworthiness as a criterion of the rigour of qualitative research, there are widely agreed-upon procedures to ensure the quality of qualitative research. For example, to better ensure transferability, qualitative researchers must provide sufficient detail of the research context and process (i.e., data collection, analysis, and interpretation) so the reader is able to decide whether the findings can justifiably be applied to the other setting (Shenton, 2004). The overall goal is essentially to assess whether the findings of a study are "worth paying attention to" (Lincoln & Guba, 1985).

MIXED METHODS

It is important not to overstate the boundaries between these two principal methodological approaches—quantitative and qualitative—as they are not as clear-cut as some suggest. Indeed, many researchers employ what is termed a "mixed-methods" approach that draws upon a combination of these methods to answer different layers or aspects of a social phenomenon using the most appropriate methodology. One method can complement another during the process of inquiry in an effort to provide a better or more thorough understanding of a social phenomenon in its totality. In general, mixed method designs are conceptually more complex because they must integrate different ways of conceptualizing social phenomenon as well as different ways of analyzing and integrating the data.

Grounded theory, an approach that moves in an inductive fashion from observation to theory development, is an example of a mixed-methods approach. While studying death and dying in a hospital setting, Glaser and Strauss pioneered the method by demonstrating how theory can be generated from the analysis of empirical data. By analyzing themes emerging from the data and comparing different analytical categories, they claimed it is possible to build a theory from the collected data (rather than to collect data to prove a theory—the traditional deductive approach) (Glaser & Strauss, 1967). Grounded theory is an iterative approach, moving from observation to theory development and back to observation to confirm or refine the theory. Observations can be made using a variety of quantitative and qualitative methods as the theory is developed, refined, and confirmed.

Some consider a mixed-methods approach as a distinctive methodology in and of itself because of the manner in which the methods and findings must be integrated into a whole. This depends, in part, on the manner in which the methods are mixed. A researcher could collect and analyze data using different methods either sequentially or concurrently in a more integrated manner. In fact, the ability to identify the same pattern across more than one methodology, known as **triangulation**, provides more strength to the findings and confidence in the results.

SUMMARY

This chapter provides a foundation on which to identify, evaluate, and compare various methodologies and research study designs commonly employed to examine the social dimensions of health and health care in Canada. It is important to realize that there are many methodologies used in health research, and while all are unified by the rigour of the investigators as they attempt to further our understanding of health, each study design has its strengths and limitations. All methodologies work in tandem with the various theoretical perspectives to examine and critical assess generally held societal beliefs and perceptions of health. While the theoretical tools provide a means to view issues from a variety of different angles (theoretical perspectives) to gain a more thorough understanding of topics, the methodological tools presented here provide the systematic techniques in which to collect and evaluate information to help confirm or reject derived hypotheses and commonly held beliefs. With these tools and the complementary theoretical tools presented in the last chapter, readers are prepared to explore a range of health and health care issues in Canada.

Key Terms

Control (including experimental control and statistical control)—keeping constant all other things that may provide an alternative explanation to the relationship between the independent variable and the dependent variable

Cross-sectional survey—the gathering of information on all variables at the same point in time

Ethnography—the close observation of and, often, participation in the social life of the group being researched

Grounded theory—an inductive approach at theory generation that moves from observation to theory development

Hypothesis—a proposed relationship between an independent variable and a dependent variable

Instrument (measurement instrument)—a set of questions or items that, when combined, accurately measure a theoretical construct

Key informants—important representatives and stakeholders involved in the policy or historical phenomenon being studied

Longitudinal survey—repeated surveys administered to the same people at multiple points in time to be able to more accurately examine change over time

Matched-group design—matching individuals or groups across as many characteristics as needed and then randomly assigning them into the intervention or comparison group

Methodology—a systematic approach of inquiry, or a structured process, to gather information and evidence on a specific phenomenon

Operationalization—the process of taking an abstract theoretical construct and defining it as an observable phenomenon, so that its presence or degree can be measured

Quasi-experiment—tests the implementation of a program or policy in the "real world"

Randomization—a process of randomly assigning subjects into either the experimental group or the control group in an effort to balance all extraneous factors

Random sample—a systematic selection of individuals from the population where everyone has a chance to be selected

Reliability—the ability to consistently measure the same construct across time, space, or persons

Sample—selection of individuals from a target population of interest

Survey—a compilation of a list of questions and instruments distributed to a population or sample of a population

Theoretical construct—conceptualized and defined concept of interest

Transferability—applicability of the results beyond the bounds of the project to similar phenomenon and settings

Triangulation—the use of two or more methodologies to examine the same phenomenon to demonstrate greater confidence in the overall findings

Trustworthiness—an assessment of the credibility of the findings of a particular study

Validity—the ability to measure what we actually intend to measure

Variable—a theoretical construct that has two or more values or categories

Critical Thinking Questions

1. Why is it important to understand the methods used to generate evidence?

2. What is the most appropriate study design in quantitative research to examine the social aspects of health and why?

3. Compare and contrast the concepts of validity and reliability used in quantitative research to the concepts of trustworthiness and transferability used in qualitative research.

4. Identify a health-related research topic of interest and discuss which methodological approach would be best to examine the topic.

Further Readings and Resources

Babbie, E. (2012). *The practice of social research*. Stamford, CT: Cengage Learning.

Bourgeault, I. Dingwall, R., de Vries, R. (2010). *The SAGE handbook of qualitative methods in health research*. Thousand Oaks, CA.: Sage.

Canadian Institute for Health Information (CIHI).
www.cihi.ca/

<odesi> (Ontario Data Documentation, Extraction Service and Infrastructure Initiative)
www.odesi.ca

Statistics Canada
www.statcan.gc.ca

Statistics Canada DLI (Data Library Initiative)
www.statcan.gc.ca/dli-idd/dli-idd-eng.htm

Chapter 3

The Development of the Canadian Health Care System

Chapter Outline

Learning Objectives

After studying this chapter, you will be able to:

1. Present a historical picture of the development of the current government-run, single-payer, Canadian health care system;

2. Discuss how various political forces, key stakeholders, and special interest groups shaped the current health care system;

3. Articulate the various federal initiatives that deal directly and indirectly with health and health services;

4. Frame the continuing discussions on health care reform, including privatization, in Canada, within the historical context of its development.

The Canadian Health Care system[1] constitutes the largest social service sector in the country. In the 1980s, it was the third-largest employer in Canada, next to manufacturing

---

[1] An earlier version of this chapter was published in Frankel, B. G., Speechley, M., & Wade, T. J. (1996). *The sociology of health and health care: A Canadian perspective*. Toronto: Copp Clark.

and trade (Iglehart, 1986). With the decline in the manufacturing sector in Canada over the past few decades, health care has become the second-largest industry after trade (Statistics Canada, 2012, October 5). The immense size and reliance upon public funds for support of a publicly funded health care system attract critical scrutiny, especially in times of fiscal pressures. Critical questions deal with the efficiency of the system, its cost-effectiveness, the distribution of its budget across services, and ways to improve the delivery of care. However, before we grapple with these questions, it is useful to examine the historical evolution of the current Canadian health care system.

We Canadians generally take our health care system for granted. When we go to the doctor or hospital, we expect to receive excellent care regardless of our ability to pay. This has not always been the case. In most provinces prior to the early 1960s, the health care system was very much a private system run like any business. If an individual did not have private health care insurance, he or she was asked to pay for services upon receipt. The cost of some care—emergency and complex medical procedures, chronic illness care, long-term care, pharmaceuticals, and so on—often resulted in financial ruin for a family. Canada has moved away from this "pay-as-you-go" structure to a system in which people are not "taxed" because they are in need of care.

This chapter provides a historical view of the development of the Canadian health care system from Confederation to today. It examines how various social and political forces moulded the system that exists today. Included is a detailed discussion of the legacy of the initial introduction of full public health insurance in Saskatchewan in 1962 and the resulting provincial doctors' strike. Finally, it discusses more recent developments at the federal, provincial, and judicial levels affecting the system and leading to change.

A timeline of the developments in health care in Canada is outlined in Box 3.1.

BEFORE MEDICARE

The original British North America Act (BNA, 1867) specified the jurisdiction of the federal and provincial governments with respect to health care. That is, according to the Constitution Act, 1982 that succeeded the BNA Act, the administration and delivery of health care is the responsibility of the provinces/territories (Section 92), whereas the federal government controls revenue transfers to the provinces (Health Canada, n.d.).

Since the beginning of the 1900s, groups had been advocating for some sort of public medical insurance program for Canadian citizens, with the strongest support traditionally being among labour and farming associations. For example, in 1914, the first municipal doctor plan in the country was introduced in Saskatchewan (Houston, 2002). In Ontario in 1914, when the Sarnia region was about to lose its only doctor, the community paid him a $1500 retainer to stay (Naylor, 1986). The practice of municipal contracts was the beginning of the Canadian movement toward public payment. Historically, the Canadian Medical Association (CMA) was against any type of intervention by the state, unless it had to do with the payment of bills for people who were unable to pay themselves. It maintained its **fee-for-service** practice, with a hierarchical fee scale based on patients' income. Seeing a threat to their autonomy after the initiation of the British health insurance system in 1912, the CMA cautioned the Canadian government to avoid such a program in this country.

During the latter stages of World War I, interest in health insurance in Canada became more widespread. In British Columbia, a major push for some sort of government health insurance system began, in part, because British Columbia suffered some of the worst labour tensions in Canada with health insurance being a particularly contentious issue. As well, with veterans returning home after the war, there was a call for an improvement in domestic conditions as a reward for overseas service. At the same time, an epidemic of Spanish influenza swept through British Columbia, claiming 3000 lives and affecting many more. In 1919, a provincial commission was established there to study the possibility of public health insurance. Such a program was seen as one possible way to reduce tensions in the province. The governing Liberals chose not to proceed with the insurance program because of fiscal concerns and the opposition of the British Columbia Medical Association (BCMA).

By the early 1920s, the Canadian economy was thriving and there was less interest in state-supported health insurance. The medical profession was prospering along with the rest of the economy. Physicians in British Columbia initiated a movement to extend Workers' Compensation Board Benefits to pay for the medical bills of injured workers, mainly because these displaced workers could not afford to pay for services themselves. The goal of is effort was to reduce revenue losses for physicians. In 1920–1921, the British Columbia Medical Association (BCMA) struck a deal with organized labour to underwrite these claims at two-thirds of the BCMA fee schedule. Both physicians and workers perceived this action was necessary, since fewer than 5% of industrial workers had any type of health insurance (Naylor, 1986, p. 47).

The worldwide economic collapse beginning in October, 1929 (beginning on 29 October, also called Black Friday) and the onset of the Great Depression saw unemployment in Canada reaching levels up to 30%. Many Canadians were unable to pay for the basic necessities of life with health care being further out of reach for more individuals. Remember that many social safety-net programs we take for granted today, including Employment Insurance (EI), welfare (social assistance), disability insurance, and the Canadian Pension Plan (CPP), did not exist. Many people relied on family, neighbours, and the local community for assistance.

Since many patients could not afford to pay for their health care, physicians, especially in British Columbia, Ontario, Alberta, and Saskatchewan, called for some sort of government supported health care insurance plan. This support by physician organizations for public health care was unprecedented and came about because their members too were affected, albeit indirectly, by the economic collapse. In 1933, finding little support for publicly funded health care from the provincial governments, the CMA met with then Prime Minister R. B. Bennett to make a plea for a national health insurance program.

Bennett sympathized with the position of the doctors, but refused to act, arguing that health care was strictly a provincial matter. This was the first and only time ever in which the CMA actively supported and promoted the development of a national public health insurance system in Canada.

Discussions returned to the provincial level and once again the major impetus for change took place in British Columbia. In 1935, the BCMA submitted a proposal to the provincial government that included many of the principles articulated earlier by the CMA (Naylor, 1986). A committee appointed by the BC government toured the province to obtain feedback on the proposed plan. As a result of what it heard, the committee altered the proposal and the BCMA rejected the revisions. One of the strongest criticisms by the BCMA of the revised plan was that physician payment was amended to be on a **capitation** model instead of the existing, and professionally supported, fee-for-service system. A capitation model provides a set payment on a per-patient basis or on a roster of patients, regardless of the number of doctor visits. Amid a great deal of opposition, the new bill including the capitation clause was passed in the BC legislature on March 31, 1935 (Naylor, 1986). The Liberal government of the day claimed that the bill would provide health insurance to more than 275 000 people of the province; the CMA argued that it left out over 100 000 of those who were truly in need of the coverage (Naylor, 1986).

Even though the bill passed in the house, its implementation was delayed. The delay was viewed as a victory by the physicians. In 1936, as the economy began to show signs of improvement, the BCMA maintained its strong resistance to the new legislation. At the same time, the political commitment of the sitting government to public health insurance began to waver (Naylor, 1986). With the approach of a provincial election, the Liberals decided to suspend implementation of the bill, and to call for a referendum on the issue. Again the physicians claimed victory. Against strong criticism from the BCMA and the business community, the legislation was submitted to a referendum during the 1937 provincial election. The plebiscite for public health insurance was supported by 59% of voters, and the Liberals were returned to office. Even with majority support from British Columbia voters and support from the opposition in the legislature (the Co-operative Commonwealth Federation [CCF]) and labour groups, health insurance was stalled in the legislature, ultimately leading to the demise of this health initiative.

Parallel to these political movements, developments in medical technology and science also had a major effect on the health care system during the 1930s and 1940s. The discovery of "magical" drugs such as sulphates and antibiotics as well as the dramatic progress in surgical techniques provided a new-found confidence in and respect for the medical community and the scientific basis of health care. These circumstances helped to maintain the dominance of the medical profession as the major force in the health care field, and accorded physicians considerable leverage over the future of health care delivery in Canada.

In 1940, the Rowell-Sirois Commission, struck to review the division of powers between Ottawa and the provinces, concluded that a national health insurance scheme might be an appropriate alternative to the current private system, but emphasized that administrative control should remain in provincial hands (Naylor, 1986). Even the CMA acknowledged that publicly funded health care was inevitable. In 1942 Jonathan Meakins, the CMA president, suggested this inevitability to members of the profession, but urged them to ensure that forthcoming legislation was tailored to their specifications. By that time, the CMA was involved in closed-door meetings with the federal government, meetings that profoundly influenced the Federal Advisory Committee on Health Insurance.

A final report was issued by the committee before the end of 1943. The economic feasibility of the plan was questioned by both the Department of Finance and the federal cabinet, and the plan was revised with input from the CMA. The revision was completed by the end of 1944, but its reading in the federal legislature was delayed by the governing Liberal party until after the election in 1945. After their re-election, the Liberals presented the final document to the provincial governments, but the two levels of government failed to agree on a mutually acceptable national health insurance program even though public support for the initiative remained high. A Gallup poll taken in 1944 found that over 80% of Canadians supported a government health insurance plan. This support was reaffirmed in another poll taken in 1949, in which respondents gave overwhelming support to the question: "Would you approve or disapprove of a national health plan whereby a flat monthly payment brought assurance of complete medical and hospital coverage by the federal government?" (Naylor, 1986, p. 135).

The next chapter of the story of the Canadian health care system was written in Saskatchewan. In the summer of 1944, Saskatchewan elected the Co-operative Commonwealth Federation (CCF) under the leadership of Tommy Douglas, the first "socialist" government to win power in North America. True to his election platform, Douglas promoted the development of Medicare in Saskatchewan. Based on his unrelenting effort, Saskatchewan led the way by implementing the first government-funded health care program in the 1940s. By January 1, 1945, a medical care plan on a fee-for-service basis was implemented across Saskatchewan that covered "2500 old age pensioners, recipients of mother's allowance, blind pensioners, and wards of the state" (Naylor, 1986, p. 138).

Refusing to stop there, the government implemented a pilot program in the Swift Current region to test the first universal hospital insurance plan. By 1947, two years after the federal failure, Saskatchewan established a universal hospital insurance program. By 1949, British Columbia followed Saskatchewan's lead with its own provincial hospital insurance plan and by 1950, two other provinces had followed suit (Houston, 2002).

In the 1950s, the general political climate in North America became much less favourable to state intervention. This turn against state involvement was, in part, a response to the McCarthy anti-Communist crusade in the United States and to the influence of the American Medical Association (AMA). In 1952, the public relations committee of the CMA launched a campaign to support alternatives to government-funded insurance from private enterprise. Not surprisingly, this campaign found a great deal of support in the business community.

Box 3.1

Timeline of Major Developments Affecting the Canadian Health Care System

1867   British North American Act (BNA Act) passed giving responsibilities for health care to pro-vincial governments for hospitals, asylums, and charitable institutions and to the federal government for marine hospitals and quarantine.

1884   National Sickness Insurance implemented in Germany under Bismarck

1912   Britain implemented the National Insurance Act of 1911 that established its first unemploy-ment benefit and national health insurance scheme

1914   First rural municipal health insurance plan introduced in Sarnia, Ontario, and in Saskatchewan

1919   British Columbia provincial committee established to study public health insurance

        Federal Department of Health created, removing health from the Department of Agriculture

1929   Beginning of the Great Depression of the 1930s

1933   Canadian Medical Association met with then-Prime Minister R. B. Bennett to make a plea for a national health insurance program

1935–37 British Columbia Insurance Act passed in provincial legislature and was subsequently supported by a provincial referendum but never implemented; a similar act in Alberta passed but also was not implemented

1940   Rowell-Sirois Commission recommended a national health insurance program as feasible

1944–45 Health insurance program based on Rowell-Sirois Commission proposed by Liberal govern-ment under Mackenzie King but failed to secure agreement from provinces

1945   Saskatchewan, under the CCF government, implemented pilot project for universal hospital insurance program in Swift Current region

1947   Saskatchewan implemented the first provincial universal hospital insurance program in Canada

1948   The federal government, through its *National Health Grants Program*, provides grants to provinces and territories for hospital and health care facility construction

1949   British Columbia, following the lead of Saskatchewan, implemented its own universal hospital insurance program

1957   Federal government passed the *Hospital Insurance and Diagnostic Services Act* (HIDS) based on the Saskatchewan model.

1958   HIDS implemented nationally by Diefenbaker's Progressive Conservative federal government

        BC, Alberta, Saskatchewan, Manitoba, and Newfoundland enter national HIDS agreement

1959   Ontario, Nova Scotia, New Brunswick, and Prince Edward Island enter HIDS agreement

1961   Quebec enters HIDS agreements and, for the first time in Canadian history, all Canadians are covered under a public hospital insurance program

(continued)

Box 3.1 *(Continued)*

Royal Commission on Health Services chaired by Mr. Justice Emmett Hall to study universal health insurance appointed by the federal government at the request of the CMA

Saskatchewan legislature passes the Saskatchewan Medical Care Act to provide universal health insurance to all residents of the province

1962   Saskatchewan Medical Care Act implemented providing universal health care coverage to all provincial citizens (July 1, 1962)

Saskatchewan physicians go on a three-week strike in an attempt to force the provincial government to rescind the Act (July 1—July 22, 1962)

1964   Royal Commission on Health Services final report recommends support for a Saskatchewan-based model of public health insurance for nation

1966   Federal Medical Care Act based on Saskatchewan model introduced in the House of Commons by the Lester B. Pearson Liberal government

1967   Medical Care Act passed in House of Commons

1968   British Columbia joins the National Medical Care Insurance Program (NMCIP)

1969   Alberta, Manitoba, Ontario, Nova Scotia, and Newfoundland join the NMCIP

1970   Quebec and Prince Edward Island join the NMCIP

1971   New Brunswick and Northwest Territories join the NMCIP

1972   Yukon Territory joins the NMCIP and for the first time in Canadian history, all Canadians are covered under universal health insurance program

1977   Federal government changes its financial commitment under the 1967 Medical Care Act from a 50/50 split with provinces to a system based on block grants and transfer payments based on the Gross National Product (GNP)

1979   Federal Conservatives appoint a Royal Commission on the current status (crisis) of the health care system to be chaired once again by Mr. Justice Emmett Hall.

1980   The Royal Commission recommends banning extra-billing practices

1983   Federal Government, under Pierre Elliot Trudeau's Liberals, introduce the Canada Health Act to Parliament to ban extra-billing practices by physicians, hospitals, and provinces through penalizing transfer payments

1984   The Canada Health Act banning user fees and extra billing passed

Saskatchewan, Manitoba, and Nova Scotia pass bills to eliminate extra-billing practices

1986   Ontario government introduces legislation to eliminate extra-billing practices and Ontario doctors go on an unsuccessful strike to oppose change

Federal Government, now under Brian Mulroney's Conservatives, reduce transfer payments to provinces in addition to previous ban on extra-billing, further compounding the financial pressure on provinces to maintain health insurance program; reductions in transfers continue until 1994

1994   Royal Commission established under the federal Liberal government by Prime Minister Jean Chrétien (National Forum on Health) to improve health systems and assess

Box 3.1 (*Continued*)

financial needs. Interestingly, this coincided with the beginning of the Federal government's cuts to address the federal deficit and Canada's reduced credit rating. The report was released in 1997.

Federal government implemented a coordinated, national population health surveillance initiative, including both the Canadian Institute for Health Information (CIHI) and the ongoing national health surveillance survey program

1995	Canadian Health and Social Transfer (CHST) federal funding mechanism for provinces further reduces health transfers and combines them for the first time with funding for social services.
2000	Establishment of the Canadian Institutes of Health Research (CIHR), successor to the Medical Research Council of Canada (MRC) and the National Health Research and Development Program (NHRDP)
2001	Royal Commission on the Future of Health Care in Canada was established, headed by Roy Romanow, former Premier of Saskatchewan.
2002	Two seminal (and some argue opposing) reports on the current state of health care in Canada are released: the Romanow Report based on the Royal Commission on the Future of Health Care in Canada, and the Kirby Report, which was the final report from the Senate Committee on Social Affairs
2003	First Ministers' Accord on Health Care Renewal
	Establishment of the Health Council of Canada to monitor Accord
	Canadian Patient Safety Institute established
2004	Liberal Prime Minister Paul Martin provides an additional $40 billion to provinces over 10 years and guarantees a 6% increase until 2016
2005	Establishment of the Public Health Agency of Canada as a result of the inquiry into the management of the SARS outbreak
2007	Establishment of the Mental Health Commission of Canada
2011	The new federal-provincial funding arrangement for health care mandated by the federal Conservative government to take effect after the expiry of the 2003 Health Accord
2013	Expiration of the First Ministers' Accord on Health Care Renewal
2014	Dissolution of the Health Council of Canada established to monitor the First Ministers' Accord on Health Care Renewal

NATIONAL MEDICARE IN CANADA

In 1957, the Federal Government unanimously passed the Hospital Insurance and Diagnostic Services Act (HIDS) based on the Saskatchewan model, paving the way for the entire country to adopt a government-funded hospital insurance plan (Health Canada, n.d.). The legislation provided for a 50/50 cost-sharing agreement between provinces and the federal government. John Diefenbaker and the Progressive Conservatives implemented the national health insurance program on July 1, 1958. In 1959, Ontario, Nova Scotia, New Brunswick, and Prince Edward Island joined the plan. With the entry of Quebec on January 1, 1961, all Canadians were covered under public hospital insurance. The 50/50 split in costs, in addition to federal grants established in 1948, funded a boom in construction of hospital and acute care centres across provinces that continued until the late 1970s when the federal government revised the cost-sharing arrangements.

Saskatchewan then turned its attention to fight for even greater health care coverage. The province began to press for a universal health care program for all residents. The plan met with resistance from the Saskatchewan College of Physicians and Surgeons (SCPS). As a delay tactic, the CMA requested a federal commission as a tactic to defuse the growing tension between the province of Saskatchewan and its physicians over the proposed universal health care plan. In 1961, the Royal Commission on Health Services, chaired by Mr. Justice Emmett Hall, was appointed by the federal government to study the concept of universal public health care insurance. Despite resistance from physicians and from some residents of the province who feared that the government plan would destroy their health care system, the Saskatchewan Medical Care Act was passed on November 17, 1961.

Members of the Saskatchewan Medical Association refused to cooperate with the province in the implementation of the new law. They argued that the legislation would turn physicians in the province into salaried servants of the state and would interfere in the doctor–patient relationship and the autonomy of physicians to provide appropriate care. Implementation was delayed until July 1, 1962, because of the lack of cooperation from the medical profession. Anticipating a strike from the doctors upon implementation, the Saskatchewan government secured replacement physicians from other provinces, Britain, and the United States to ensure a continuation of health care delivery in the province.

During the final days before the July 1 deadline, provincial physicians, with the support of the CMA, devised a strike plan. On July 1, 1962, the Act took effect and the majority of doctors closed their offices in protest. Some Saskatchewan doctors provided emergency service at hospitals, but only 35 of over 500 members of the Saskatchewan Medical Association actively practised under the Act. This number was augmented by the replacement physicians.

The striking physicians, with support of the press, managed to gain some public support for their position, but it remained problematic; they realized that the Saskatchewan public was expecting some sort of comprehensive public health insurance. The striking physicians and their supporters organized a rally on July 11, 1962, on the steps of the provincial legislature to show their strength in opposing the Act. Despite a great deal of publicity, the rally to demonstrate support for the striking physicians failed, drawing a crowd of less than 10% of how many had been expected. The physicians resumed negotiations with the province. The former made some concessions and the government agreed to some amendments, including a fee-for-service reimbursement structure and allowing

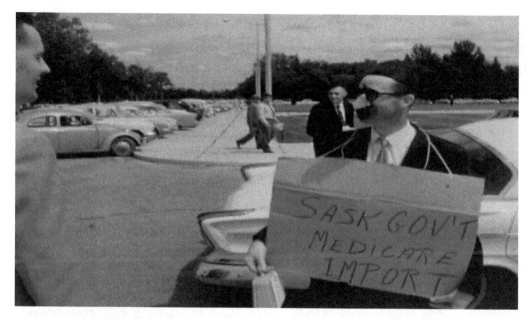

Figure 3.1 Protester Picture

This protestor of the Saskatchewan Medical Care Act depicts a stereotypically racist image—with a large nose and long ponytail—of the imported doctors whom the Saskatchewan government would allegedly recruit to replace striking physicians.

Source: The Canadian Broadcasting Corporation

individual physicians to opt out of the program and bill patients directly. The physicians began their return to work on July 23, 1962. Badgley and Wolfe (1967) wrote a detailed analysis of the Saskatchewan strike (see Researcher Profile 3.1).

Other provinces were examining alternatives to the Saskatchewan plan. Alberta, British Columbia, and Ontario considered working in conjunction with private insurance companies and using subsidies. Members of the medical profession endorsed the idea of multiple insurance carriers. Such a scheme would allow physicians to protect their fee structure since no single agency could exert sufficient power to control the market for their services (Starr, 1982). Because of initiatives subsequently undertaken by the federal government, this approach never really gained much currency in Canada.

In 1964, the Royal Commission on Health Services released its report. Although originally requested by physicians as an attempt to hold back the growing tide of public health insurance, the report supported the government plan whole-heartedly. The report recommended a wide-ranging health insurance program based on the Saskatchewan model, disagreeing with the contention of the CMA that any type of universal public insurance would erode the autonomy of practising physicians. Opposing most of the recommendations of the CMA, the commission did support a fee-for-service payment system and the dominance of the medical profession over competition from podiatric, optometric, and chiropractic services.

Robin Badgley

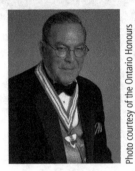

Photo courtesy of the Ontario Honours Awards Secretariat, Ontario Ministry of Citizenship, Immigration and International Trade

Robin Badgley (1931–2011) received his Masters' degree from McGill and his PhD from Yale. He began his formal career at the University of Saskatchewan in 1959. At that time the CCF government in the province was planning to introduce a government-run medical plan, the forerunner of Medicare. Badgley was a great proponent of Medicare and provided much needed support to the pro-Medicare movement. Badgley and Sam Wolfe, a physician from the United States, later wrote the famous and definitive analysis of the doctor's strike in their book, *Doctor's strike: Medical care and conflict in Saskatchewan*, published in 1967.

In 1968 Badgley became the founding chairman of the Department of Behavioural Science at the University of Toronto, the major initial task of which was to teach social sciences to medical students. He made the department a major national resource for social science and health research training a new generation of scholars in the social sciences and health area in Canada.

Badgley chaired two royal commissions, the first on the functioning of the law on abortions and the second on the sexual abuse of children and youth. He ended his formal university career in 1996 receiving the Order of Ontario in 2005, he continued to publish scholarly work until his death in 2011.

Source: Excerpted from the biography written by David Coburn for the Canadian Society for the Sociology of Health website www.cssh-scss.ca

The 1966 Medical Care Act

In 1964, the federal Liberal government of Lester B. Pearson recommended the creation of a national medical plan based on the Saskatchewan model. The plan was presented to the provinces in 1965 at a federal–provincial conference. Some of the provincial premiers viewed the proposal as an intrusion into provincial jurisdiction. There was even some trepidation within the Liberal party itself, but with a minority government and the New Democratic Party (NDP) holding the balance of power, the government was committed to see the Hall plan through to fruition. In 1966, the Medical Care Act, Bill C-227, was introduced in the federal House of Commons for its first reading.

The principles of the Medical Care Act of 1966 included:

1. **Universality**—one of the five principles of Canadian Medicare—guarantees health care coverage for all Canadian citizens regardless of age, condition, or ability to pay for service;

2. **Accessibility**—refers to the ability to access services regardless of geographic location or financial means;

3. **Comprehensiveness**—covers all necessary services provided in hospital or by physicians;

4. **Portability** across the provinces/territories; and

5. **Public administration** by a non-profit entity responsible to the provincial/territorial government.

As the bill moved to second and third reading, the CMA described it as a threat to the autonomy of physicians and as bringing to an end the traditional doctor–patient relationship. On December 8, 1967, by a vote of 177 to 2, the bill was passed by the Canadian parliament. The CMA warned that the legislation would impose difficult restrictions. The only part of the legislation the doctors supported was the opt-out clause that allowed physicians to bill their patients directly, leaving patients to seek reimbursement from the province (Blishen, 1991). In this way, physicians were not restricted to the provincial fee-schedule.

In 1968, British Columbia joined the National Medical Care Insurance program, followed in 1969 by Alberta, Manitoba, Ontario, Nova Scotia, and Newfoundland. In 1970, Quebec and Prince Edward Island joined. By 1972, when the Yukon Territory entered the plan, Canadians had universal health care coverage that was portable across the country. Under the plan, the federal government continued to share the costs of providing health care with the provinces, contributing about half the cost. While there is some debate as to the underlying political motive for implementing Medicare, it was now a national, universal program (see Box 3.2). (The term *Medicare* is unofficial in Canada, even though it is used on Health Canada's website. Our plan officially is the National Health Insurance Plan. Medicare is an official term only in the United States.)

By 1977, the federal government, finding the financial commitment of a fifty-fifty split too burdensome, revised the cost sharing arrangement with the provinces. Through the Federal-Provincial Fiscal Arrangements and Established Programmes Financing Act, the federal government changed the cost-sharing arrangement to a system based on block grants and transfer payments of personal and corporate taxes. This linked the financial commitment of the federal government to the growth of the Gross National Product (GNP), and created financial pressure for the provinces to meet the extra costs of a burgeoning medical system.

Interestingly, despite their outspoken opposition, the introduction of the Act increased the incomes of physicians immediately in seven of the ten provinces (Iglehart, 1986). However, physicians continued to express concern about the system. Over the next decade, with rising inflation and the continued dissatisfaction of physicians, the main focus for physician discontent was the right to extra-bill. The Medical Care Act gave physicians the right to bill patients directly but, sometimes, the amount they billed was in excess of what the provincial plan would reimburse the patient. Although limited in amount to the fee schedules negotiated by provincial medical associations, **extra-billing** was practised by over 20% of Canadian physicians. The argument by physicians was that extra-billing only helped them to recoup income lost to inflation and to provincial restrictions on fees. This did little to defuse growing public resistance toward extra-billing in the late 1970s (Blishen, 1991).

Two Views on Class and Medicare

There are two main positions regarding the conflicts and accommodations that led to the creation of the Canadian health care system. Swartz (1977) argued that it was a response to working-class pressure and a resolution of class conflict. This was reflected in the collective lobbying efforts of farmers and labourers in Saskatchewan to establish publicly funded hospital and medical care and the responsiveness of the social democratic party in power in the province over those years—the Cooperative Commonwealth Federation, which later evolved into the New Democratic Party. By way of contrast, Walters (1982) argues that there was little evidence of major class conflict or massive pressure by labour. One could equally interpret the accommodations made by the government as acting in the long-term interests of the capitalist class to increase the productive capacity of labour, to reduce the economic costs of illness, and to appease the working classes.

Whatever the case, there are two key outcomes of the negotiations to establish publicly funded health care in Canada. Medicare has helped to reduce the crippling financial burden of serious illness and to equalize access and utilization. However, these repercussions are far from equal in a system across such a large geographic area. A recent Alberta inquiry has also made it clear that there is considerable queue jumping through the utilization of social network ties.

Structurally, Medicare includes coverage of the costs of some of the most expensive forms of care—hospitals and physicians' services. There is little or no consistent coverage of extended health services that include residential long-term care, home care, adult residential care, and ambulatory health services across provinces. This leaves a much more fragmented and privatized system of health care for those in need of long-term care, which has a broad range of consequences for an aging population.

The accommodations made to establish Medicare in Canada serve to institutionalize, or as Larkin (1983) argued in the case of the British National Health Service, crystallize the status quo of medical dominance with doctors as the gatekeepers to access many aspects of the system. That is, there is a structural embeddedness of medical dominance in the various forms of legislation that govern health care (Bourgeault & Mulvale, 2006). With no comprehensive changes to the organization and delivery of health care, this increases the difficulty to implement changes to make the health care system more responsive to changing population health needs.

Source: Republished with permission of Wiley-Blackwell, from Canada: Healthcare Delivery System, Encyclopedia on Health and Illness. Excerpted from Bourgeault, I.L. (2014); permission conveyed through Copyright Clearance Center, Inc.

The 1984 Canada Health Act

In 1979, the federal government established another commission, this time to study the effects of extra-billing. The commission concluded that extra-billing by physicians along with hospital user charges (another form of extra-billing at an institutional level), posed a direct threat to the integrity of universal health care, because it eroded equal accessibility to health care. By this time, health care was a cherished Canadian institution. As a result of public support, the Liberal government under Pierre Trudeau used the extra-billing issue to gain voter support. In 1980, the government proposed compulsory arbitration to resolve fee-setting disputes between physicians and provincial ministries of health, a proposal rejected by the physicians. In 1983, with an election imminent, the Liberals made extra-billing an election issue. The proposed ban on extra-billing practices and hospital user fees was rejected by the CMA and by all the provinces. The CMA argued that such a ban would infringe on the professional rights of its members while the provinces reminded the federal government that health was a matter of provincial jurisdiction (Blishen, 1991). Still suffering from changes in federal-provincial transfers that had moved from a cost split to block grants based on GNP, some of the provinces saw extra-billing as a way to offset lost revenue.

Despite the rejection by the provinces and the CMA, the Liberals pursued their plan, introducing Bill C-94 to Parliament under the Minister of Health, the Honourable Monique Bégin (see Researcher Profile 3.2). The Canada Health Act banned extra-billing and punished provinces that did not comply by penalizing them one dollar in their block grant funding transfers for each dollar taken in by physicians and hospitals in extra-billing charges. The bill was also designed to reassert federal power over provincial health plans. The Progressive Conservative opposition under Brian Mulroney supported the physicians and the provinces, fighting unsuccessfully against the bill in committees and the house. Once the bill was submitted

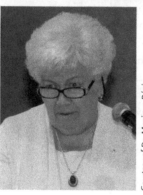

for final reading, the Progressive Conservatives voted unanimously to pass the bill, even though they opposed its principles. The fact that the bill passed unanimously in the house is a reflection of the mood of Canadians at the time, and the sensitivity of Canadian politicians to the voters in an election year. Since the Liberals had turned the Canada Health Act into an election issue and the Act had strong public support, the Conservatives were not willing to jeopardize their chances in the upcoming election by opposing it.

In response to the legislation, Saskatchewan, Manitoba, and Nova Scotia took immediate steps to eliminate extra-billing, which in Saskatchewan provoked rotating strikes by physicians. The resistance by physicians was greatest in Ontario (Iglehart, 1986). The Ontario government implemented legislation to prohibit extra-billing in that province on June 20, 1984. If extra-billing was not stopped by April, 1987, the province would be ineligible to "recoup the $4.4 million per month being withheld by the federal government as a consequence of physicians' use of the practice" (Iglehart, 1986, p. 208). The Ontario Medical Association (OMA) and the Ontario Liberal government could not agree on this issue. The OMA argued that it was a direct threat to their autonomy as professionals, and to demonstrate their opposition, most of the physicians in Ontario launched a two-day strike on May 29 and 30, 1984, refusing to perform any non-emergency services. Physician support for the OMA position was very high, but the support had no effect on the provincial government. On June 9, 1984, the OMA called on its 17 000 member physicians to strike once again on June 12. Only about half of the members responded to the strike call. Despite attempts to explain their side of the issue, there was little public support for the physicians. The overwhelming majority of people in Ontario approved of the ban on extra-billing and saw the strike as a fight over money as opposed to a fight over professionalism and autonomy. The strike ended 25 days later. The bill was passed in the Ontario provincial parliament by a vote of 69 to 47, ending the right of Ontario physicians to extra-bill.

The provinces, while required to eliminate extra-billing, were dealt another blow by the new federal government. After winning the 1984 federal election, the Progressive Conservatives, under the leadership of Brian Mulroney, during their first year in office reduced transfer payments to the provinces in an effort to address the growing fiscal deficit. This double-barrelled attack on block grant funding to provinces and health care funding specifically created a huge financial burden for the provinces, leaving them no way to recoup losses short of raising taxes or cutting services. (The law prohibiting extra-billing pertained only to government-insured services. Physicians and other health professionals were still able to bill patients directly for other services, such as medical notes and insurance forms, and continue to do so.)

RECENT DEVELOPMENTS IN HEALTH AND HEALTH CARE

Despite the central role that the federal government played in establishing universal Medicare, under the BNA Act, 1867, and continued under the Constitution Act, 1982, the federal government still does not have jurisdiction over the delivery of health care services to most Canadians. The only health care services falling under federal control focus on Aboriginal peoples, members of military services, new immigrants and refugees, and those in the federal penitentiary system. Other than that, the federal government *coordinates* the provision of health care and partially funds the system. The federal government has taken on additional roles in health, some of which are outlined in Box 3.3. Because of the historical distribution of responsibilities between the federal and provincial levels, provincial governments have considerable autonomy in all matters related to delivery of health care services, leading some scholars to suggest that Canada has not one, but 13 health care systems (Fierlbeck, 2011). Provinces have no *legal* obligation to adhere to the Canada Health Act of 1984. The only leverage that the federal government has to ensure adherence is the threat of financial penalty by reducing block transfer grants for a breach in the obligations outlined by the Act (Fierlbeck, 2011).

Box 3.3

Additional Federal Health Initiatives and Organizations

Although the federal government is only a funder for provincial health care, it does have an important role to play in health and health care in Canada. Specifically, it helps maintain the national health infrastructure, invests in research and development, and promotes public health initiatives. Due to the structure of the system existing across 13 jurisdictions, successive federal governments have implemented a number of initiatives in the past few years to facilitate the exchange of information and to invest in health promotion and public health.

Canadian Institute for Health Information (CIHI)

Until recently, health service information across jurisdictions was often scattered, and the standardized collection and exchange of information was not easy. To address this deficit, the Canadian Institute for Health Information (CIHI), a federal-provincial-territorial initiative, was established in 1994 as an independent, arms-length organization to facilitate the sharing and distribution of health utilization information. It collects, collates, and synthesizes Medicare data on billing, hospital

and physician visits, diagnoses, and so on for all billable claims across all jurisdictions. This provides information for the oversight of delivery of services across provinces and policy decisions.

National Health Surveillance Survey Initiative

Beginning in 1994, the federal government also initiated a coordinated, on-going, national population health surveillance initiative (discussed in detail in Chapter 2 on methodology) to collect and track Canadians' health status and health utilization based on self-report surveys. Before the survey, there was no coordinated, on-going national initiative to track health and health care at a population level. This survey initiative, in concert with CIHI, provides important population data to assess how changes to the health care system affect Canadians.

Canadian Institutes of Health Research (CIHR)

Created by legislation passed by Parliament in June, 2000, the Canadian Institutes of Health Research (CIHR) became the national funding

(continued)

Box 3.3 (*Continued*)

agency for health research in Canada. The focus of CIHR is based on four pillars of research: basic biomedical, clinical, population health, and health systems and services. It grew originally from the amalgamation of two previous national research funding agencies, MRC (Medical Research Council of Canada) and NHRDP (National Health and Research Development Program). One of its primary goals is to assist in the knowledge transfer of research into improving health and health services for Canadians.

Health Council of Canada (HCC)

Established by the First Ministers [the provincial and territorial Premiers and the Prime Minister of Canada] in 2003 through the First Ministers' Accord on Health Care Renewal, the HCC provides a coordinated voice to defend and strengthen health care in Canada. The Council's focus is on identifying innovative and best health care practices for health care improvement.

Public Health Agency of Canada (PHAC)

Another relatively new development in Canadian health care policy was the establishment of the Public Health Agency of Canada. During the 2003 SARS outbreak, it became evident that poor coordination of public health care can pose a very real threat. In 2005, the Public Health Agency of Canada was established to coordinate initiatives aiming to control the spread of infectious diseases, address health emergencies at a national level, and to promote health and reduce health inequalities.

Mental Health Commission of Canada (MHCC)

The 2006 Kirby Report on mental health, *Out of the Shadows at Last*, was the first comprehensive look at mental health status and health care services in Canada. The report made 118 recommendations on how to improve the current situation in mental health and called for a national, coordinated strategy to address the needs of Canadians (Standing Committee on Social Affairs, Science and Technology, 2006). As part of the recommendations in the report, in 2007 the federal government established the Mental Health Commission of Canada. The goals of the commission are (1) to develop a national mental health strategy; (2) to share the knowledge across provincial jurisdictions; and (3) to promote public campaigns that will fight the stigma attached to mental illness (Standing Committee on Social Affairs, Science and Technology, 2006). In 2009, the Commission published the very first Canadian mental health strategy (Mental Health Commission of Canada, 2009).

But the federal threat of financial penalty was beginning to lose its effectiveness. In 1986, 1989, and 1991 under the Conservative government, there were successive reductions in provincial transfers. As the national debt closed in on 72% of Canadian GDP with continued annual deficits, and in response to various credit downgrades by international credit rating agencies because of the increase in the Canadian national debt between 1992 and 1995, further budget cuts were implemented by the Liberal federal government under Jean Chrétien. The credit rating downgrades forced the hand of the government. Under the direction of Paul Martin as finance minister, in 1995 the government introduced a new block funding transfer mechanism, the Canadian Health and Social Transfer (CHST), to gain control over the country's fiscal problems. After severe spending cuts and some tax increases, the government successfully eliminated the federal deficit and began to run surpluses by 1998, reducing the accumulated national debt from about 72% of national GDP in 1995 to less than 50% a few years later. The reductions in transfer payments reduced the effect of the federal financial lever used to ensure provincial adherence to the Canada Health Act. Some provinces began to explore additional ways to reduce costs that flouted the Act, including privatization of some services.

National Forum on Health

In 1994, to address the ongoing concern over Medicare, Prime Minister Jean Chrétien established a National Forum on Health (NFH). It identified two important aspects for innovation in health care: (1) to improve health information systems and (2) to provide cash transfers to the provinces that would address their health needs. Released in 1997, it recommended funding for pharmacare and home care. As a result of the improved fiscal landscape in Canada, in 2000, the Liberal government negotiated a new health accord with the provinces to inject $23 billion dollars of new funding into health over five years (Rachlis, 2005). The government drew upon the 1997 NFH and targeted resources to help begin to refocus the health care system away from expensive, acute hospital care to home care, primary care, and diagnostics. However, there was little federal control over the funding in the first few years and much of it went to increases in salaries and physician fee-for-service schedules.

Royal Commission on the Future of Health Care in Canada

To address the funding directions, in 2001, the federal government and Governor General Adrienne Clarkson appointed Roy Romanow to head the Royal Commission on the Future of Health Care in Canada. This Royal Commission was an extensive, fact-finding mission costing over $15 million dollars and involving coast-to-coast-to-coast public consultation, expert hearings, contracted research, reports, presentations, and discussion papers. In 2002, the *Romanow Report* was released proposing widespread changes to the system to ensure both short- and long-term sustainability. Reaffirming the five principles of Medicare, it contained 47 recommendations addressing the federal–provincial fiscal relationship, its public nature, and the need to shift the system to address long-term, non-acute care based on three themes: the need for strong leadership and improved governance to keep Medicare a national asset; the need to make the system more responsive, efficient, and accountable to Canadians; and the need to make strategic investments over the short term to address priority concerns, as well as over the long term to place the system on a more sustainable footing (Romanow, 2002). While not opposing privatization directly, the report did recommend that diagnostic services (such as MRIs and CAT scans) be defined as medically necessary and be covered under the Act, and proposed that Workers' Compensation Boards be prohibited from purchasing medical services privately (Rachlis, 2005).

One of the specific recommendations of the *Romanow Report* for the creation of the Health Council of Canada was to depoliticize federal–provincial relations regarding health and to ensure monitoring, performance evaluation, and public accountability:

> To provide national leadership, the mandate of the Health Council of Canada should be to:
> - Act as an effective and impartial mechanism for the collection and analysis of data on the performance of the health care system;
> - Provide strategic advice and analysis to federal, provincial and territorial health ministers and deputy ministers on important and emerging policy issues; and
> - Seek ongoing input and advice from the public and stakeholders on strategic policy issues. (Romanow, 2002, p. 54)

Standing Senate Committee on Social Affairs, Science, and Technology (Kirby) Report

In addition to the Royal Commission, the federal Senate also produced a report to achieve a better coordination of health care services provided to Canadians, and to some degree re-establish the leadership of federal government in health care. The Standing Senate Committee on Social Affairs, Science, and Technology undertook to review the provision of health services in Canada. The Kirby Report, named after the chair of the commission, Michael Kirby, argued that the five principles of health care outlined in the 1984 Canada Health Act were not consistent with the two overarching federal objectives of health care, namely:

- To ensure that every Canadian has *timely* access to all medically necessary health services *regardless* of his or her ability to pay for those services.

- To ensure that *no* Canadian suffers *undue* financial hardship as a result of having to pay health care bills. (Standing Committee on Social Affairs, Science and Technology, 2006, pp. 307–308)

The Kirby report identified some of the gaps in the provision of health care services, including poor coordination of human resources and competition among provinces in planning and delivering health care services. Kirby recommended building a pan-Canadian health human resources strategy. The federal government was to take leadership in health human resources planning and work with the provinces to ensure that we have information about their human resources needs; that we train sufficient health care providers; that Canada addresses the health care needs of Aboriginal and remote/rural communities; and that there is better coordination in training and licensing of health care professionals. The report outlines that before any expansion of public funds for coverage of current gaps in services, such as pharmacare and homecare, additional principles need to be followed, specifically transparency and accountability. Moreover, it argues that there is an obligation to specify how any new program will be financed and that the government should not necessarily follow the "first dollar coverage" model, but keep the principle objectives in mind (Kirby, 2002). Some have criticized the report as opposing the Romanow report by supporting private health care. This criticism is based, in part, on Senator Kirby's business connections to private health care. (At the time, Senator Kirby was on the board of directors of Extendicare Inc., a for-profit health corporation that owns a major home-care division called ParaMed (McBane, 2002).)

First Ministers' Accord on Health Care Renewal

These two reports laid the groundwork for the subsequent 2003 First Ministers' Accord on Health Care Renewal. The Accord provided $34.8 billion in funding to the provinces over five years, even though there was debate between levels of government as to whether this constituted new money or some of it was money that had already been promised in the 2000 Accord (Rachlis, 2005). The 2003 Accord established federal–provincial priorities for the health care system and identified a number of areas in which the provision of health care services should be improved. While the needs of each province may have been somewhat different, all provinces were struggling to sustain their health care systems and improve the quality of health care. The Accord identified primary care, home care, and drug coverage as especially challenging issues, but it also highlighted the need to invest in diagnostic services and establish better information technology. Other important goals of the Accord were to establish a better system of communication among the provinces in setting the course for the health care system and to make the decision making in health care more transparent to the public. First Ministers agreed to produce annual reports, available to the public, in which they would use indicators that demonstrate how the health care systems are working and if they are achieving the established goals.

In 2004, the new Liberal Prime Minister Paul Martin promised an additional $42 billion over 10 years and a guarantee to increase health care spending by 6% until 2016/17 in the "10 Year Plan to Strengthen Health Care" (Health Canada, 2004). While there was fanfare about how this would address issues such as wait times and home care, there were very few restrictions on these additional monies. This agreement suffered from the same deficits as the previous 2000 and 2003 accords with respect to lack of accountability and transparency (Canadian Health Coalition, 2004). As such, it is questionable as to how much this new money, coupled with the previous accords, assisted in helping the system evolve to address the changing health care needs of Canadians versus retaining the status quo (Rachlis, 2005). The Canadian Health Coalition (2004) argued, moreover, that the new plan did not address the on-going move toward privatization of health care.

In the 2006 election, the new Conservative Party of Canada, under the leadership of Stephen Harper, won a minority government replacing the Liberals who had been in power since 1993. The Conservatives have remained in power since then, gaining a majority government in 2011. Stephen Harper had been an elected Member of Parliament (MP) for the Reform Party (which changed its name to the Canadian Alliance Party and then amalgamated with the Progressive Conservative Party to form the new Conservative Party of Canada in December, 2003) and also was the leader of the National Citizen's Coalition

(NCC), a conservative think tank, from 1998 to 2002. As leader of the NCC, Harper actively argued in support of private health care as a solution for problems with Medicare.

Changing Political Winds over Federal and Provincial Jurisdictions

The new governing Conservative Party changed the focus of the federal government. Whereas the Liberals dealt more with social programs, the Conservatives have focused more on tax cuts and crime, being careful not to step into provincial jurisdictions. Although the Conservatives have honoured the previous financial agreement of a 6% increase in spending until 2016/17, their approach to health care and federal–provincial negotiations has been quite different. In fact, in a First Ministers' meeting in December, 2011, instead of negotiating with Premiers as had been done in the past, the Federal Minister of Finance Jim Flaherty provided a non-negotiable provincial health care funding arrangement pegged at the economic growth rate of the country, but not to drop below 3%. Romanow criticized the new approach, arguing that the federal government was abandoning health care by not getting more involved in negotiations with the provinces to ensure the adherence to the 1984 Canada Health Act and its five principles (Romanow, 2012).

REFORMS AND THE FUTURE OF MEDICARE

The Canadian health care system is a source of pride for many Canadians, but it is also often criticized for being too expensive and unresponsive to people's needs. Many individuals are dissatisfied with long wait times and lack of access to certain services. In recent years, we increasingly hear the criticisms levelled against the Canadian health care system and the need to reform the system to be more cost-efficient and accessible.

These sentiments are reflective of a new vision of management of public health care systems that is rooted in the **New Public Management** reforms (NPM) implemented by the Thatcher Conservative government in the United Kingdom in the 1980s. The United Kingdom health care system, National Health Services (NHS), was established in 1948. Just like Canadians, most Britons are very proud of their health care system, but they were also concerned with raising health care costs. Seeking to reduce the spending on health care and make it more efficient, the NPM reforms introduced a new model of managing health care. These reforms adopted a businesslike model of management of health care services that sees the free market as the ideal set of relations that help to increase competition, to reduce costs, and to increase efficiency (Fierlbeck, 2011).

The NPM reforms identified three major routes for restructuring health care. First, it called for the detachment of policy making from health services delivery. Those who promote NPM see competition in service delivery as an essential step for reducing costs and providing services more efficiently. NPM reformers believed if two hospitals are competing for patients, the hospitals would have to strive to provide better services at reduced costs. The second goal of NPM was to establish a service delivery business model that highlights transparency and accountability. As with business, the health care sectors are expected to produce business plans and to develop a set of performance indicators that allow evaluation of the achievement of goals identified in the business plans. The final goal of NPM was to empower citizens as consumers of health care services. Citizens are expected to take an active part in health policy making and to participate in decision making related to health care policy (Fierlbeck, 2011).

The NPM resonated in many developed countries that were starting to look for ways to increase efficiency and reduce costs in health care and other social services. The cuts in health care services and other social programs are a hallmark of a *neoliberal* economy. Another hallmark is the adoption of a market model and market ideology in the provision of health care and social services. Canada has not been immune to those changes. When we discuss the health care system today, there is talk about "annual reports," "benchmarks," "performance indicators," "efficiency," "consumers," and "managers." Some argue that we have to privatize health care services or allow a two-tier health care system—one tier to provide free-of-charge services to Canadians and another to offer private services to those who can afford to pay for it (see Box 3.4 on a recent Canadian Supreme Court ruling on private services). Many provinces in Canada implemented the NPM approach to varying degrees and increased the amount of contracted-out health services based on the premise of cost savings. The provinces established the benchmarks for waiting times and compare these based on jointly agreed-upon performance indicators (such as waiting times in certain areas).

Box 3.4

Supreme Court Case for the Privatization of Health Care in Quebec and Canada

Chaoulli v. Quebec (Attorney General) [2005] 1 S.C.R. 791, 2005 SCC 35

In 1997, Jacques Chaoulli, a physician from Quebec, and his patient, George Zeliotis, who had to wait almost a year for his hip replacement, launched a case against Quebec's government. They claimed that a ban on private health insurance results in long waiting times for essential medical services (such as hip replacement), and ultimately, violates the constitutional rights of Canadian citizens.

The Quebec court, and later an appeal court, suggested that they did not see a violation of the constitutional rights by the ban on private insurance. Furthermore, the judges in Quebec saw this violation, even if it existed, as necessary for the benefit of all the people of Quebec who have a right to receive universal health care services. Appealed to the Supreme Court of Canada, and after much deliberation and testimony, the court ruled in favour of Chaoulli on violation of Quebec's Charter of Rights and Freedoms but was evenly split on any violation of Canadian Charter of Rights and Freedoms. The Supreme Court agreed with the claimants that the ban on private health insurance contributes to long waiting times, and thus, ultimately, violates the rights of Quebecers.

The proponents of privatization saw the Chaoulli case as a pioneering case for legalizing private

(continued)

Box 3.4 (*Continued*)

health insurance. Those who were critical of the decision referred to the language ambiguity of the ruling, which did not really "ban" the exclusive right of public insurance, but conditioned it on "adequate care and waiting times." The court never properly defined what actually constitutes "adequate care" (Fierlbeck, 2011). Moreover, since the ruling was framed in conditional terms (e.g. if/when . . . then), it was open for interpretation (e.g., If the provinces do not reduce waiting times, then it should provide private health insurance—but what if they do reduce waiting times?).

Another problem that critics saw in Chaoulli's case ruling was the assumption that private health insurance would actually reduce wait times. While some experts on health policy testified that was the case, other expert witnesses argued that a two-tier system (public and private health insurance) does not reduce waiting time, and can even increase it. Finally, the ruling of the court implied that the private health care system would benefit individuals who have the right to receive necessary medical treatment. Looking at the US, however, we witnessed that sick people are often denied medical coverage by private insurance companies. Moreover, when public health insurance is a viable option, private insurance principally benefits the wealthiest among the population.

Ironically, Mr. Zeliotis, an older man with limited means and serious medical conditions, would probably not benefit from the implementation of private insurance (Fierlbeck, 2011).

So far, however, the implications of the Chaoulli case have been minimal. Since the judges did not agree on whether or not there was a violation of Canadian Charter of Rights and Freedoms, the decision of the Supreme Court only concerns Quebec. Already working with other provinces on reduction of waiting times, Quebec released a statement guaranteeing reduced waiting times for certain treatments. It allowed the establishment of private insurance for some medical services but at the same time it prevented physicians from practising in public and private health care systems. Thus, if physicians decide to work for private sector, they would be unable to work for the public system as well (Fierlbeck, 2011). However, it is possible that the true implications of the case are yet to follow. In recent years, legal actions have been launched in British Columbia, Alberta, and Ontario to challenge the monopoly of public health insurance and the Chaoulli case is often cited in support of private health care in these matters.

Source: Chaoulli v. Quebec (Attorney General) [2005] 1 S.C.R. 791, 2005 SCC 35. Reproduced with the permission of the Supreme Court of Canada, 2013.

Whether these reforms are actually beneficial to our health care system is being hotly debated among scholars, politicians, and stakeholders. Some argue that these reforms will improve the health care systems while others see it as a move toward the privatization of health care services that will threaten public health care, the social solidarity of Canadians, and the safe working conditions of health care professionals (Armstrong & Armstrong, 2002; Fierlbeck, 2011; Gibson & Fuller, 2006). Robert Evans, one of the nation's leading health economists, argues that the recent push toward privatization is based on a series of myths regarding the efficiency, quality, and sustainability of the current system (see Box 3.5). The views of Canadians over the next decades might certainly change, but today the majority of Canadians see our publicly funded, universal health care system as an important part of Canadian identity.

Box 3.5

Current Myths about the Sustainability of Canadian Public Health Care

Myths	Facts
Our aging population will make health care unaffordable.	Private health care services, not an aging population, are driving health care spending. (Only 0.8% of increasing health care spending is due to an aging population. Private spending on services not covered such as prescription drugs, dental care, and home care is responsible for the increase.)
The cost of health care is eating up provincial budgets and crowding out other services.	Medicare spending takes up about the same share of provincial revenues as it did 20 years ago. (The drop in provincial revenues due to large tax cuts increases the percentage of health care on overall budgets.)
Public health care spending is skyrocketing and out of control.	Public health care spending is stable. Spending on private health care, as described above, is driving up costs. (From 1975 to 2009 Medicare spending has been stable, from 4 to 5% of GDP.)
Privatization of health services will control health care costs.	Public health care is the best way to control health care spending. Privatization is not sustainable. (Shifting from public to private spending shifts the cost burden from the wealthy to the sick. "Unsustainable" public spending cannot be magically sustainable when shifted from taxpayers to patients.)

Source: Evans, Robert. Sustainability of health care. Myths and Facts. Published by the Canadian Health Coalition, *Just the Facts* newsletter, June, 2010.

SUMMARY

One of the principal concerns expressed by physicians about a publicly administered health care system was that the profession would lose its ability to set fees. They viewed this as a first step in reducing the profession to the status of government employees, with no control over the labour process. Not only would such a status reduce their autonomy, it would also reduce their power within the system. Despite the sometimes intense opposition of the medical profession, none of the developments related to the implementation of the public system or the ban on extra-billing appear to have jeopardized professional autonomy or the sanctity of the physician–patient relationship. In fact, the organization of the health care system in Canada under public control may be one of the major factors that prevented the erosion of the position of members of the medical profession (Naylor, 1986).

It is interesting to compare their position with their American physician counterparts. American physicians have been very successful in resisting any type of national health insurance. Starr (1982) suggests that there are consequences to the failure to rationalize physician services under the public umbrella in the United States. Ultimately, physician's services were rationalized under a corporate umbrella, creating conflicts between corporate demands for profit and physicians' right to practise medicine. Conversely, the health care system in place in Canada has removed the corporate profit motive, and this may be the major factor that has maintained physicians' autonomy in Canada. While negotiating fees with the province is difficult, the provinces do not interfere in any physician decision-making. If a test or treatment is recommended by the physician, there is no second guessing or approval required at the administrative level, which is often done private health care companies because their primary motives are profit and shareholder return. It appears that members of the Canadian medical profession have been successful at maintaining both their autonomy and their income.

The report by the Royal Commission on Medicare chaired by Hall in 1964 concluded that the private insurance industry would be unable to provide adequate, affordable health care coverage to the entire Canadian population. Specifically, the commission believed that the poorest and unhealthiest groups would be excluded from private health insurance programs. Thus, the federal and provincial governments would have an obligation to insure the highest-risk categories without being able to take advantage of cost averaging by including low-risk groups.

Finally, we must remember that social policy will always be influenced by the values and priorities of the policy makers and society at large (Sutherland & Fulton 1990). The development of a health care system takes place within the larger arena of the social structure. As Starr (Starr, 1982) notes, those with power have the ability to impress their agenda upon others, whether or not that agenda is consistent with the common good. In the case of the Canadian health care system, we can see this play out over time as various groups and political ideologies influence the decision-making process. The only constant over time has been the ongoing support by the overwhelming majority of Canadians for public health care.

Key Terms

Accessibility—one of the five principles of Canadian Medicare, each province must provide reasonable access to health care services regardless of geographic location or financial means

Capitation—the payment of a set (negotiated) annual flat fee per patient to a physician for providing all necessary health care

Comprehensiveness—one of the five principles of Canadian Medicare, all services defined as medically necessary will be provided in hospital or by physicians

Extra-billing—additional fees charged on top of what was reimbursed by the province for health care services

Fee-for-service—the payment of a set (negotiated) fee for every individual health care service provided by a physician

New Public Management—a model of managing health care that adopts a business-like model of management of health care services. The free market provides the ideal model: by increasing competition, costs are reduced and efficiency increased

Portability—one of the five principles of Canadian Medicare, coverage will be accepted across any province or territory without cost to the patient

Public administration—one of the five principles of Canadian Medicare, Medicare is to be managed by a non-profit entity responsible to the provincial/territorial government

Universality—one of the five principles of Canadian Medicare, guarantees health care coverage for all Canadian citizens regardless of age, condition, or ability to pay for service

Critical Thinking Questions

1. What are the positive and negative aspects of having a single-payer, public health care system?

2. How did various key stakeholder groups influence the shape of the Canadian public health care system and what are some of the consequences?

3. How might the system have evolved differently if other stakeholder groups had been more influential?

4. Discuss how the health care debate in Canada is has evolved since the inception of Medicare.

5. Is privatization a solution for the reorganization and reform of the Canadian public health care system?

Further Readings and Resources

Badgley, R., & Wolfe, S. (1967). *Doctor's Strike: Medical Care and Conflict in Saskatchewan.* New York: Atherton Press.

Canadian Institute for Health Information. (2013, May). *Lifetime distributional effects of publicly financed health care in Canada.* http://bit.ly/10Mn9sp

Canadian Museum of History. (2010). *Making medicare: The history of health care in Canada, 1914–2007.* www.civilization.ca/cmc/exhibitions/hist/medicare/medic00e.shtml

Marchildon, G. (Ed.) (2012). *Making medicare: New perspectives on the history of medicare in Canada.* Toronto: University of Toronto Press.

Marchildon, G., & Campbell, B. (Eds.) (2007). *Medicare: Facts, myths, problems, promise.* Toronto: James Lorimer and Company Ltd.

Rachlis, M. (2005). *Prescription for excellence: How innovation in saving Canada's health care system.* Toronto: HarperPerennialCanada, HarperCollins Publishers.

Shandel, T. [Director]. (1983). *Bitter medicine, Part 1: The birth of medicare.* [Motion picture]. Available from the Canadian National Film Board and the Canadian Broadcasting Corporation, www.nfb.ca

Canadian Health Coalition
http://healthcoalition.ca/

Health Council of Canada
www.healthcouncilcanada.ca

Chapter 4

Health Professions and Health Policy in Canada

Chapter Outline

Learning Objectives

After studying this chapter, you should be able to:

1. Compare and contrast the functionalist, trait, and process approaches of early professionalization theory;

2. Distinguish between neo-Weberian and neo-Marxist theories of professionalism;

3. Differentiate among subordinate, limited, and excluded health occupations, and provide one example for each category;

4. Describe the impact of health care reforms and cutbacks on *who* provides *what* various forms of health care;

5. Examine the various elements of health human resource policy, planning, and management.

The role of health professions in the health and broader social system have been a critical concern of sociologists studying health beginning perhaps with Talcott Parsons' analysis of *The Social System* (1951). In this chapter, we focus on the work of health care professionals; how their domains of practice have developed; and the more recently related issue of health human resource policy, planning, and management. We include a discussion of the health care division of labour from both historical and current perspectives; the training requirements for various health professionals and how they are related to professionalization, licensing, and regulation; and how the medical profession has emerged as dominant in the hierarchy of health professions, subordinating, limiting, or excluding others. It is within this important historical, social, political, and economic context that we situate contemporary health human resource concerns about the supply, distribution, and mix of health professionals to meet population health needs.

THE HEALTH CARE DIVISION OF LABOUR

To understand the present situation for health professions and health policy in Canada, it is important to first gain an appreciation of some key sociological concepts. At the most basic level, it is important to appreciate how health professionals work within a **health care division of labour**. This is not just the space occupied by all of the personnel involved in the provision of health and illness care—both formal and informal. It also involves the work arrangements and the control of both the work setting and the social relationships among personnel (Storch, 2010). This includes both recognized (i.e., regulated) and unrecognized (i.e., unregulated) professions and occupations. What is inherent in this description is that different personnel not only have different roles but these roles have differing statuses and legitimacy that have evolved over time.

The historical health care division of labour in Canada (long before Confederation in 1867) was quite eclectic and unregulated. It included Aboriginal healers and midwives, care providers in religious orders—usually nuns as nurses—and barber-surgeons (Connor, 1989; Laforce, 1990; Mason, 1988). There were large differences between urban centres in Upper and Lower Canada (Ontario and Quebec) and the more rural and remote areas, including the "Western Territories" where there was largely a reliance on self-care or lay models of care (Mason, 1988). Waves of immigration also brought health care providers trained in a wide variety of countries, some of whom initially practised only within their immigrant communities before extending services to members of the broader community (Biggs, 2004). Local health education and training programs were also established, including the first medical school, in Montreal in 1824, and the first nursing school, in St. Catharines, Ontario, in 1874 (Coburn et al. 1983; Coburn, 1988).

Much like other divisions of labour, the health care division of labour is highly segregated and hierarchical. Due to a variety of factors that we will discuss, the medical profession emerged as the dominant actor in the Canadian health care division of labour, consolidating its power between World War I and the early 1960s (Coburn et al. 1983).

This brings us to a conversation about the difference between an occupation and a profession, and how, historically, certain health care occupations became professions.

PROFESSIONALIZATION

Scholars working within the theoretical domain of the sociology of the professions define an **occupation** as an activity in which a person is formally engaged for the purposes of some form of pay whereas a **profession** is defined either as an occupation based on advanced knowledge, or alternately, as a means of controlling an occupation (Johnson, 1972). The orientation of these definitions varies depending on the theoretical perspective. In some cases, the question that emerges is how an occupation becomes a profession, a process referred to as **professionalization**. This too varies depending on the guiding theoretical school of thought, such as early trait and functionalist approaches or the more critical social closure and Marxist perspectives.

Trait and Functionalist Approaches

Early professionalization theory began within the *functionalist* approach, identified largely with the work of Parsons (1951), who emphasized the distinctiveness of the professions among occupational categories based on their higher education and service ethic. The key question Parsons asked was what part professions play in the established order of society. He differentiated professions as being ethically positive and embodying the *central values* of the society. Because of this, they were accorded a great deal of social, political, and economic power.

The *trait* approach, which was developed later, involved describing the criteria or attributes of a profession (Barber, 1963; Goode, 1969; Greenwood, 1957; Hughes, 1963). Some of the key attributes of a profession cited by these theorists include:

- A high level of skill that was based on theoretical knowledge
- A professional culture sustained by an association
- An altruistic service orientation
- An adherence to an ethical code of conduct
- An authority recognized by clients and sanctioned by society

In this "taxonomic" approach (Klegon, 1978), the process of professionalization is conceptualized simply as the achievement of a specified number of attributes, principally prolonged and specialized training in a body of abstract knowledge, and a client-service orientation. There was never much agreement, however, on how many attributes were important and which were more critical than others.

Others have proposed a somewhat related *process approach*. Wilensky (1964) described a sequence of events in the process of professionalization, including (1) becoming a full-time occupation; (2) establishing a training school, ideally within a university setting;

(3) forming a professional association, locally at first and then nationally; (4) embarking on persistent political agitation to win the support of the law in the form of licensing to protect job territory; and (5) establishing a formal code of ethics to eliminate the unqualified, protect clients, and reduce internal competition. Not all occupations seeking professional status necessarily achieve it. Barriers to the process of professionalization include employment in bureaucratic organizations that threaten professionals' autonomy and their service ethic, and a knowledge base that is too general and vague or too narrow and specific threatening the ability to claim exclusive control over the domain.

This early conceptualization of professionalization has been criticized for taking the claims of professionals at face value (Johnson, 1972). Others have argued that there is no such thing as a 'natural' process of professionalization (Brante, 1988; Freidson, 1970a, 1970b; Saks, 1983). Freidson (1970a, 1970b), for example, noted that for many would-be professions, work domains are dominated by more established professions that are unwilling to share control. Any focus on the 'naturalness' of the development of professions misses the power struggles involved in the competing process of professionalization among occupations (Saks, 1983).

Neo-Weberian/Closure Theories

Neo-Weberian scholars critiqued previous approaches, focusing instead on the importance of power in the process of professionalization (cf. Johnson, 1972). Within this perspective, professions were regarded as self-interested, monopoly-seeking groups. Because power is an essential attribute of closure, many of these theorists either explicitly or implicitly drew on Weber's theory of **social closure** (Brante, 1988; Saks, 1983). Weber employed the concept of closure to refer to the monopolization of opportunities by social groups in order to maximize their own rewards and privileges by limiting others' access (Brante, 1988; Parkin, 1979).

Parkin (1979) was one of the first to explicitly expand upon the theory of social closure. He stated that, "[t]he distinguishing feature of exclusionary closure is the attempt by one group to secure for itself a privileged position at the expense of some other group through a process of subordination" (p. 45). He identified two generic types of closure action, exclusion and usurpation. **Exclusion** was power directed downward through the subordination of socially defined inferiors, usually through legalistic procedures such as state-sponsored licensure. **Usurpation** was power directed upward, oriented at improving the position of a subordinate group at the expense of a dominant group, usually through solidarity tactics such as lobbying and group protest. Exclusionary strategies are based predominantly on property ownership and academic or professional qualification and credentials but can also be based on other factors such as gender or race. Usurpation is both a consequence of and a collective response to exclusion.

Closure and Professional Dominance Professionalization involves occupations marking out the territory they wish to control and monopolize. Components of control include a system of self-government, restricted recruitment, and legal sanctions for a professional domain (Parry & Parry, 1976). Registration and membership are other strategies employed to achieve and maintain social closure. Professions control terrain to limit the dilution of power and prestige by limiting association with subordinate groups, and regulating relationships and the distribution of power within their occupation (Macdonald 1985; MacDonald & Ritzer 1988). Freidson (1970a, 1970b), implicitly drew on social closure theory in discussing **professional dominance**, the ultimate stage of professionalization. **Medical dominance** was achieved by establishing a powerful professional organization through the control of the production of medical knowledge and the sponsorship of medicine by a societal or strategic elite persuaded of the trustworthiness of the profession. Medical dominance consists of:

1. self-regulation over the content of medical work;

2. regulation over the terms, conditions, or context of medical work;

3. control over other health occupations; and

4. control over clients.

Professional dominance over other professions leads to **occupational imperialism**, the occupation-based monopolization aimed at conserving particular skills, "poaching" skills from other occupations, and establishing advantageous relationships with allied groups (Larkin, 1983). Occupational imperialism involves a continual process in "an *arena of tension* [italics added] and conflict between groups that is largely shaped in outcome by the differential access of each group to exterior power sources" (Larkin, 1983, p. 17). Abbott (1988) expanded upon the idea of an arena of tension describing how professions interact through a *system of professions*. The *system* is a complex, dynamic, and interdependent structural network of professions within a given domain of work that constantly compete over jurisdictions of knowledge and skill expertise. Professions develop from interrelations with other professions when jurisdictions become vacant in response to external system disturbances, such as technological or organizational change, or because a previous tenant has abandoned it. A profession's success in occupying a jurisdiction is based on its efforts as well as the situation of its competitors. Subordination of one professional group by another occurs when a profession vacates a jurisdiction but maintains control over it through such strategies as supervising the new tenant.

In sum, neo-Weberian theorists portray professions as powerful occupations through the process to control a particular field of work by monopolizing a legitimate knowledge base (see also Researcher Profile 4.1). This perspective is more sophisticated than traditional approaches but it is not without its flaws. For example, Murphy (1986) criticized social closure theory for overrating the power and market position of professionals. Larson (1977) criticized this approach for not linking the closure process to the broader social structure. Saks (1983) also criticized the neo-Weberian approach for devoting too little attention to how and why legal enforcement for exclusion is obtained from societal elites. Although many neo-Weberian scholars assert the importance of social, economic, and political factors, few clarify their influence.

Everett C. Hughes

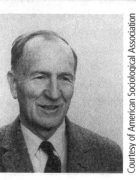

Courtesy of American Sociological Association

Everett C. Hughes (1897–1983) was born in Ohio, married Canadian sociologist Helen McGill-Hughes, and undertook his first work on *French Canada in Transition*. Some of his key publications on the professions included *Men and Their Work (1958)* and *Good People and Dirty Work* (1962). Examining professions, Hughes spoke in terms of action as opposed to structure:

> I passed from the false question "Is this occupation a profession?" to the more fundamental one "what are the circumstances in which people in an occupation attempt to turn it into a profession and themselves into professional people?" (Hughes, 1958, p. 45)

He argued that work situations are based on systems of interaction where various occupations, professions, and lay persons interact in defined relationships that are both technical and social. For example, he described a *moral division of labour* or a hierarchy of the delegation and conduct of "dirty" work/the cleanliness of tasks.

He also distinguished between the concepts of *licence* and *mandate*. An occupation consists of the implied or explicit licence that legitimates one to carry out certain activities for remuneration. Licence is generally given through specific legal permission to pursue the occupation. A professional has a licence to deviate from lay conduct in action and in every mode of thought. It is an institutionalized deviation, for example, a surgeon being licensed to cut someone. The situation is one of *credat emptor*—where the client is to trust the professional, which is in contrast to *caveat emptor*—buyer beware.

Professions also claim a broad legal, moral, and intellectual mandate. *Individually*, a professional exercises a licence; *collectively*, the profession dictates what is good and right more generally for society. The mandate flows from the legitimized claim to professional knowledge and high skill.

Neo-Marxist/Class Theories

An explicit analysis of the wider sources of power underpinning professionalism has been pursued by scholars working from a neo-Marxist perspective. Moving away from the neo-Weberian approach in his later work, Johnson (1977) argued that theorizing professional power as based on its knowledge is not an adequate explanation. Neo-Weberian scholars do not show what *kind* of knowledge is socially valuable enough to bestow power. Johnson argued that a neo-Marxist perspective puts the relations of production and the division of labour at the centre of the analysis, identifying what knowledge is more valuable and which positions in the social formation possess the potential to exercise power on the basis of knowledge.

Boreham (1983) argued that many of the conclusions drawn about the autonomy, legitimacy, and power of professionals overlook the fact that professionals can only achieve and maintain their position through the "identification with appropriate recognized norms and values in the context of the capitalist organisation of the labour process" and by following "rules [that] originate primarily from the superordinate structural level of economic relationships worked out through the capitalist mode of production" (pp. 713–714). Professionalization, as a form of occupational control, can only arise when it "*coincides with requirements of capital* [italics added]; that is where core work activities fulfil the global function of capital with respect to control and surveillance, including the specific function of the reproduction of labour power" (Johnson, 1977, p. 106). In other words, the tasks of surveillance and control are carried out by professions as agents of the dominant class; professional workers "become both agents of capitalist control and also the professionally trained servants of capitalism" (Esland, 1980, p. 229). For example, Navarro (1976, 1986) and Waitzkin (1983) asserted that the medical profession acts on behalf of the dominant class by obscuring or excluding the social causes of much illness to mask the economic patterns of activity and inequality that damage health (see Chapters 7 and 12). Boreham (1983) further asserted that capitalist hegemony is maintained through the integration of the professions into class alliances, in that professions not only attune themselves to the value of capitalism, they are also rewarded for their allegiance through membership into the upper strata of society (Macdonald & Ritzer, 1988).

Despite the intuitive appeal of neo-Marxist professionalization theory, some have argued that because of its high level of abstraction, there have been few applications of this theoretical approach. Larkin (1983) and Saks (1983), for example, criticized this field for not fully substantiating their arguments with empirical evidence. Saks (1983) stated about Johnson, for example, that "[he] is open to the charge of not fully articulating the constituents of the control and surveillance functions in which the professions are said to be engaged" (p. 15).

Nonetheless, the concerns raised by neo-Marxist scholars about the neo-Weberian approach should not be discounted simply because of problems with their own lack of conceptual clarity and evidentiary base. Neo-Marxist scholars make an important contribution by prompting us to take a broader, societal level analysis of professional power and the factors and forces influencing it. We should not confine ourselves to an either/or perspective debating neo-Weberian *versus* neo-Marxist and recognize the importance of both; the *meso* level of analysis taken by neo-Weberian theorists and the *macro* level of analysis taken by neo-Marxist theorists. Several professionalization theorists have stressed the importance of linking professions to their sociopolitical context and argue that the neo-Weberian and neo-Marxist approaches need not be mutually exclusive (Crompton, 1987; Larkin, 1983; Larson, 1977; Macdonald & Ritzer, 1988; Witz, 1992).

Combining Critical Approaches

One scholar who attempted to respond to criticisms of both the neo-Weberian and neo-Marxist approaches and reconcile their differences is Larson (1977, 1979) examining the development of British and American medical professions. She introduced the concept of a **professional project** that involves two interrelated processes: (1) control over a market

Box 4.1

Studies of Medical Socialization

One of the earliest studies of professional socialization into medicine was conducted by Dr. Oswald Hall (1924–1976), a Canadian sociologist who studied medical doctors in Providence, Rhode Island. Examining the life of doctors in this relatively small community, Hall identified a number of stages that form a medical career: (1) generation of ambition, (2) gaining access to the medical establishment, (3) acquiring a clientele (patients), and (4) generating relationships with other medical professionals (Hall, 1948). He suggested that the decision to become a doctor is tied to ambition, since the training for the profession is quite extensive and expensive. This ambition is usually *social in nature* and generated by social networks, family, and friends who motivate the candidate to pursue a career in medicine. Hall also noticed ethnic differences and hierarchical relationship within the medical establishment where the prestigious schools and positions within the hospital formed a professional hierarchy.

The works of structural functionalists on medical socialization were informed by Parsons (1951), who saw medicine as a profession that gained privileged and penetrating access to people's bodies. Many times, people share with their physicians the very intimate details of their private lives; they reveal their bodies. Therefore, the physician–patient relationship should maintain some emotional distance. The work of Merton et al. (1957) elaborated on this process of emotional detachment, describing the ways in which medical students learned to disassociate themselves from the patients and deal with constant uncertainty related to outcomes of the treatment through the adoption of shared values. Fox (1959)

described the sources of this uncertainty, suggesting that the vastness of medical knowledge, the gaps in medical knowledge, and doubts about the lack of knowledge as stemming from personal ignorance or the limitation of science shape the uncertainly experienced by medical students. It should be noted that since Fox (1959) conducted her research, the area of medical research has grown even more, which has furthered the dilemma of medical students having to deal with uncertainty.

Symbolic interactionist researchers have studied medical students, examining how, over the course of their training, they assume the identity of a medical doctor. The classical work by Becker et al. (1961) in *Boys in White* depicted how, over the course of their training, medical students learn to "get through" the program. The initial idealism with which the students start the program slowly gives way to cynicism toward medicine. The work of Haas and Shaffir (1987), who studied students at McMaster Medical School, suggested that the students developed a *cloak of competence* or impression management tactics to convince others and themselves that they are competent and confident to face the immense responsibilities of their privileged role as a doctor.

More recent critical studies of medical students focused on some of the problems related to the recruitment of medical students. In *Getting Doctored*, Shapiro (1978) described how the selection of medical students was skewed to certain groups of individuals. Similarly, Columbotos (1988) argued that there are persistent class-based characteristics in medical students that may result in tensions in subsequent doctor–patient relations.

for expertise and (2) a collective process of upward social mobility. An upwardly mobile occupation must create a need for its services and at the same time create a scarcity of resources—i.e., *its own members*. Through the process of professionalization, a monopoly of expertise in the market and a monopoly of status in a system of stratification are both accomplished through professional licensing and certification following a standardized, mandatory system of professional training and evaluation. The latter was accomplished through the reform of medical training and education that privileged scientific training and allopathic approaches, controlling recruits to the profession (excluding women, racial, and ethnic minorities), producing a uniform body of knowledge, and socializing students to increase professional cohesion (see Box 4.1 for other sociological analyses of medical socialization).

Market conditions alone, however, are insufficient to guarantee professional power, and here Larson highlighted a link to capital. As a profession attempts to rise upward, it

> must form "organic" ties with significant fractions of the ruling class (or of a rising class); persuasion and justification depend on ideological resources, the import and legitimacy of which are ultimately defined by the context of hegemonic power in a ruling class society. (1977, p. xv)

In the case of medicine, she asserted that its collective rise was facilitated by the fit between its emerging doctrines and the ideology that was being used to justify the increasing power of the corporate capitalist class (Coburn et al., 1983). Thus, professionalization results when an occupational group seeks upward mobility by controlling its knowledge base within a socio-political context defined by capitalist relations of production. What remains unclear from Larson's analysis, however, is whether it is mainly through the efforts of an upwardly mobile occupational group organized around a certain knowledge base to form ties with the ruling class that leads to professional power and status, or whether it is simply the *logic* of capitalism that enables an occupation with a knowledge base that fits with capitalist ideology to become powerful.

HISTORICAL EVOLUTION OF THE HEALTH CARE DIVISION OF LABOUR IN CANADA

The Rise and Fall (?) of Medical Dominance

Drawing upon the concepts of professional projects and its outcome, professional dominance, Coburn et al. (1983) described the rise (1795–1912), consolidation (1912–1962), and potential decline (from 1962) of medical dominance in Canada through a case study of the province of Ontario. Dominance of the Canadian medical profession was first achieved by establishing a professional organization that successfully lobbied for protective legislation to place limits on who would be legally allowed to practise medicine. Although this began in 1795 with the establishment of the first Medical Act in Ontario (Upper Canada), it was difficult to enforce because of the small number of medical practitioners at that time. The profession was not able to start to consolidate its power until the turn of the twentieth century when increasingly powerful medical associations and their leaders were able to exert stronger control over the production of medical practitioners through entrance to medical schools. These activities were bolstered by the Carnegie Foundation sponsorship of medical school reform in the United States and Canada in 1912, culminating in the *Flexner Report* (named after the lead reviewer). Although the Flexner Report did not recommend closing any medical schools in Canada, as was the case for several schools in the United States (particularly those dedicated to women and ethnic and visible minorities), the report signalled an era of increased power of the medical profession to secure state sponsorship for its efforts, in part through its appeal to elite members of society.

The event that initiated the beginning of the decline of medical dominance, according to Coburn et al. (1983) argument was the doctors' strike in Saskatchewan in 1962 (see Chapter 3). In making this argument, Coburn drew upon a growing literature indicating the demise of near hegemonic medical power. Specifically, the bureaucratization of medical practice and **proletarianization** of physicians (McKinlay, 1982) was eroding the control of both the context and content of medical work by the profession. Proletarianization may be defined as a situation in which professions work in contexts where none of their privileges remain and the content, control, and location of the work are managed by outsiders (Leicht & Fennell, 2001). McKinlay (1982), however, defines proletarianization in more neo-Marxist terms as being when professionals become more like other workers (the *proletariat*). Key indicators of proletarianization include (1) a growth of professional employment in bureaucratic settings on salary or contract; (2) fragmented work that is subordinated to the interests of capital (their employers); and (3) the standardization and systematization of medical knowledge through, for example, clinical practice guidelines (Coburn, Rappolt, & Bourgeault, 1997).

Alternatively, the **deprofessionalization** thesis suggests that medical professionals are losing control vis-à-vis their clients (patients), reflecting the increasingly consumerist environment (Haug, 1979). Deprofessionalization denotes how increasingly educated and consumerist clients narrow the knowledge gap (and therefore the prestige gap) between professional and client, for example, through accessibility of medical knowledge on the internet and the increasing use of internet-based knowledge in medical encounters.

Coburn's (1988) examination of the decline of medical dominance in Canada argues that an analysis of the history of the conflicts between the Canadian government and the medical profession provides evidence that medical dominance has declined. He does not, however, feel that there is sufficient evidence to support the thesis of proletarianization due to the relative power of the medical profession within the Canadian health care division of labour. Much of that power still remains in the control of physicians via their professional associations (see Researcher Profile 4.2).

Another strand of the decline of medical dominance thesis is its loss of power to its neighbouring or competing professions. That is, although scholars such as Wardwell (1992) and Willis (1989) have described the professionalization process of a range of health occupations in terms of their ultimate relationship to the dominant medical profession, these are constantly shifting. Let us examine three case studies of the (1) *subordinate* professions,

David Coburn

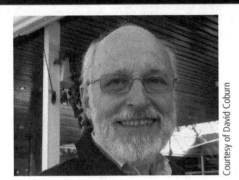

Courtesy of David Coburn

David Coburn, formerly of the School of Public Health at the University of Toronto, could easily be considered the father of the sociology of health professions in Canada. His early work mapped the professionalization of medicine in Canada with a particular emphasis on the rise and fall of the professional dominance thesis (Coburn 1988, 1999, 2006) within the context of a changing capitalism. He has also analyzed the professionalization of nursing (1988) and, along with a number of his students, has examined chiropractic (Coburn & Biggs, 1986) and naturopathy (Gort & Coburn, 1988). He has carried out research on the continued dynamics of medical dominance vis-à-vis the state through a case study of the control over fees and clinical practice guidelines (Coburn, Rappolt & Bourgeault, 1997). More recently he has described the influence of neo-liberalism on global health trends and inequalities. His current research, with Elaine Coburn, focuses on the changing ideology of the World Bank and the IMF.

which originally functioned only under direct supervision of the medical profession; (2) *limited* professions, which practise independently of medical supervision but with a limited scope of practice, in terms of a specific part of the body or through a range of treatment modalities; and (3) *excluded* professions, which practised outside of the mainstream medical system (those that are captured by the term *complementary and alternative medicine*). We also examine a fourth case that encompassed all three statuses: midwifery.

The Rise of Subordinate Professions—The Case of Nursing

Coburn (1988) described the development of the nursing profession beginning with lay nursing and the efforts to control it from organization and registration to the move to hospital duty and finally to the push toward unionization. The first acts regulating nursing were passed in 1913 in Manitoba and 1922 in Ontario, much later than those for physicians. These early efforts did not secure nurses a monopoly, but they did garner the exclusive right to use the title *nurse* or *RN* to indicate that they were registered nurses.

Historically, the nursing elite sought to raise the standards and status of nursing by excluding untrained nurses and by strictly controlling the behaviour of nurses to coincide with the prevailing ideal of femininity (see Box 4.2). Nursing leaders sought the ideal of professionalism, which focused on the altruistic, selfless orientation, and escalating educational credentials. The move from private duty to hospital duty during a time of high nursing unemployment marked a change in orientation, especially by the rank-and-file, toward nursing as work. Increasingly the rank-and-file pushed for unionization and collective bargaining in response to what they felt was the timidity of their leaders who viewed such a direction as contrary to their professionalization efforts. It is at this point, Coburn (1988) argued, that nursing came to be characterized by the twin goals of professionalization by an elite and unionization by the rank-and-file. Increasingly, this division created a bifurcation or separation of nursing into two orientations: the professionalizing elite were somewhat successful in attaining occupational recognition and autonomy similar to medicine, while the unionized rank-and-file were still struggling over control of the nursing labour process.

One of the key vehicles for the professionalization of nursing has been the form and content of its education and training programs. Intent on increasing the recognition of nursing, leaders of the profession managed to shift the credential to practise nursing from a two- to three-year hospital-based program to a four-year college- and university-based baccalaureate program (for an RN). To be sure, this increase in education should also be regarded as reflecting the increasingly complex nature of modern nursing. Some feel, however, that the professionalization of nursing is still incomplete. They argue that nurses' focus on the jurisdiction of "care" by way of contrast to physicians' focus on "cure" is not yet fully developed.

There is also strong evidence of the proletarianization of nursing, particularly of the rank-and-file. Nursing has followed a trajectory moving from self-employment to wage labour, and, in doing so, has become increasingly fragmented, bureaucratized, and under managerial surveillance. That is, the professionalization of nursing is not only influenced by medical dominance, it has also been subordinated by hospital management and control. Because nursing human resources are one of the primary hospital budgetary items, nurses are constantly targeted by cost-cutting measures in times of fiscal restraint. As a direct result of hospital cost cutting, the nursing profession has experienced a dramatic loss of jobs and replacement of RNs by staff with less nursing training. Nursing layoffs were exacerbated by the trend toward the replacement of RNs with Registered Practical Nurses (RPNs) and Unregulated Care Providers (UCPs). Concurrently, more full-time positions have been converted to part-time as a means of increasing management's control over the nursing workforce.

As noted in Box 4.2, those examining the status of nursing through a feminist lens argue that, because nurses are predominantly women and the profession developed at a time of negligible female power, gender serves to both hinder the professionalization and foster the proletarianization of the profession. They argue that the nature of "skilled" work is socially defined and valued along gender lines and nurses' work is viewed as a natural extension of the caring work that women provide for their families in the private sphere. As such, it was not generally seen as the product of rigorous training (Coburn, 1987; Kazanjian, 1993). As a result, it is easier to delegate their tasks to lesser-trained workers (a process that has been described as **deskilling**). Canadian sociologists Pat and Hugh Armstrong and their colleagues have been key contributors describing these trends (see Researcher Profile in Chapter 5).

The Gendered Nature of the Health Care Division of Labour

One of the key consequences of the strategies to achieve medical dominance has been the gendered exclusion and segregation of the health care division of labour by assigning a secondary status to women. Historically, gender was used as an exclusionary criterion by the medical profession in its quest for professional status. This began with efforts to exclude women from medical school, and failing that, from medical practice and/or hospital admitting privileges. Prior to the mid-twentieth century, only a handful of women under the most unusual circumstances managed to receive medical training in Canada (Strong-Boag, 1979). Even when female students were admitted, they were made to feel very uncomfortable, they lacked female role models, and many experienced subtle and not-so-subtle sexual harassment.

Women's involvement in the health care division of labour was largely channelled into support and subordinate occupations—such as nursing, dental hygiene, and dental and legal assistant work—with limited scopes of practice, lower status, and little autonomy (Adams & Bourgeault, 2003) or excluded altogether in the case of midwifery. Indeed, female-dominated professions have been regarded by some as achieving only "semi-professional" (Etzioni, 1969) or subordinate (Willis, 1989) status, often only able to function under the direct supervision of more powerful professions dominated by men. Thus, while women made up the bulk of health care providers within the health care division of labour, their employment was relegated to a subordinate role.

Source: Excerpted and revised from Bourgeault, I. L. (2006). The provision of care: Professions, politics and profit. In Raphael, D., Bryant, T. & Rioux, M. (Eds.). *Staying alive: Critical perspectives on health, illness, and health care* (pp. 263–282). Toronto: Canadian Scholar's Press.

By way of contrast with the proletarianization and deskilling trend in nursing, there is a parallel trend toward expanding its scope of practice in the form of nurse practitioners. Basically, nurse practitioners (or NPs) are registered nurses with advanced training (typically at a Master's level) who are able to provide an expanded range of services, including taking the patient's history; performing a physical exam, and ordering appropriate laboratory tests and procedures; diagnosing, treating, and managing acute and chronic diseases; providing prescriptions and coordinating referrals; and promoting healthy activities in collaboration with the patient. These expanded tasks have historically been within the domain of the medical profession. Indeed, the development of NPs in Canada has occurred in the face of sometimes fierce opposition from medical organizations (Angus & Bourgeault, 1998/99). As a consequence of this opposition, these tasks have been constrained, making NPs nearer to *limited professionals* discussed in the next section.

The development of NPs also has an interesting gender dimension. Some argue that the reasoning behind the push toward NPs is that they are cheaper than physicians. For example, the delegation of technical skills provided to women has long been justified on the basis of driving down the cost of labour (Wajcman, 1991). However, the notion that people are paid on the basis of their skills obscures the very nature of skilled work as a socially defined and socially evaluated set of characteristics that varies according to the gender, ethnicity, and power of workers, as well as with historical and economic context (Gaskell, 1987). Specifically, female health care providers operate within a social system of health care that is inherently gendered to devalue their skills and knowledge.

The Expansion of Limited Professions—The Case of Pharmacy

Pharmacy provides an excellent case of a limited profession. Other examples include podiatry, optometry, and psychology. It is noteworthy that each of these professions have recently expanded their scope of practice to include very limited practice of prescribing that overlaps even more fully with the traditional domain of medicine.

The history of pharmacy and its relationship to the medical profession has been a quintessential story of professional competition. Prior to any strict form of regulation, pharmacists used to diagnose minor disorders for which they stocked the "cure" and physicians used to regularly dispense similar "cures" from their clinics following diagnosis. Following Larson's interest in the social class of those undertaking professional projects, it is notable that historically the class background of physicians was higher of that of pharmacists. Indeed, there were also class dimensions relevant to each of these professional's clientele—with their clients coming from similar class backgrounds to themselves.

It is due, in part, to potential economic conflicts of interest that the act of *prescribing* medicines (following diagnosis) was divided from *dispensing* medicines. The task of prescribing fell within the domain of medicine whereas that of dispensing was within the domain of pharmacy. In Canada, this was first delineated in 1871 when the concern was with the control of the sale of drugs. Until most recently with the limited expansion of prescriptive privileges of pharmacists (e.g., in the case of smoking cessation products in Ontario), the scope of practice of pharmacy included only ". . . the custody, compounding and dispensing of drugs, the provision of non-prescription drugs, health care aids and devices and the provision of information related to drug use." (Pharmacy Act of Ontario, 1991). That is, pharmacists have always "prescribed" over-the-counter medication within the context of their community-based pharmacies but were controlled by medicine from dispensing those drugs that were restricted by prescription.

Some could regard the recently expanded scope of pharmacy practice as a contemporary dimension of their continued professional project. To be sure, there has been a revamping of their educational programs across Canada to reflect this more clinical dimension to pharmacy, which has been coined *pharmaceutical care*. The new curriculum focuses on a more patient- or client-oriented approach to the provision of pharmaceutical services but many of the courses have been grafted onto existing curricula so that the strong biochemical focus continues. There is also an overarching concern that continuing education programs are supported by pharmaceutical manufacturers (another potential conflict of interest—see Chapter 12).

Linda Muzzin

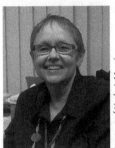

Courtesy of Linda J. Muzzin

Linda Muzzin, a professor at the Ontario Institute for Studies in Education at the University of Toronto, has tackled an issue of great concern but little evidence—the feminization of pharmacy and its link with concerns about workforce shortages. (The same argument has been applied to the feminization of medicine. According to this argument, the increasing number of women in a profession will result in shortages because of their tendency to work part-time, especially during their child-bearing and -rearing years. In a series of articles (1994; 1995), Muzzin and her colleagues not only challenge this limited view by arguing that these fears are overstated but also further speculate about the actual consequences of women's massive movement into the pharmacy profession on its professionalization process. Because more women are drawn into chain-based pharmacies, it could provide an opportunity to move pharmacy toward *pharmaceutical care* and away from the entrepreneurial, business orientation. Thus, they argue that female pharmacists may actually be helping to guarantee the survival of the profession and the success of their professional project.

Beyond this, there has been a rapid decline in pharmacist-owned community pharmacies in the face of an increase in large chain or franchise pharmacies. Commercially oriented, chain-based pharmacies now make up 75% of pharmacy practice, which makes pharmaceutical care difficult to put into practice (CIHI, 2010b). Beyond the expanded scope of practice of pharmacy, another contemporary issue facing the profession has been a rather rapid *feminization* (see Researcher Profile 4.3). Similar to the bureaucratization argument for medical dominance, these developments may serve as a challenge to pharmacists' professional autonomy.

The Recognition of Once Excluded Professions—The Case of Naturopathy

We now turn to the case of excluded professions or those considered under the umbrella concept of **complementary and alternative medicine**, or CAM. The term CAM encompasses two somewhat distinct elements. Specifically, whereas the term complementary implies supplementation, the term alternative implies substitution. This can be a very important distinction. Moreover, there is a problem applying this label to different forms of therapies and practitioners, lumping together very different modalities into a residual category of 'other':

> ... definitions of medicine and CAM (i.e. what is considered mainstream, complementary or alternative) differ according to nation-state, culture, regulatory environment and financing arrangement. Many of the notions of CAM that we have in the West, for example, reflect the influence of medical hegemony, are value-laden, exoticize these therapies, and tend to define them as little more than a residual category ... (Hirschkorn & Bourgeault, 2005, p. 166)

This tends to reinforce the marginalization or perception of "otherness" of CAM in relation to the public, other health professions, and the state. A helpful distinction is made by Wardwell (1994) between marginal or parallel practitioners and quasi-practitioners. *Marginal* or *parallel practitioners* are "those who treat a wide range of human diseases but whose philosophy or theory of health and disease conflicts with that of orthodox medicine" (p. 1063). Examples include acupuncturists, homeopaths, and naturopaths. By way of contrast, *quasi-practitioners* are "those who reject the medical model of the doctor-patient relationship yet assist people in obtaining relief" (p. 1063). Examples here would be paranormal healers, mental therapists, and anthroposophical medicine. Although the health care division of labour encompasses both marginal and parallel practitioners, it is the professionalizing activities of these practitioners that have been of particular interest in the study of health professions.

Naturopathy offers us an interesting case in the Canadian context. Briefly, **naturopathy** is

> a distinct system of primary health care that addresses the root causes of illness and promotes health and healing using natural therapies. It supports [the] body's own healing ability using an integrated approach to disease diagnosis, treatment and prevention that includes: acupuncture, ... botanical medicine, physical medicine ..., clinical nutrition, homeopathic medicine [and] lifestyle counselling. (Canadian College of Naturopathic Medicine, n.d.)

This includes the CAM domains of botanical medicine, homeopathy, Traditional Chinese Medicine or TCM, acupuncture, clinical nutrition, and massage, among other modalities. The emphasis of naturopathic care is on treating the "whole person" (Boon, 1998). The regulation of naturopathy in Canada has largely reflected its residual characteristic and exclusion from the mainstream. Initially excluded under the Drugless Practitioners Act of 1925 that included chiropractors, chiropodists, drugless therapists, masseurs, and osteopaths, it was finally included under the revision of the Act in 1944. A more recent effort was made to include naturopathy in omnibus legislation regulating a number of health professions in Ontario in 1994 that originally did not include naturopathy. Although the government agreed in principle with the need to regulate naturopathy, there was a concern about the breadth of naturopaths' proposed scope of practice. The province continued to review the request for regulation by the Naturopathic Association, in addition to separate submissions for TCM and acupuncture. These efforts culminated in 2007 legislation, the Health Systems Improvements Act, 2007, a new health profession act to regulate the profession of naturopathy along with homeopathy, kinesiology, and psychotherapy.

Gort and Coburn (1988) examined the unsuccessful attempts of naturopathy to gain state legitimacy and become incorporated into the health care system in Ontario. They attributed this lack of success to several factors. Naturopathy lacks internal unity. Its professional association was only established in 1949 and few naturopaths belonged. As a parallel system of care, naturopathy faces fierce opposition from the medical profession. The relationship of naturopathy to chiropractic has also been influential. Although chiropractors initially sought dual registration in naturopathy to overcome their limited scope of practice, more recent efforts on the part of the chiropractic elite have been to disassociate itself from naturopathy in order to legitimize chiropractic practice. This left naturopathy without the support of many of these dually registered professionals.

Studies of the form and evolution of naturopathy education offer some interesting insights on parallel systems of care. One of the key issues highlighted by Boon (1998) is how the structure of naturopathy emulates the traditional structure of medical education. Boon noted the degree of integration of Western biomedical knowledge into the curriculum. It is not surprising that these shifts in education paralleled the profession's on-going struggle for regulatory recognition, representing another example of how control of training is a critical element in the professionalization process. Some within the profession express concern, however, over the potential loss of professional identity and the uniqueness of the naturopathic profession as a result of these shifts (see Researcher Profile on Heather Boon in Chapter 10).

The Unique Case of Midwifery in Canada

The case of midwifery in Canada represents a mixture of each of the types of health professions described by Wardwell (1994). It was initially subordinated, then excluded, and most recently has re-emerged as a limited profession. The Canadian history of midwifery contains elements similar to other countries with one unique twist—Canada became the only Western industrialized nation not to have any provisions for midwifery care until it was re-integrated in the province of Ontario in 1993.

Before the turn of the twentieth century, midwives in Canada, as in many other countries, were the predominant attendants at childbirth. Prior to European contact, traditional Aboriginal midwives played a fundamental role in the childbirth process, often also serving as midwives to new Canadian settlers (Carroll & Benoit, 2004; Rushing 1991). Colonial governments also appointed midwives, an indication of the importance of midwifery to early colonial life and the respectability of such a position (Rushing, 1991). For example, in New France midwifery was considered a profession in its own right and a distinctive branch of medicine (Laforce, 1990). Because midwifery in English Canada was not as formally organized, this system of midwifery rapidly deteriorated after the British conquest. Childbirth, particularly in rural areas, was considered a community affair often handled by female neighbours of the pregnant woman (Mason, 1988) with services rendered in kind (Connor, 1994). Training was derived less from formal study and apprenticeship than from participation in a birth culture that expected neighbouring women to help each other out (Mason, 1987). Although women whose primary function was being a midwife were rare, some women in certain communities did emerge as midwives and were regarded and called upon for their special knowledge and skills in childbirth attendance (Biggs, 2004).

This early, informal system of midwifery care in English Canada and the more formal system that existed in French Canada were soon eclipsed by various factors and forces. First was the rise in medical interest in childbirth attendance toward the end of the eighteenth century. The medical profession in Canada was relatively late to develop and was not initially interested in the practice of midwifery or the exclusion of midwives. Toward the end of the eighteenth century, when their numbers grew, however, and as they began to organize as a profession, the first male medical practitioners entered the childbirth scene, primarily as an entrée into family practice (Barrington, 1985; Rushing, 1991). Thus midwives became the "victims" of increasingly restrictive medical licensure laws dating back to 1795, even if they may not have been the main target (Connor, 1994). The demise of midwifery was also influenced by changing societal attitudes toward childbirth with hospitals being marketed as modern institutions that could provide women relief from suffering. It is interesting to note that at the time of these efforts, hospitals were statistically much more dangerous places to give birth due to a range of infectious elements. Finally, midwives themselves, many of whom were illiterate and from different ethnic/immigrant communities, did not have the resources to organize into a professional association as was possible for other professions, including medicine and nursing.

There were some early attempts to institute a form of nurse-midwife in remote outposts of the Red Cross. Despite "catching" several babies, this form of care was never institutionalized and the increased practice of flying women south to give birth in urban hospitals led to its demise. There were remnants of midwifery on the island of Newfoundland that were sustained by its late entry into the Canadian federation, but here too there was a move toward hospital-based births attended by physicians (see Researcher Profile 4.4).

The rebirth of midwifery in Canada emerged from the counterculture movement that gave rise to debates about the cons of medical control and medicalization particularly of women's lives (see Chapter 12). Out of this movement came a group of sometimes self-taught or informally taught midwives who began to practise what at the time was considered radical—home births. Similar to other professional projects, these midwives formed a professional association that would successfully lobby a number of provincial governments for regulation and inclusion in the formal health care division of labour, beginning with the province of Ontario in 1993. The form of their regulation has been like other professions—self-regulation—with multiple routes of entry, the ability to practise not only at home but also in hospitals through having admitting privileges, and in most places, with public funding for their services to ensure client

Cecilia Benoit

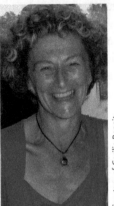

Courtesy of Cecilia Benoit

Cecilia Benoit is a Professor of Sociology at the University of Victoria. Cecilia completed her doctoral training in sociology at the University of Toronto with Oswald Hall in 1989. For her thesis, she examined the remnants of midwifery in Newfoundland by interviewing a number of the granny midwives who remained in the province. Because Newfoundland joined the Canadian federation much later than other provinces, Benoit was able to trace how midwifery developed a unique trajectory from a community-based, home birth practice to a system of local maternity units staffed by midwives to the evolution into large district hospitals that ultimately resulted in the demise of independent midwifery.

Apart from ongoing research focused on the occupation of midwifery and the organization of maternity care in Canada and internationally, Benoit is involved in a variety of projects that employ mixed methodologies to investigate the health of vulnerable populations, including Aboriginal girls and women in Vancouver's Downtown Eastside, female adolescents confronting health stigmas associated with obesity and asthma, homeless female and male youth, frontline service workers in female-dominated low-prestige and stigmatized occupations, women and men involved in the sex industry, and pregnant women using addictive substances. She has been a visiting professor in Sweden, Finland, and Japan. Her native ancestry is Qalipu Mi'kmaw First Nation of Newfoundland.

accessibility. Their scope of practice, as defined in this case by the Midwifery Act (1991) in Ontario, includes, "the assessment and monitoring of women during pregnancy, labour and the post-partum period and of their newborn babies, the provision of care during *normal* [italics added] pregnancy, labour and post-partum period and the conducting of spontaneous normal vaginal deliveries." It is the limitation of midwifery practice to *normal* pregnancy, labour, and birth that makes it more akin to a limited profession (see Bourgeault, 2006).

In sum, the health care division of labour in Canada is a complex, dynamic system influenced by a broader gendered, historical context. When efforts arose to reshape the health care division of labour following the inception of Medicare in the 1960s, the various professional groups were at different starting points. Medical dominance, Coburn et al. (1983) argue, was beginning to decline. The status of largely female health professions, such as nursing, was just beginning to climb, propelled in part by the women's movement and labour movement. All professions, however, were and continue to be subject to the **rationalization** process that focuses on the most efficient use of health care resources, or the assignment of tasks to the "most appropriate" professional. Two key issues involved in the rationalization process include flexibility and cost. *Flexibility* means the ability to respond to shortages and surpluses through the substitution of health labour. Some would argue, however, that the primary concern is with *keeping costs low* so that the least expensive worker performs tasks at the lowest unit cost. These reforms have led to some dramatic changes in *who* does *what* in the provision of health care (Bourgeault, 2006). In the next section, we reflect on these dynamics by discussing some key elements of the broader literature on health human resource policy.

HEALTH HUMAN RESOURCE POLICY

The domain of health human resources (HHR) addresses concerns with preparing, regulating, deploying, and assigning tasks to people who work in health care. It asks, "What types of workers will exist?" "What will each type of worker do?" and "What training and educational requirements will there be?" Because of the historical legacies of the development and institutionalization of a range of professions, it is difficult to ask those questions in a way that people might pose if they had a clean slate with which to work. Therefore, an appreciation of the historical context of health care professionalization and existing professional practice is critical to informed HHR policy.

In general, in the field of HHR policy there are three basic problems to be addressed. The first is the problem of *supply*, or concern about the *number* of health care professionals providing services to a population. The second is the problem of *distribution*, or concern about the *location* or deployment of health care professionals across geographic areas. In a country as big as Canada, this latter issue is a particularly vexing policy problem. Third, there is the problem with *mix*, or concern about the relative numbers of health care professionals providing various types of *specialty* services.

Problem with HHR Supply

Two key concepts within the HHR supply literature are *shortages* and *surpluses*. Shortages exist when persons with legitimate needs for care must wait long times or travel long distances or do without. Areas with shortages of providers are sometimes called *underserviced areas*. This term reflects not only a supply issue but also a distribution issue. Surpluses exist when health professionals are un-employed, under-employed, or, they are self-employed but do not have enough legitimate work to keep them busy or sustain their practice. There are no agreed upon definitions of what constitute shortages or surpluses, and determination of shortages or surpluses tends to reflect the interest of the parties making the claim. As Larson noted in the case of professional projects, there is a role that shortages play in the overall control and prestige a profession is able to attain. Therefore, it may be helpful to adopt a social constructionist perspective and talk of *perceptions* of shortages and surpluses.

Over the last 10 to 20 years there has been a shift in the perception of a range of policy government decision-makers from a situation of surplus to a concern over shortages. Indeed, in the case of medicine, perceptions about the supply of physicians in Canada have taken a 180-degree turn over the past decade. Many Canadians now report difficulty finding family doctors, and stories of waiting lists for specialist services are common. Yet, just 10 years ago, medical school positions were cut, physicians were encouraged to retire, and doctors from other countries were discouraged from coming to Canada. According to the CMA, the current state of the physician shortage reveals that:

■ Almost 5 million Canadians do not have a family physician and 5 million more could be in the same situation by 2018.

■ Canada will need 26 000 more doctors to meet the OECD average of physicians per population. (CNW, 2008, January 15)

These reports are bolstered with data from the Canadian Institute of Health Information (CIHI, 2010b) that confirm that there has been a 5% drop in physician supply since 2000[?]. Some of the reasons for this drop is the aging of the physician population, the more intense use of health care services by the elderly, and the growing number of female physicians who, on average, work fewer hours than their male colleagues (i.e., the feminisation of medicine) (Chan, 2002). A sizeable proportion of the decline (22%) was due to fewer foreign doctors entering Canada, 17% was due to more physicians retiring, and 11% was due to medical school enrolment cuts (Chan, 2002) (see Box 4.3). The biggest factor behind the drop, however, was an increase in the amount of time doctors spend in postgraduate training. Prior to 1993, graduating medical students could enter practice after a one-year rotating internship. After 1993, doctors wanting to enter family practice needed two years of extra training after graduation instead of one. This essentially took one entire cohort out of the system. Also after 1993, there were many more specialists being trained compared to family physicians, and specialists spend more time in training.

Problem with HHR Distribution

The health care division of labour is not only gendered, it contains inherent inequities in access along geographic lines. Urban residents have far greater accessibility to a wider range of health care services than rural residents. For example, although approximately 30% of Canada's population lived in rural areas and small communities of up to 10 000 people, only 14% of family or general practitioners and less than 5% of specialists are in rural practice (Sutherns, 2005). Several factors are behind these disparities, including the lifestyle and nature of work for physicians (i.e., it is considered to be of poorer quality in rural settings), the changing needs of the population, the high degree of specialization within the medical profession, and government cost-cutting of services in areas of less need. Some policy solutions provincial governments have attempted include regulating the billing numbers for physicians, discounting fees in areas not considered underserviced (often only for new registrants), and the substitution of alternate care providers (e.g., NPs

Box 4.3

What is the Role of Internationally Educated Health Professionals in the Canadian Health Care Division of Labour?

Health care workers have long been nationally and internationally mobile. While some have lamented the health care brain drain from Canada to the United States, it is important to note that we are not just an exporter of health labour, but a significant importer as well. Indeed, Canada has historically relied extensively on foreign health labour to help solve a range of problems with the overall supply and distribution of certain health professionals.

A recent report from CIHI (2010b) reveals the extent to which we rely on internationally educated health professionals. Of all of the occupations examined (excluding pharmacists for whom data are not yet available), physicians and physiotherapists had the highest percentage of internationally trained professionals (22% and 15%, respectively). Although those percentages are high because of the sheer size of the nursing profession, the numbers of internationally educated nurses that make up 7% of the profession eclipses that of other professions.

CIHI also declares that the United Kingdom is the top source country for internationally educated professionals. Specifically, for the six health occupations examined, internationally trained health care workers were most likely to have received their education in the United Kingdom, the United States, India, the Philippines, South Africa, Ireland, and Hong Kong. Although this is true, it is important to tease out how this differs across health professions. The number of physicians from South Africa will soon exceed the number from the United Kingdom and nurses from the Philippines make up by far the largest demographic in that profession.

At the same time, we hear of numerous accounts of internationally trained providers not being able to practise their profession. This is particularly the case for international medical graduates. Recent research (Jablonski, 2012) reveals that there are over 5000 internationally trained physicians in the province of Ontario who are not practising medicine. Although there are growing international concerns with the brain drain from low to high income countries, or from countries that are in greater need of health workers, the situation in Canada is akin to a brain waste where the skills of health workers are lost both to their country of origin and their country of destination (CIHI, 2010b).

for GPs) in rural and remote locations. Other than the last strategy of substituting NPs, most of these policy attempts have been unsuccessful.

Not only is there a problem of the disparity between urban and rural communities within a province, there is also significant interprovincial migration. CIHI reports that, between 2003 and 2007, Alberta and British Columbia were the only two provinces that experienced net gains from the interprovincial migration of physicians. Provinces that tend to have a larger outmigration of health workers—Newfoundland and Labrador, Manitoba, and Saskatchewan—tend to also be those provinces that disproportionately recruit internationally educated health professionals to bridge the gap (see Figure 4.1).

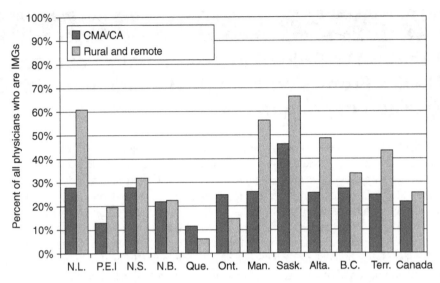

Figure 4.1 Percent of All Physicians in Canada Who Are IMGs by Community Size (CMA/CA or Rural and Remote) by Province, 2007

Note: CMA/CA refers to census metropolitan area (CMA–population of 100,000 or more) and census agglomeration (CA–population of 10,000 to 100,000). Rural and remote refers to smaller communities, rural areas or the territories.

Source: Figure 11, "Percent of All Physicians in Canada Who Are IMGs by Community Size (CMA/CA or Rural and Remote) by Province, 2007," found on page 18 of the CIHI publication "Analysis in Brief, August 20, 2009, International Medical Graduates in Canada: 1972 to 2007." Reprinted by permission of the Canadian Institute for Health Information.

Problems with HHR Mix

Concern about the mix of health professionals addresses issues both within and among professions. In the case of medicine, for example, there are continued debates as to the appropriate distribution of generalists (GPs and family physicians) and the number and types of specialists. This is linked to concerns about the shortages of specific types of physicians, with anestheseologists, obstetricians, oncologists, radiologists, emergentologists (emergency care physicians), and psychiatrists typically topping that list. There are also broad concerns about super-specialization and even specialization within general or family practice. The traditional policy response in the short term has been to increase fees and recruit internationally. Longer term, the response is to increase speciality training positions. There has also been a shift to other providers that has included the expanded scope of practice of family physicians, such as GP-anestheseologists and GP-obstetricians, which are more typical in rural areas. The shift to other providers can also include other health professionals as we discussed in the case of nurse practitioners. The use of NPs is bolstered by arguments that nurses can perform between 30 and 70% of the tasks performed by doctors, with equivalent outcomes (Richardson & Maynard, 1995). Some provinces have also established physician assistant roles—health professionals who work under the direct supervision of physicians and support physicians in a range of tasks.

There is also a growing interest in collaborative models of health care—or what has been referred to as **interprofessionalism**—as a means to address a range of concerns within health care systems, including shortages of health care professionals (Irvine et al., 2002). Interprofessionalism or collaborative practice involves the continuous interaction of two or more professions or disciplines, organized into a communal effort to solve or explore common issues. It is designed to promote the active participation of a range of health professionals in patient care, provide mechanisms for continuous communication, optimize participation of all team members in clinical decision making, and foster respect for the contributions of all professions. Some examples of interprofessional practices are Family Health Teams and Community Health Centres (see Chapter 5 on Health Institutions). It has been described as patient-centred because it enhances patient- and family-centred goals and values.

Sociologists who study such collaborative arrangements are particularly interested in the everyday work of managing professional boundaries. Several researchers call attention to how professional boundaries are constructed, maintained, and negotiated through the everyday actions and rhetoric used by health care providers (Griffiths, 1997; Hindmarsh & Pilnick, 2002; Mizrachi et al., 2005). Allen (1997, 2001, 2002), for example, describes how the boundary between nurses' and physicians' work in the hospital has blurred in that some of the tasks undertaken by nurses, such as prescribing medicine, were clearly within the traditional domain of medicine (see also Hughes, 1988). Physicians, by way of contrast, have rarely been noted as taking up the traditional tasks of nursing.

Overall, collaborative models of practice are viewed as an important tool for increasing the flexibility of the health labour force. In a recent report on medical human resources, it is argued that "bringing together physicians and other health professionals to work in teams can be an important part of the solution to challenges such as access to care, wait times for patients, shortages and burn out for professionals." (Task Force Two, 2006, p. iv). This reflects the broader view that increased interprofessional collaboration can address HHR shortages both by using existing resources more efficiently and by making the provision of care less demanding on practitioners, thereby improving retention. This has been particularly salient in rural areas where these problems are experienced most acutely (McNair et al., 2005). In addition to helping solve problems of supply, mix, and distribution, interprofessional collaborative care arrangements are said to be a more satisfying work arrangement for a range of health professionals.

SUMMARY

In this chapter we have described some of the key historical trends and contemporary concerns of a number of professions that represent not only different functional but also different conceptual spaces in health care division of labour. This has centred in particular on the role of the dominant medical profession and how this role emerged historically. We have also examined how some of the strategies and concepts applied in the case of medical professionalization can be similarly applied to other health professions. Indeed, we find that there are several key, cross-discipline issues revealed from this examination:

the important influence of gender how typical health human resource policy concepts of supply and distribution fit into the more sociological conceptualization of how the health care division of labour is configured, and the need to attend to the broader international context that involves the migration of health workers.

Key Terms

Complementary and alternative medicine (CAM)—often defined in a residual fashion to refer to anything outside of mainstream medicine, it encompasses two somewhat distinct elements: *complementary* that implies supplementation, and *alternative* that implies substitution

Deprofessionalization—how increasingly educated and consumerist clients narrow the knowledge gap (and therefore the prestige gap) between the professional and the client resulting in a decline of power and dominance

Deskilling—a process by which tasks are delegated from more highly trained (and higher-paid) health care workers to lesser-trained and paid workers; the value of the tasks are highly influenced by gender

Exclusion—power directed downward through the subordination of socially defined inferiors

Health care division of labour—work arrangements and social relations of the various personnel providing health and illness care, both formal and informal

Interprofessionalism—a collaborative practice involving the continuous interaction of two or more professions or disciplines, organized into a communal effort to solve or explore common issues

Medical dominance—the ultimate stage of professionalization within the health care division of labour (see professional dominance)

Naturopathy—"a distinct system of primary health care that addresses the root causes of illness and promotes health and healing using natural therapies . . ."

Occupation—an activity where a person is formally engaged for the purposes of some form of remuneration

Occupational imperialism—occupation-based monopolies aimed at conserving particular skills and establishing advantageous relationships with allied groups

Profession—either an occupation based on advanced knowledge or alternately a means of controlling an occupation

Professional dominance—the ultimate stage of professionalization dominating through the control of the production of knowledge and the sponsorship of medicine by a societal or strategic elite persuaded of the trustworthiness of the profession

Professionalization—process by which an occupation becomes a profession

Professional project—a concept that combines closure and class dimensions of professionalization as involving two interrelated processes of (1) control over a market for expertise and (2) a collective process of upward social mobility

Proletarianization—professionals losing their control over the labour process, becoming more like other workers (the proletariat)

Rationalization—(in the context of the health care division of labour)—the process of assigning tasks to the "most appropriate" health care provider and an overall focus on the most efficient use of health care human resources, with the implicit or explicit purpose of controlling rising health care costs

Social closure—the monopolization of opportunities by social groups in order to maximize their own rewards and privileges by limiting access to others

Usurpation—power directed upward with the goal of improving the position of a subordinate group at the expense of a dominant group

Critical Thinking Questions

1. How do neo-Weberian and neo-Marxist theories of professionalism differ from the functionalist, trait, and process approaches?

2. What does the literature on the impact of feminization on traditionally male professions highlight regarding the longstanding issues facing predominantely female health professions? How does this relate to subordinate, limited, and excluded health occupations?

3. If the fall of medical dominance is bona fide, what are the consequences for patients, other health professions, and society? How does this relate to health care reforms and interprofessional models of practice?

4. What are the ways in which the typical concerns of health human resource policy can be informed by the sociological literature on the form and content of professional projects?

Further Readings and Resources

Bourgeault, I. L. (2006). *Push! The struggle to integrate midwifery in Ontario*. Montreal/Kingston: McGill-Queen's University Press.

Coburn, D., Torrance, G., & Kaufert, J. (1983). Medical dominance in Canada in historical perspective: The rise and fall of medicine? *International Journal of Health Services, 13*, 407–432.

Canadian Health Coalition
www.medicare.ca

Canadian Institute for Health Information
www.cihi.ca

Canadian Medical Association
www.cma.ca

Chapter 5

Health Institutions and Organizations in Canada

Chapter Outline

- **Learning Objectives**
- **The Evolution of the Social Organization of Health Care**
- **Hospitals**
  - *Hospital Governance and Administration*
  - *Hospital Patients*
  - *Hospital Restructuring and Reorganization*
- **Long-Term Care Facilities and Nursing Homes**
- **Health Care in the Community**
  - *Community Health Centres*
  - *Evolution of Family Practice Models*
- **Challenges to the Organization of Health Care in Canada**
  - *Managing Health Risk in Society*
  - *New Medical Technologies*

Learning Objectives

After studying this chapter, you should be able to:

1. Describe the evolution of the social organization of health care in Canada;

2. Provide a description of the current organization of hospital care and the challenges faced by hospitals;

3. Recognize the role of community health care services and identify some of the challenges faced by these providers;

4. Identify some of the possible future directions for health care institutions and organizations in Canada.

If you were asked to summarize schematically the health care system in Canada, what would you include in your presentation? Hospitals? Nursing homes? Doctors' offices? Medical laboratories? Canadian Blood Services? The health care system includes all these and much more. When you go to the hospital, for instance, you not only receive assistance from the attending physician or a team of nurses, there are many other workers such as health care aids, pharmacists, technicians, clerks, kitchen staff, laundry operators, janitorial staff, administrative staff, and even volunteers who make your stay in the hospital possible. All the people in these professions and occupations are engaged in complex relationships, and all of them are working within the **medical–industrial complex**—a set of private and public institutions that provides health care. Just as there are interactions between people and occupations within health care organizations, there is also a web of interactions among organizations providing health care services, businesses engaged in the health care industry, and individuals within these organizations. Some of the organizations within the medical–industrial complex work for profit (such as private cosmetic surgery clinics, private long-term care facilities), while others provide services without the goal of generating a profit (such as the majority of hospitals in Canada). Regardless of the goals of these businesses and corporations, they all are part of the system of health care in Canada.

Due to its enormous size and complexity, we cannot fully describe the medical–industrial complex in Canada in a single chapter, but we will map out some of its institutional dynamics and present some of the major health care organizations. We will briefly discuss the evolution of health care organization and talk about hospitals—one of the biggest fiscal and organizational challenges of our contemporary health care system. As the demographics of our country change and we shift our focus from acute to chronic conditions, our health care system moves away from acute to community care (Rockwell, 2010). As such, we will also discuss how health care in the community is organized and discuss other key health care institutions, including long-term care facilities and nursing homes. Finally, we will identify some of the pressing challenges faced by our health care system today. This includes how budget cuts and privatization affect the operation of health care institutions, and how advances in medical technology may influence the future development of the medical–industrial complex.

THE EVOLUTION OF THE SOCIAL ORGANIZATION OF HEALTH CARE

The short history of our contemporary social organization of healing and medicine and the emergence of our current health care system have witnessed significant changes. Jewson (1976) described the change in social relations of healing that parallels the evolution of the social organization of health care, identifying three distinct stages— Bedside Medicine, Hospital Medicine, and Laboratory Medicine. During the era of Bedside Medicine, which Jewson (1976) dates around the mid-1700s, care was delivered in the homes of the ill or through local community services. Nurses provided around-the-clock care at the bedside and various types of physicians visited patients in their homes. This was when medicine began to emerge as a profession and had not yet achieved its dominant status among other providers.

During this period, doctors practising what we now call Western, allopathic medicine faced serious competition from a range of other health care providers, and the lack of advanced medical knowledge made them particularly aware of the importance of impression management in the healing process. Relying heavily on the medical history of the patient, who conveyed to the doctor the nature of the ailment, the symptoms, and the response to the suggested treatment, the healing process was organized around a holistic view of the patient. As such, the medical encounter at the bedside was of utmost importance to the process of healing.

The Hospital Medicine era began during the nineteenth century. Hospitals in Canada started out small, operating through the charity of wealthy benefactors and the church. Located in cities and local communities, they were populated by clients predominantly from the lower classes (those who could not afford home care from a physician). Some hospitals, particularly in large urban settings, became the sites for production of medical knowledge, where medical doctors achieved increasing power and control over the healing process. Many medical historians detail how the evolution of the hospital from warehouses of the sick to *temples of science* paralleled the rising dominance of Western allopathic physicians.

During this hospital era, subjected to what Foucault termed the **medical gaze**, patients ceased to be important in diagnosing disease and their bodies became dehumanized objects for the generation of medical knowledge (Foucault, 1975). Many patients who received care in these new hospitals did so in exchange for being "material" for medical training. Medicine moved from a holistic view of the patient to a preoccupation with the classification and diagnosis of symptoms and diseases. Physicians were expected to find the diseased organ within the body, a pathology, rather than focusing on the holistic view of the body and mind.

The power imbalance between patient and provider in the healing encounter shifted during the hospital era with physicians becoming the holders of specialized medical knowledge, ordaining, with almost complete authority over their patients in the medical decision-making process. Women and other marginalized populations, such as members of visible minorities, were often compelled to receive medical treatment. One of the most vivid examples of the abuses of power by North American doctors can be found in many cases of sterilization of African-American women in the United States and Aboriginal women in Canada, many of whom were sterilized without their consent (Browne & Fiske, 2001).

The third era, Laboratory Medicine, can be traced back to Germany in the middle of the nineteenth century, where, at the University of Berlin, scientists inquired into the role of cell pathology as a source of disease (Jewson, 1976). Rather than focusing on the organs, the new direction for the expansion of medical knowledge took place in the laboratory, under the microscope, where pathology could be examined and analyzed at the cellular level. This completed the removal of the patient from the generation of medical knowledge. It also created a new hierarchy in the field of medicine, elevating both the scientist-physician who produces new knowledge in the medical laboratory and the practising physician who introduced this knowledge into medical practice.

This evolution of the production of medical knowledge had a distinct effect on the organization of our health care system. The emergence of the hospital as a site for medical care and developments in laboratory medicine, to a large extent, shaped the structure and work of health care institutions. In the next section, we look more closely at the work of hospitals, starting with the historical developments of hospitals in Canada and moving to identify the current structure and organization of hospital care.

HOSPITALS

The hospital, as we know it today, bears very little resemblance to the first hospitals established in Canada and in Western Europe. Up until the end of the nineteenth century, hospitals were mainly the domain of the poor and the homeless, serving the function of social housing and social service, rather than the place where disease was to be treated and cured. Founded mostly by religious institutions and various community groups, hospitals largely housed more unfortunate members of society (see Box 5.1 on Bedlam).

Due to lack of proper sanitation (e.g., the infamous Bedlam was built over a sewer), the spread of diseases within the hospital was relatively rapid and many of those who stayed in hospitals were not likely to leave alive (Edginton, 1989). Prior to the recognition of **asepsis**, or the protection against infection through the process of removing pathogenic microorganisms, physicians, who rarely washed their hands, were key vectors of transmission of infection. Thus, hospitals were considered places where one went to die rather than a place to go to get cured. By the late 1800s and early 1900s, with improved sanitation, availability of medical technology, and better accommodations, hospitals in Canada began to open their doors to individuals from the middle and upper classes. Gagan (1989) described how the higher classes were enticed into hospitals through the use of "hoteling" services such as private rooms and the reconceptualization of hospitals as necessary embodiments of modern medical science. Concurrently, doctors were also enticed into using hospitals rather than their own community clinics largely because of the availability of nursing and laboratory services, new diagnostic and surgical technology, and medical expertise and specialization (Torrance, 1998).

So, although in the nineteenth century hospitals were sad, unsanitary places that many people saw as their last stop before death, by the early twentieth century, the hospital came to be seen as the centre for advanced treatment and cures and the location for both nursing and medical training (Wotherspoon, 2009). As a result of this shift, a large number of hospitals were constructed across Canada (see Box 5.2). According to the Canadian Museum of History (2010), by 1929 there were around 950 hospitals in Canada of which about half (481) were public general hospitals and just over a quarter (269) were private. The other hospitals included mental institutions (42), tuberculosis sanatoria (31), hospitals for incurables (33), as well as Red Cross hospitals and convalescent homes.

The services and new medical technologies now available in hospitals were expensive. The general population's increasing confidence in medical knowledge and treatment made medical technologies a necessary hospital service. Hospitals became more and more expensive, and because hospitalization of the indigent was seen to be a community responsibility, these rising costs were largely subsidized by paying clients. With an admission to a hospital resulting in a potentially severe financial burden for individuals

Box 5.1

The Infamous Bedlam Hospital

The Bethlem Royal Hospital, known to most as Bedlam, was established in the late 1300s as the first hospital to "treat" the mentally ill. Such treatment, as depicted in this woodcut, included being chained to beds, whipped, or plunged into ice-cold water to achieve submission. Thus, the word *bedlam* became synonymous with a state of madness or utter chaos.

Later, within the new Bethlem Royal Hospital, the public was invited in to "view" the patients, as is depicted in the image from *The Rake's Progress*. It was soon thereafter that many hospitals came to build theatres to display patients to a paying audience now largely made up of medical students.

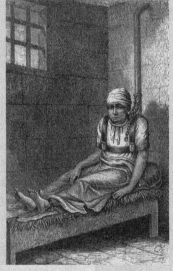

Stock Montage/Archive Photos/Getty Images

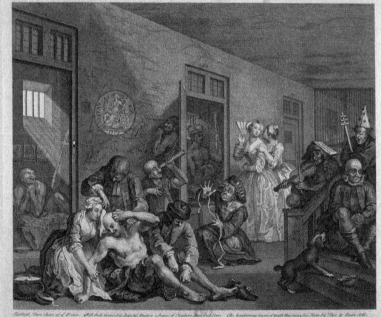

Heritage Image Partnership Ltd/Alamy

Source: The Rake's Progress by William Hogarth 1730s

Cottage Hospitals into "Health Factories" in Canada

In his essay "Hospitals as Health Factories," Torrance (1998) details how general hospitals in Canada were usually founded by religious orders, groups of prominent citizens, or by municipalities, while mental hospitals were established by provincial governments. Most of the care was provided by unpaid providers, such as nuns in religious institutions and student nurses who lived on-site in residences in teaching hospitals.

In most rural areas such care was absent until the advent of the **cottage hospital** system. Newfoundland and Labrador adopted a system of small cottage hospitals, a concept that originated in rural Scotland. From 1936 to 1954, 19 cottage hospitals were opened strategically around coastal areas of Newfoundland. Funding for construction was provided by the government, but local residents were expected to contribute by donating building material, labour, and even land (Collier, 2011).

In 1948, the federal government introduced the hospital construction grant allowing provinces to invest in building new hospitals (Fierlbeck, 2011). This resulted in a wave of capital expansion.

Two key changes in the staffing of hospitals followed this rapid expansion in the size and infusion of new technologies. The first was an increase in the intensity of staffing based on the number of staff per patient or per hospital bed. The second was an increased differentiation among occupations and specializations. This was particularly apparent between the ranks of allied professional and technical workers. As Torrance (1998) details:

> Bigger hospitals were being built, and into them were pouring the flood of innovations which have made moderns hospitals the centre of high-technology medicine. New diagnostic tests and equipment, new monitoring machinery for critically ill patients, new therapies and surgical techniques were introduced at an unprecedented rate. These not only required more staff, but a more highly trained and specialized staff. The new technologists staffed units such as emergency services, intensive care, diagnostic laboratories and rehabilitation medicine which were arising both within and outside the traditional four-service structure of medicine, surgery, obstetrics and pediatrics. (p. 441)

and their families, the coverage of services in hospitals became a prominent political issue. Provincial governments tried to implement various social programs for low- and middle-income families to address this financial burden (see Chapter 3).

Hospital Governance and Administration

Today, hospitals are large, complex organizations, with their distinct administration and organization of patient care (Torrance, 1998). In 2011, there were an estimated 1172 hospitals in Canada (Statistics Canada, 2001) providing various health care services (see Table 5.1) (CIHI, 2011). From 1997 to 2003, between 3.1 and 3.3 million people were admitted annually to Canadian hospitals (CIHI, 2005).

The majority of hospitals in Canada are operated privately by not-for-profit religious organizations or not-for-profit voluntary corporations (Fuller, 1998). Some hospitals were

Table 5.1 Number of Hospitals and Hospital Beds by Region and Type, 2010–2011*

	Number of Hospitals	Number of Hospital Beds							
		Intensive Care	Obstetrics	Paediatrics	Psychiatric	Rehabilitation	Long-Term Care	Other Acute	Total
Alberta	136	661	328	1978	914	225	5209	5281	13348
British Columbia	188	375	473	135	1190	458	5431	5071	14226
Manitoba	66	221	196	31	316	444	412	2841	4461
New Brunswick	44	141	163	92	439	83	332	1603	2853
Newfoundland and Labrador	40	127	121	28	237	63	713	1101	2405
Nova Scotia	53	177	178	24	371	162	309	1952	3173
Northwest Territories	13	4	13	10	10	0	13	30	169
Ontario	315	1653	1758	530	4724	2278	5971	14412	31326
Prince Edward Island	3	—[1]	—[1]	—[1]	—[1]	—[1]	—[1]	—[1]	594
Saskatchewan	72	66	125	71	82	38	237	1454	3676
Yukon Territory	1	—[1]	—[1]	—[1]	—[1]	—[1]	—[1]	49	49
Total	1172	3425	3355	2899	8283	3751	18627	33794	76280

*These numbers show beds available and staffed and in operation. Residential facilities within hospitals are not included.

[1]Data not identified or is missing

Sources: Statistics Canada. (2011, December). *Canadian business patterns database.* Available at www.ic.gc.ca/cis-sic/cis-sic.nsf/IDE/cis-sic622etbe.html

Canadian Institute for Health Information. (2011). *Hospital beds staffed and in operation, fiscal year 2010–2011.* Retrieved from www.cihi.ca/CIHI-ext-portal/internet/EN/Quick_Stats/quick+stats/quick_stats_main?xTopic=Spending&pageNumber=1&resultCount=10&filterTypeBy=undefined&filterTopicBy=14&autorefresh=1

designated as teaching hospitals to provide learning opportunities for future health care providers and locales where they could conduct medical research. These are often associated with universities, providing medical and nursing education to students. The other hospitals are community hospitals with the mandate to provide health care services to local communities and sponsor patient education programs (CIHI, 2005)

Although hospitals receive most of their funding from the government, they are usually governed by a board of directors and a CEO, not a government official. The dynamic within the hospital makes the decision-making process about funding and service delivery complicated. Goss (1963) defined the hospital as having a **dual authority**. The administration of the hospital is nominally responsible for governance, administration, and staffing; physicians are the ones who admit patients to the hospital and discharge them, define the treatment and the types of diagnostic procedures to be undertaken, and establish the course of treatment. Since the majority of practising physicians in Canada do not receive remuneration from the hospital but are reimbursed directly for their services by provincial health plans and have their own private practices that operate independently from the hospitals, the hospital administration does not have full authority over medical doctors.

Nurses and other health care support and facility staff, on the other hand, fall under the direct supervision of the hospital administration. They are employees of the hospitals. Their wages and duties of service are directed by hospital administration and the hospital can alter them to a considerable degree (Turner, 1995). The dependent position of nurses has become especially visible during past years of "restructuring" in health care, followed by the cutbacks in funding provided to hospitals and other health care services (Armstrong & Armstrong, 2002; Varcoe & Rodney, 2009).

Hospital Patients

Although many of us would agree that hospitals provide good medical care, most of us also dislike being in the hospital. What makes hospitals so unpleasant? Clearly, the state in which individuals seek medical care in the hospital does not contribute to a sense of happiness and optimism, with the possible exception of maternity wards. When we go to the hospital, the illness and uncertainty of medical diagnosis make us particularly vulnerable. Although today the patient is envisioned as an active participant in the decision-making process in medical encounters (Fisher, 2009), in real life, many patients intentionally or unintentionally do not assume this "active" role (Bury, 2000; Lupton, 2003).

In his work on *Asylums*, Goffman (1961) (see Chapter 1) coined the concept **total institution**, which refers to "a place of residence and work where a large number of like-situated individuals, cut off from the wider society for an appreciable period of time, together lead an enclosed, formally administered round of life" (p. xiii). A concept that applies to all hospitals, one of the important aspects of the total institution is *depersonalization*—whereby striving to create a group from a collection of individuals (e.g., soldiers, students, patients), the institution works on making individuals similar to each other by wearing the same clothes, haircuts, and behaviours. Although stays in acute care hospitals are relatively short, it is not hard to draw some parallels with the process of depersonalization that characterizes total institutions. First, patients are stripped from their identity both symbolically and physically—they are assigned numbers (that sometimes are placed on a band around the patient's wrist) in hospital databases; their clothes are replaced with hospital robes (which could be construed as demeaning); patients are assigned to specific wards and their mobility is restricted; and certain places, such as staff lounges, are off-limits. Similar beds, clothing, blankets, food, and protocols of care transform people from *individuals* into *patients*.

At the same time, it would be wrong to assume that all patients receive the same care in the hospital. Cultural biases and beliefs of patients and staff are often evident in the type of care provided (Fisher, 2009). For example, Glaser and Strauss (1967) documented how the perceived social worth of the patient affected the work of medical personnel in the hospitals. Young patients and those who were considered to be socially worthy often received better care than older individuals and those who were believed to be less worthy of the heroic efforts of contemporary medicine (Collier & Haliburton, 2011). The social characteristics of the patients often become a silent motivator for providing more or less care in the hospital. For example, the inquest into the death of Brian Sinclair, who came to Winnipeg's Health Sciences Centre emergency department to receive care but was found dead 34 hours later, found that his Aboriginal and low-income status played a role in his death (Puxley, 2013).

Hospital Restructuring and Reorganization

Hospitals consume the largest proportion of the health care budget both nationally and provincially (see Figures 5.1 and 5.2) (Tholl, 1994). Provincial health care budgets during the

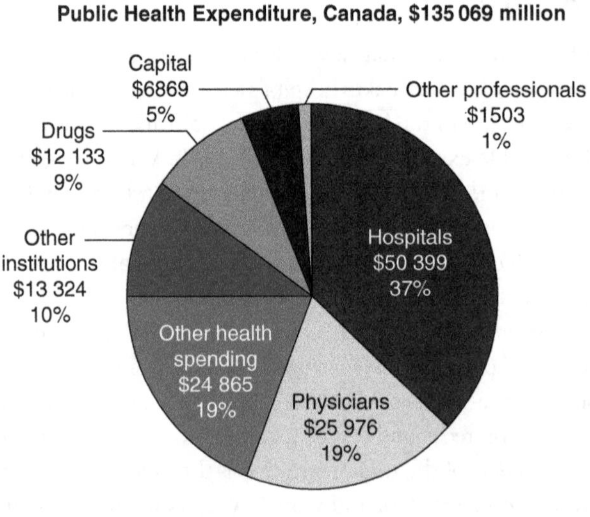

Public Health Expenditure, Canada, $135 069 million

Capital
$6869
5%

Other professionals
$1503
1%

Drugs
$12 133
9%

Other
institutions
$13 324
10%

Hospitals
$50 399
37%

Other health
spending
$24 865
19%

Physicians
$25 976
19%

Figure 5.1 Public Expenditure on Health, by Type of Spending, Canada 2010

Source: National Health Expenditure Database, Canadian Institute for Health Information, 2010. Reprinted by permission.

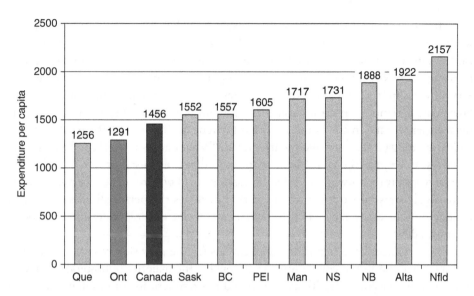

Figure 5.2 Hospital Expenditure per Capita by Provincial Governments, by Province, 2010

Source: Ontario Hospital Association. Reprinted by permission.

neo-liberalism era of the past few decades have made hospitals an easy target for budget reductions. This neo-liberal narrative is based on state reductions in economic and social activities and interventions, the deregulation of labour and financial markets to liberate the enormous creative energy of the market, and the stimulation of commerce and investments by eliminating borders and barriers to the full mobility of labour, capital, goods, and services (Navarro, 2009). Implementation of these neo-liberal policies in the health sector favours market relations and individual responsibility creating a new policy environment that emphasizes the need to reduce public responsibility and funding for the health of individuals and populations and increase individuals' personal responsibility. Even the discourse is changing: patients are referred to as clients and consumers of health care.

These neo-liberal political pressures have resulted in hospital mergers and closures (Fierlbeck, 2011) and in the restructuring, re-organization, and marketing of services provided in the hospitals (Armstrong, 2002). Under pressure to cut spending, hospitals started to redefine their provision of services in order to find alternative means to provide care to patients. These measures include cutting the number of acute care and emergency room beds, shortening the average length of stay in hospitals, and offering same-day surgery and out-patient follow-up services. Another strategy was to cut salaried hospital employees and contract out non-medical services (Armstrong, 2002). The so-called hotel services provided in the hospital (laundry, food preparation, and maintenance) were increasingly contracted out to private firms in an effort to reduce expenses (Armstrong, 2002).

The number of nursing positions has also been reduced and the nature of nursing work has been redefined and restructured (Armstrong, 2002). A *standardization* of care results in increased attention paid to following specific protocols of care, documenting the physical tasks done by nurses, and neglecting other aspects of care. It is easy to measure the efficiency of manual tasks (e.g. how many pills were given to how many patients), but critics argue it is difficult to measure the efficiency of holding a patient's hand in the minute of crisis (Varcoe & Rodney, 2009). As Armstrong and Armstrong (2002) have eloquently stated, "What counts is what can be counted" (see Researcher Profile 5.1). Since hospital policies refocused on measurable outcomes, work protocols were oriented on tasks instead of care, exposing nurses to an increasingly stressful work environment that devalues the personalized approach to patients and the ethos of care that is fundamental to the nursing profession (Varcoe & Rodney, 2009).

These changes have significant implications for the provision of care not only in hospitals, but also in the community. Traditionally, the majority of hospital employees were women (nursing or health care aids) and the restructuring of hospitals has had a

Researcher Profile 5.1

Pat and Hugh Armstrong

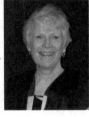

Courtesy of Pat Armstrong/ York University

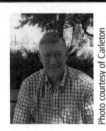

Photo courtesy of Carleton University

Pat Armstrong is a Distinguished Research Professor in Sociology at York University in Toronto, and a Fellow of the Royal Society of Canada. She held a prestigious Chair from CHSRF/ CIHR entitled Women and Health Services: Policies and Politics. Initially her focus was on women's work and social policy but her more recent publications cover a wide range of issues related to women's health and health care work. Hugh Armstrong is a Distinguished Research Professor and Professor Emeritus of Social Work, Political Economy and Sociology at Carleton University in Ottawa. Together Pat and Hugh have conducted research focused on women and work and on health care. Their most recent publications include *Critical to Care: The Invisible Women in Health* (UTP, 2008, with Krista Scott-Dixon); *About Canada: Health Care* (Fernwood Publishing, 2008); "Contradictions at Work: Struggles for Control in Canadian Health Care" in Panitch and Leys (eds.), *Morbid Symptoms: Health under Capitalism* (Merlin Press, 2009); and "Gendering Work? Women and Technologies in Health" in Balka, Green and Henwood (eds.), *Gender, Health and Information Technologies in Context* (Palgrave Macmillan, 2009, with Karen Messing). In 2010, Oxford University Press republished two of their previous books (with new prefaces): *The Double Ghetto: Canadian Women and Their Segregated Work*, first published in 1978, and *Wasting Away: The Undermining of Canadian Health Care*, first published in 1996. Their combined work has formed a critical contribution to the medical sociology literature on nursing, health care, and women's work from a critical gender perspective.

direct negative impact on their job security, employment opportunities, and job satisfaction (Armstrong, 2002). Moreover, transferring services to the community basically meant transferring care to *women* in the community, because women remain the major providers of both paid and unpaid care in our society. The reduction in hospital stays means that people with more health problems and needs are being discharged more quickly into the community. Some argue the lack of appropriate community care has made women more vulnerable to the stress of providing unpaid care for their loved ones (Armstrong, 2002).

To summarize, the transformation of the modern hospital has witnessed a transition from the place of refuge for the socially disadvantaged to the centre of provision of most advanced medical care and utilization of new medical technology. More recently, threatened by the restructuring in health care services, hospitals re-organized their administration and care. The emphasis on protocols, standardization of care, and cost-reduction initiatives affected not only hospitals but also other health care institutions. In the remainder of this chapter, we take a closer look at these institutions.

LONG-TERM CARE AND NURSING HOMES

As we discuss in Chapter 9 on aging, the increased life expectancy and the associated chronic health problems of our population poses a challenge to our health care system and its ability to deal with patients who have health conditions that limit their capacity to live independently. Although the majority of older adults live at home and prefer this arrangement to any other accommodations (Connidis, 2010), close to 14% of approximately 4.7 million of older Canadians need assistance with the activities of daily living, such as dressing, bathing, and eating (Statistics Canada, 2010c). Although the majority of them receive care at home from family or paid caregivers, the lack of adequate long-term care is a significant barrier for older adults who need care in an institutional setting.

Long-term care cannot simply be defined as a place but as a complex system of care for persons who are at significant risk of having progressive and/or chronic conditions and require services to meet their long-term functional needs (see also Grignon & Bernier, 2012). Long-term care includes both facility/residential-based care as well as home care services. The lack of available facilities results in supplementing our long-term care needs through acute care hospital beds and home care services. On any given day in Canada, **alternate level of care** (ALC) patients occupy the equivalent of approximately 7550 beds in acute care hospitals. ALC refers to patients who are receiving care in the wrong setting, such as those in acute care who are waiting for a transfer to a more appropriate long-term care facility or a rehabilitation facility. In 2008–2009, there were more than 92 000 hospitalizations and more than 2.4 million hospital days involving ALC stays in Canada (CIHI, 2010c). Hospital acute care beds are expensive. According to the North East Ontario Local Health Integration Network (LHIN), for instance, the daily cost of a hospital bed was $842 while the long-term care bed cost only $126 per day and home care cost $42 (North East LHIN, 2011).

Given the differences in costs in providing home care, long-term care, and acute care, and the fact that the majority of seniors would prefer to stay at home, it seems reasonable to expect that more effort would be placed on establishing good home care services, and that long-term care facilities would be a priority over acute hospital care. Although economically such an arrangement would make sense, in real life there are historical and systemic barriers to its implementation. Home-care services and long-term care services are not covered by the 1984 Canada Health Act, and eligibility to receive government assistance in covering these services is often determined by income/means-testing (Grignon & Bernier, 2012). Moreover, unlike hospitals, long-term care and nursing homes often operate on a for-profit basis and there are considerable costs to people through out-of-pocket payments and private spending on long-term care (Grignon & Bernier, 2012). The annual out-of-pocket costs of stay for patients also varies by provinces, ranging from a maximum of $12 157 in Quebec to $33 600 in Newfoundland and Labrador (Grignon & Bernier, 2012).

When health care services operate on a for-profit basis, there is a concern that the health needs of individuals will be compromised in pursuit of profits (Fierlbeck, 2011). In the context of long-term care facilities, this quest for profit is especially alarming, as the majority of residents often lack the power and ability to demand the appropriate services and good care due to old age, vulnerability, or dependence on caregivers (Connidis, 2010). In addition, there is the challenge of providing continuity of care in for-profit settings (Armstrong, 2002). When the facility is no longer profitable, it can be closed because private companies are less accountable to local communities than not-for-profit corporations.

These compromises can also be seen among staff. People working in for-profit long-term residential care in Ontario often work in more hazardous environments and experience more workplace injuries and less job security than those in not-for-profit facilities (Armstrong, 2002). Because the majority of employees providing care in long-term care facilities are women (Armstrong, 2002), they are paid less for their services and are also less skilled than nurses working in the hospitals. Generally, the lack of nursing skills among long-term care workers should not be a problem. But since individuals are now being discharged from acute care hospitals earlier, the type of care provided in long-term care facilities by paid caregivers as well as at home by paid and unpaid caregivers is becoming more complex (Armstrong, 2002).

While Canadians prefer home care services over nursing homes, the working conditions of home care workers are also not ideal. Home care workers report high levels of job stress and dissatisfaction (Denton, Zeytinoglu, Davies, & Lian, 2002). The funding for home care services is fragmented and varies by province (Grignon & Bernier, 2012). As the number of elderly requiring care increases concomitant with the continually shrinking social safety net, it becomes more difficult for individuals to pay for long-term or home care services. However, given the current fiscal pressure on health care spending, the introduction of any nationally coordinated insurance plan for long-term health care services seems extremely unlikely, even though more and more scholars and policy makers recognize the need for better government funding of home service provision (CLHIA, 2012; Grignon & Bernier, 2012).

COMMUNITY HEALTH CARE

Community health care is health care that is delivered in the community rather than in an institutional setting. Although home care is often included under the umbrella of community health care, because we have already discussed home care services, we focus here on the provision of primary care services in the community. **Primary care** is typically defined as one's first point of contact in the health care system (typically family physicians or nurse practitioners or midwives), which is in contrast to *secondary care*, that is, acute care in hospitals or hospital-based clinics, and *tertiary care*, which is rehabilitative care either in institutional, community, or home settings. The term *primary health care* is a broader concept that includes primary care services, health promotion and disease prevention, and population-level public health functions consistent with the World Health Organization 1978 *Alma Ata Declaration* (WHO, 1978). We begin with a description of the more traditional arrangements for primary care through private family physicians working through fee-for-service and then focus on alternative models, including community health centres and the range of new organizational models of primary care.

Private, Fee-For-Service Medical Practice

Primary care has long been thought of as being provided by family physicians working in solo or group practice funded through a *fee-for-service* (FFS) model; that is, each service that a physician provides from an ear examination or throat swab to the writing up of a prescription has a specified fee attached to it. The province or territory pays each of these based on a fee negotiated between the provincial or territorial ministry of health and the provincial medical association. Naylor (1986) described this situation as public payment for private practice.

Historically, this has been the predominant form of primary care delivery but the number of physicians in individual fee-for-service practice has been declining. This is due, in part, to a new generation of physicians who are more interested in balancing work–life demands and avoiding a business approach to medical practice that involves many hours of work and being on-call. Moreover, some physicians prefer working in a team with other health professionals and some prefer working on salary or through alternative payment plans. From a systems perspective, the traditional approach to practice has also raised concerns about the lack of coordination of services due to physicians working in silos as well as an undue focus on FFS medical reimbursement to physicians for acute care at the expense of prevention and chronic disease management. As a response to these concerns, a variety of models of primary care delivery have been developed and implemented. In Ontario, for example, Health Service Organizations and Community Health Centres were developed in the 1970s. During the 1990s, other models, including family health groups, networks, and teams were developed. Table 5.2 presents an overview of these various models.

Table 5.2 A Comparison of Primary Care Models (Ontario)

	Fee-for-Service System	Health Service Organizations (since 1975)	Community Health Centres (began c. 1980)	Family Health Networks (since 2001)	Family Health Groups (since 2003)	Family Health Teams (since 2004)
Number of Physicians	7,439	160	146	393	2,536	650 (projected)
Physician remuneration	FFS	Capitation	Salary	FFS, blended	FFS	Capitation or salary
Patient rosters?	No	Yes	No	Yes	Yes	Yes
Group practice	Optional	Mandatory	Mandatory	Mandatory	Mandatory	Mandatory
24/7 access?	Optional	Mandatory	Mandatory	Mandatory	Mandatory	Mandatory
Funding for other care providers?	None	Some	Significant	Some	Some	Significant

Source: Hogg, W. n.d. *Comparison of primary care models in Ontario.* C.T. Lamont Primary Health Care Research Centre. Elisabeth Bruyère Research Centre, Ottawa. Reprinted by permission.

Community Health Centres

Community health care is based on an ideal model of health care services where care is provided in the community, is *integrated*, and is focused on *health promotion* and *prevention*. Currently, community health centres (CHCs) serve over 2 million Canadians although there is unequal distribution of this service across provinces and territories (Canadian Association of Community Health Centres, 2012). While the names of the centres may vary, all community health centres are based on the model that incorporates the following features:

- They are not-for-profit publically funded;
- Services are provided by a team of health care professionals, including physicians, nurses, nutritionists, and other health care professionals;
- They focus on primary care, health promotion, and prevention;
- They are designed to address the needs of the community in which they are located (Canadian Association of Community Health Centres, 2012).

The idea of Community Health Centres (CHC) is not new—such centres were founded in some provinces even before the introduction of Medicare, including the Saskatoon Community Clinic in 1962 and the Sault Ste. Marie Group Health Centre in 1963. In fact, Tommy Douglas' original vision of publicly funded health care services was based on the community health centres model (then called *community clinics*), where the residents can receive a variety of services from the team of *salary-paid* health care providers (Shandel & Johnson, 1983). Known as the "Second Stage of Medicare," this vision was never implemented although community health centres did operate in some parts of Canada. Throughout the 1970s and 1980s, a number of policy reports suggested the integration of community care centres into health services delivery (Epp, 1986; Hall, 1980). Despite convincing evidence of the promising outcomes of such centres, there was very little government action in this direction. That is because the expansion of the CHC model across the country has faced some key cultural and medical obstacles both in their perception but, more importantly, from resistance by provincial medical associations (Canadian Alliance of Community Health Centre Associations, 2009). The original model of community clinics, supported by Tommy Douglas, was blocked by the resistance of physicians. They supported fee-for-service private practice over community-based clinics because the clinics were perceived to infringe on physician autonomy and doctors' perception of themselves as businessmen [sic] (Canadian Alliance of Community Health Centre Associations, 2009).

With respect to cultural barriers, although community health care centres have been successfully providing services for many people in Europe and other parts of the world, many Canadians are more familiar with the private-office format of receiving primary care. Community health centres are often perceived as serving marginalized members of society, such as the poor and disadvantaged, and there is little public recognition of the many potential benefits of the CHCs for the health of the broader population. This is less of the case in Quebec where the CLSC model has been more fully integrated into the health care system.

An additional criticism levelled against CHCs was the lack of data on cost effectiveness. CHCs redirect their focus to address preventive care and health promotion by providing the services of various professions, including dieticians and health promotion specialists who are not covered under Medicare. While this is a concern about overall cost, it is not necessarily an issue of cost effectiveness. Cuts to health care spending and the emphasis on restructuring health care services in policy debates in the late 1980s and early 1990s have caused the interest in development of CHCs to re-emerge. Many provincial health care systems sought to establish community health care centres to serve the local population and reduce acute care costs. In addition to cost effectiveness of community care, CHCs were seen as integrated primary care settings that take a more holistic approach to care integrating health promotion and prevention with treating the already sick (Fierlbeck, 2011).

Today, there are over 300 CHCs across Canada. Since the health infrastructure is managed by provincial governments, the availability of community health centres varies from province to province. The investment in social services in the province of Quebec, for instance, resulted in a well-developed network of 149 community health clinics (CLSCs). The McGuinty-led Liberal government in Ontario placed an emphasis on expanding community health clinics and today Ontario has 101 community health centres (Ontario Ministry of Health and Long-Term Care, 2012).

Evolution of the Organization of Family Health Care

In addition to the development of interdisciplinary CHCs, two other recent models of care are the family health network (FHN) and family health team (FHT), both of which are funded through the rostering of patients rather than fee-for-service. Briefly, FHNs are groups of family physicians who work together in the delivery of care to their patients. There is modest inclusion of other health care providers in FHNs but physicians make up the majority. The FHT, by way of contrast, is usually locally driven and includes a wide range of other health care providers, including nurses and nurse practitioners, mental health professionals, specialist physicians, diagnostic services, dieticians, and so on. Funding for FHTs requires that they provide some form of access to care 24/7. Although FHTs have different types of governance—sometimes led by physicians, sometimes by the community, and sometimes by a mix of physicians and community members—this model generally favours physicians as the central figures in making the FHTs work (Rosser, Colwill, Kasperski, & Wilson, 2011). The lack of a clear model of professional relations in FHTs makes it difficult for other health care professions to negotiate their status on the health care team. Hanna (2007), for instance, noted that nurses are often reluctant to accept a leadership role over the physician and perceive a physician as a supervisor, rather than the leader of the team.

Nurse-Practitioner Led Clinics

Starting in 2007, the Ontario government also invested in Nurse Practitioner-led Clinics (NPLCs), in which nurse practitioners assume the role of the leader of the interdisciplinary health care team. However, the team must include a consulting physician (Haydt, 2012). In this model, all members of the team receive salaries, and the governance of the clinic is equally divided between nurse practitioners and community members (Haydt, 2012). The development of NPLCs has not been without controversy. The Ontario Medical Association, for example, responded to the expansion of NP-led clinics in 2009 as infringing on their domain within collaborative health care teams (Ontario Medical Association, 2009).

In sum, it is currently not clear which model might be best suited for which community. Moreover, developing a new primary health care infrastructure is expensive and requires considerable political commitment. The political climate of various provincial governments can often facilitate or impede implementation of community care. Referring to the example of Ontario, the McGuinty Liberal government not only actively lobbied for the expansion of community care services, but also invested a large sum of money in establishing this initiative. Haydt (2012) estimated that between 2005 and 2008 FHTs received approximately $600 million, CHCs $300 million, and NPLCs $38 million from the provincial budget (p. 9). In British Columbia, the government invested in the education of nurse practitioners but the lack of community health centres and clinics led by nurse practitioners left many of them having to work in a setting where their skills are not fully utilized (Watts, 2010). In 2011, there were 30 nurse practitioner-led clinics in Alberta, and the government was looking to further expand the services provided by nurse practitioners (Alberta Health Services, 2011; NPAA, 2013). In addition to providing funding, however, governments need to provide incentives for the health care practitioners to work in community care. Given that many provincial ministries are looking to reduce spending or limit expanded spending on health care, the long-term benefits of such services may be overlooked by the policy makers seeking to save money.

One interesting area of community care thought to both reduce costs and improve the patient experience is midwifery and home births and birthing centres for normal, uncomplicated pregnancies (see Box 5.3).

CHALLENGES TO THE ORGANIZATION OF HEALTH CARE IN CANADA

So far, we have described some of the major changes in organization of health care delivery in Canada. In this section, we analyze some of the Canadian health care system's new concerns brought about by advancements in medical technology. We do so by drawing upon the field of *biomedical ethics*—which enquires into the moral and ethical dilemmas faced by health care providers and health policy. First, we discuss the notion of risk society and its impact on provision of health care services and health care delivery. Then, we briefly describe how the technological advancements in medicine challenge the provision and organization of health care services.

Box 5.3

Home Birth and Birth Centres

The relatively recent reintroduction of midwives into the Canadian health care system has come with a concomitant increase in the practice of home birth. As noted by the Association of Ontario Midwives, "Birth is the leading reason for the hospitalization of women in Ontario, yet there is no medical reason to be hospitalized for a healthy, normal labour and birth." (Association of Ontario Midwives, n.d., p. 3) Indeed, a comprehensive study of all home births attended by midwives in British Columbia found that "Planned home birth attended by a registered midwife was associated with very low and comparable rates of perinatal death and reduced rates of obstetric interventions and other adverse perinatal outcomes compared with planned hospital birth attended by a midwife or physician." (Janssen et al., 2009) Medical associations, such as the Society of Obstetricians and Gynecologists of Canada, do not take a specific stand on the safety of home births, but, rather, call for more research.

In some provinces, free-standing birth centres separate from hospitals have also been established. This began in Quebec with the Maison de naissance established by the passage of midwifery legislation in 1998. Today there are over 16 birth centres in Quebec with a promise of 20 more. One already exists in Manitoba (November 2011) and in 2014 two birth centres opened in Ontario—in Toronto (**www.torontobirthcentre.ca**) and Ottawa (**www.ottawabirthcentre.ca**). Midwifery-led birth centres provide women and their families with another option to home or hospital birth and one that is argued to be both safe and cost effective.

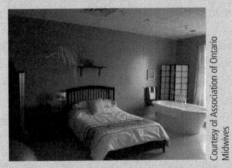

Maison de naissance in Blainville, Quebec

Source: Association of Ontario Midwives, Birth Centres: Ottawa, Toronto, and Six Nations. Available at www.ontariomidwives.ca/care/birth/birth-centres

Managing Health Care in Risk Society

The concept of *risk society* was introduced to sociology by Ulrich Beck (1992) and Anthony Giddens (1991). According to these scholars, individuals in our society are increasingly aware of the many risks that shape our existence and make us vulnerable to the dangers of living. This awareness shapes our response to these risks and changes our perceptions about the world around us as unsafe and potentially hazardous place. In the context of the health care system, the discourse on *risk* often makes it to the front of the health policy agenda. That is, although some of the risks, such as lifestyle choices, are managed at the individual level; others become a source of concern for the provision of health care and for health policy makers. Two key examples of organizational and policy-relevant risk factors are those that led to the creation of the Canadian Blood Services and the "super bugs" confronting hospitals at an increasingly alarming rate. Box 5.4 describes the social organization of the provision of blood services in Canada, the scandal that resulted from the utilization of tainted blood, and the Krever Inquiry (Krever, 1997) that examined the factors surrounding the scandal.

In addition to blood, there is an increasing need for human organs for transplantation. The rate of this medical procedure has increased exponentially since experimental organ

Box 5.4

Tainted Blood Scandal— The Krever Commission

Although today almost everyone is aware of the deadly impact of HIV (Human Immunodeficiency Virus) and AIDS (Acquired Immunodeficiency Syndrome), in the early 1980s, this disease was still unknown to the public. After people donated their blood, the collecting agency and recipients of that blood were not concerned about HIV infections.

The operation of what is known today as Canadian Blood Services can be traced back to World War II, when the Canadian Red Cross Services and Connaught Laboratories found a way to manufacture blood products and supply them for those in need, first, in the battlefield and later, to the Canadian population (Smith & Fiddler, 2009). The Red Cross had in place a number of measures to protect blood products from contamination (Krever, 1997) and Canada always relied on unpaid donors, which reduces the risk of contamination. However, between the time that new screening and testing procedures for HIV and HCV (Hepatitis C virus) in blood products were available for use and were then introduced by the Canadian Red Cross, more than 2000 Canadians had been infected with HIV and thousands were infected with HCV. Most of these individuals were hemophiliacs who rely heavily on blood donations.

Canada was not alone in its use of tainted blood—similar cases were faced by many countries, including the United States, the United Kingdom, and Japan (Feldman, 2000). Each country was also outraged by the inability of its government to prevent contamination and to protect its citizens.

In Canada, the federal government established a Royal Commission in 1993 to examine the use of tainted blood. The Krever Inquiry (1997) found fault at all levels from the federal and provincial governments and Health Canada, to hospitals and physicians, to the Canadian Red Cross and manufacturers. For instance, although the United States had already implemented more cautious donor screening, the Canadian Red Cross was very late in introducing new measures, which resulted in more people being infected (Smith & Fiddler, 2009).

Krever recommended a set of five basic principles for the Canadian blood supply system including:

> blood is a public resource; donors should not be paid; sufficient blood should be collected so that importation from other countries is unnecessary; access to blood and blood products should be free and universal; safety of the blood supply system is paramount. (Norris, 2008, p. 8)

Since 1998, Canadian Blood Services and Héma-Québec have been collecting, manufacturing, and distributing blood products. Today, the chance of contamination of blood products is considered to be miniscule, but, for far too many people, the tainted blood scandal is still a relatively fresh memory.

transplantations have become more successful. We have individuals who are in dire need of hearts, livers, kidneys, lungs, retinas, and other body parts that can be donated (harvested) by others, such as accident victims.

There are a number of complicated ethical dilemmas and risks in relation to organ donations. For example, should we pay organ donors or their families? After all, there is a considerable shortage of available organs, and some people argue that introducing payment into the current system of organ harvesting could make more organs available for those in need (Collier & Haliburton, 2011). The majority of Western countries regulate this market heavily and insist on voluntary donations. However, there is growing organ black market where kidneys, livers, and other body parts are for sale (Collier & Haliburton, 2011). Some argue that paying for organs will only increase social inequality and can increase the black market for organs (Collier & Haliburton, 2011). There are those who criticize individuals who travel to underdeveloped countries (medical tourism—see Chapter 10) to speed up the process of receiving an organ. Others believe that this practice reduces pressures on the health care system by eliminating from the waiting list those who have means to pay for travel and for an organ in another country (Collier & Haliburton, 2011).

To further complicate the discussion of risk surrounding organ transplants, there is increasing research on the use of animal-to-human organ transplants, or xenotransplants. The first reported procedure was in 1992 by Thomas Starzl who transplanted a baboon liver into an HIV patient suffering from Hepatitis B. The patient survived 70 days (Starzl et al., 1993). Due to a number of concerns, such as infectious disease transfer between primates, the pig has been identified as the most promising donor species for humans, moving science to focus on pigs (Schuurman & Pierson, 2008). Aside from the philosophical issues of humanism and the body, there continue to be other issues, such as inter-species transfer of diseases and the rejection of the organ by the body. However, research continues and there is even a journal dedicated to publishing research on inter-species transplants, called *Xenotransplanation.*

Finally, there are also those who claim that organ transplants should not be performed at all because of its relatively low success rate and the vast amount of resources invested in these operations (e.g. operating rooms, surgeons, staff, drugs, recovery period) (Collier & Haliburton, 2011). Although approximately 80% of those who have had kidney transplants and approximately 75% of those with heart or liver transplants survive the next five years (Collier & Haliburton, 2011), some analysts suggest that the money spent on these operations should be invested in other areas, such as health promotion or the establishment of long-term care facilities. After all, such operations benefit relatively few people while there are many Canadians who cannot receive needed health care services due to lack of funding.

The second example of *risk society* is the increasing problem of antibiotic-resistant strains of MRSA (*methicillin-resistant Staphylococcus aureus*) and C. diff (*Clostridium difficile*) as discussed in Box 5.5. The impact of these virulent strains on the health care system are directly related to the practices of health care professionals and institutions. A recent report on Global Risks by the World Economic Forum refers to this as the risk of hubris to health (World Economic Forum, 2013). Essentially, medicine is in a constant battle against mutation. Previous medical developments, such as vaccines, antibiotics, and antivirals, are in

Box 5.5

Iatrogenesis in Hospitals: MRSA and C. *diff*

Two key examples of iatrogenesis in hospitals currently are MRSA—short for methicillin-resistant Staphylococcus *aureus*—and C. *diff*—short for *Clostridium difficile*. The risk of both have been exacerbated in the context of hospital cutbacks (PHAC 2008; 2011). In Chapter 12, we present a detailed discussion of iatrogenesis, briefly defined as a physician- or hospital-induced illness.

According to the Public Health Agency of Canada (PHAC) fact sheet on MRSA (2008), it is described as being primarily spread by skin-to-skin contact or through contact with items contaminated by the bacteria. Those with weakened immune systems and chronic illnesses are more susceptible to the infection and MRSA has been shown to spread easily in health care settings. PHAC also notes that there are a number of reasons for a rise in MRSA:

> Screening techniques are more effective now than they were in the past. More hospitals are actively screening for MRSA, and as a result, we are seeing a higher number of reported cases of MRSA. Laboratory tests to diagnose MRSA are now more rapidly completed, which means more cases are diagnosed early. We also know that the misuse of antibiotics in both hospital and community settings can cause infections like MRSA to become more virulent and more difficult to contain and treat. If antibiotics are prescribed to treat infections unnecessarily or when individuals do not complete their prescriptions, infections can develop a resistance to antibiotics. (PHAC, 2008)

According to the PHAC fact sheet on C *diff* (PHAC, 2011), it is described as a bacterium that causes mild to severe diarrhea and inflammation of the colon. This occurs when antibiotics destroy a person's good bowel bacteria, which enables C. *difficile* bacteria to grow and produce toxins that can damage the bowel and cause diarrhea. Health care workers can easily spread the bacteria to their patients if their hands are contaminated. The elderly and those with other illnesses or who are taking antibiotics are at a greater risk of infection. C. *difficile* is the most frequent cause of infectious diarrhea in Canadian hospitals and long-term care facilities.

a continual state of flux as pathogens continue to evolve and mutate. Our confidence in medical science innovation as the white knight always riding to our rescue may be misplaced. For example, the more we use a specific antibiotic, the greater the chance of a selective bacterial mutation to become resistant to it. As we quickly go through our arsenal of effective antibiotics, we are left with fewer and fewer alternatives and are falling further behind in our ability to generate new antibiotics to treat more virulent, drug-resistant bacteria. This is one of the principal reasons behind the recent move by the Federal Drug Agency (FDA) in the United States to restrict routine use of antibiotic use in livestock (see Chapter 13).

New Medical Technologies

Today's scientific knowledge provides almost infinite possibilities to experiment with new treatments and technologies, but the moral and policy implications of these innovations are not always clear (Collier & Haliburton, 2011). Once in a while, we hear in the news about life-saving medications that are not approved by Health Canada and about new medical technologies that will revolutionize the previous approach to certain medical problems. The availability of medical technologies has been intricately connected with the development and expansion of hospitals, as we have already discussed. Medical technologies have enabled advancements in the safety and efficiency of many medical and surgical procedures in hospitals, so much so that many of the services that previously required an overnight stay in hospital can now be accomplished on the same day through outpatient clinics. There has also been an expansion of free-standing clinics that provide a range of surgical procedures, including laser eye surgery and cosmetic surgery. As such, medical technologies have an important impact on the social organization of health care.

Two recent innovations are worth particular mention, specifically telemedicine and the electronic health record. Telemedicine technologies enable patients and practitioners in rural and remote locations to consult with urban-based medical specialists. Telemedicine has been used for consultations for a wide range of health care from the more social—such as *telepsychiatry*—to those that are much more technical—such as *teledermatology*. These technologies also enable remote access that supports emergency medical care. Significant advances in telemedicine have enabled basic surgeries to be conducted remotely through the use of robotics. These technologies better enable us to achieve true accessibility to health care services despite Canada's vast geography, addressing one of the five principles of Medicare (see Box 5.6).

The development of the electronic health record (EHR) is another innovation that has been central to the reform of primary care and has enabled continuity of care across primary, secondary, and tertiary care systems. As is described in the 2010 Report of the Office of the Auditor General of Canada, 2010, Spring), the EHR is

> . . . secure and private lifetime records that describe a person's health history and care. They are made up of information from a variety of sources, including hospitals, clinics, doctors, pharmacies, and laboratories. This information is critical for treatment and is accessible to health care professionals. . . . A fully functional electronic health record (EHR) will allow health care professionals to view and update a patient's health record. Ideally, to support the provision of high quality care, an individual's EHR will be available to their authorized health care professionals anywhere and anytime. . . . EHRs are intended to solve a number of persistent problems in Canada's health system, some of which may be caused by the use of paper health records. In particular, electronic records are more likely to be legible and available when needed, and can be retrieved more easily and quickly. Potential benefits for patients include improved health care and decreased risks (such as adverse drug reactions or duplicate, invasive, or expensive tests). Health care professionals should be able to make better decisions, thanks to up-to-date, comprehensive patient information. Overall, EHRs are expected to reduce costs and improve quality of care. (pp. 1–3)

We increasingly rely on changes and advancements in technology in all aspects of our lives, including health care. However, in health care especially, we are also suspicious of new technologies and the potential individual and social risks that come with the new technology. These risks, such as developments in the science of genetics, research into cryogenics, and medications that improve performance, make us more and more aware of

How the Cell Phone Is Transforming Health Care

In the influential *Harvard Business Review*, blogger David Aylward (2011) argues that our cell phones can play a key role in transforming the future of health and health care. As he states,

> It can empower both patients and practitioners by providing them with the information they need to make informed decisions about health issues from healthy living habits, to health care provision, and monitoring of diseases. The rapid expansion of wireless networks represents a particularly exciting opportunity to reach those who are currently isolated by distance and lack of communication, using mhealth (mobile health) programs.

For example, Alberta and British Columbia have each built an app that can be downloaded to residents' smart phones to locate the closest health care centre or to receive an update on waiting times in hospitals or health alerts (Alberta Health Services, 2013; Health Link BC, 2013). There are apps that offer response from a health care provider to medically related questions. Apple's app store offers endless apps in the health and fitness category, including apps for a personalized electronic health record, management of diabetes, lab test results, sleep analysis, and much more.

Is it possible that one day soon, you will be able to enter an office of a health care provider with your complete medical record stored on your smart phone, receive an update on your most recent blood work, and show your cell phone containing a stored prescription app to a pharmacist.

the many challenges of our health care system. The potential of access to our personal information through these new advances, such as telemedicine and electronic health records, increases risks to confidentiality and personal security. For example, advancements in genetics might allow us to know if we have an increased risk for various disorders. That may help us to take steps to reduce personal risk but it may also provide ammunition for insurance companies to refuse coverage or void existing policies based on a person's identified genetic profile.

SUMMARY

There has been a steady evolution of the social organization of health care and health care institutions in Canada. Recently this has accelerated as a result of fiscal and political pressures, including lobbying from various professional associations as well as the rapid expansion of technology and health care innovations. There are some longstanding or recurring themes—such as hospital-acquired infections—that were salient before the period of asepsis but now are quite prevalent, and perhaps more lethal. There are also some interesting shifts back to forms of care that echo more traditional approaches to health care, such as midwifery and home birth and birth centres. We can see interesting and challenging social dimensions within and across each of the institutions and organizations involved in the provision of health care in Canada.

Key Terms

Alternate level of care—patients in acute care who are waiting for a transfer to a more appropriate setting, such as long-term care or a rehabilitation facility

Asepsis—protection against infection through the process of removing pathogenic microorganisms

Cottage hospital—a small hospital usually in a rural setting that has a small number of hospital beds

Dual authority—the twin lines of authority in a hospital: a medical line of authority and an administrative line of authority, the latter of which involve the supervision and control of salaried hospital staff such as nurses

Medical gaze—the depersonalizing and dehumanizing inspection of disease by medical experts based on their expertise of knowledge about human conditions

Medical–industrial complex—a set of private and public institutions that provide health care

Neo-liberalism—a perspective that favours market relations and personal responsibility and devalues intervention by the state in matters of economic and social policy

Primary care—typically defined as one's first point of contact in the health care system

Total institution—according to Goffman, a place with a large number of like-situated individuals, leading an enclosed, formally administered life that is cut off from the wider society

Critical Thinking Questions

1. What are the consequences of the hospital remaining the centre for the delivery of health care in Canada?

2. What types of changes could be made to the health care delivery system to address the shift in focus from acute to chronic health conditions?

3. Compare and evaluate the value of various community-based models to better direct health care resources.

4. What things do we need to account for when we evaluate the risk-reward equation for the implementation of new medical technologies?

Further Readings and Resources

Armstrong, P., & Armstrong, H. (2002). *Wasting Away: The Undermining of Canadian Health Care* (2nd Ed.). Toronto: Oxford University Press.

Canadian Institute for Health Information. (2005). *Hospital trends in Canada. Results of a project to create a historical series of statistical and financial data for Canadian hospitals over twenty-seven years.* Ottawa: Author.

Canadian Museum of History
Making Medicare: Community Health Centres www.historymuseum.ca/cmc/exhibitions/hist/medicare/medic-6c04e.shtml

Chapter 6
Population Health in Canada

Chapter Outline

Learning Objectives

After studying this chapter, you will be able to:

1. Understand the importance of examining health at a population level and identify both the benefits and the challenges of such a perspective;

2. Introduce the basics of epidemiology and demonstrate how it is used to examine both risk and the distribution and burden of disease;

3. Describe the characteristics of the Canadian population and how it has evolved over time;

4. Provide a snapshot of variations in health status across various groups of Canadians based on differential mortality rates.

Health has been defined in various ways based on various perspectives. As introduced previously, the biomedical perspective focuses on individual physical components of the body as being healthy or in need of repair or replacement. Taking this mechanistic perspective, the person is simply as healthy as the components of the body. For example, once damaged arteries have been replaced through a surgical bypass, the person is on the road to a healthy recovery. More recent definitions of health have moved past this mechanistic approach to include other factors important for health. These definitions generally maintain their focus on the individual, moving the concept of health from a traditional biomedical perspective that focuses on the physical body and the mere absence of disease to include the person as a whole, his or her perspective, and the context of the person's life.

In this chapter, we build upon our knowledge of theory and methods to examine health and the distribution of health status at a population level. First, we discuss what is meant by population health, its importance, and how it is measured. Next, we introduce the discipline of epidemiology as a science based on understanding risk factors and the causes of health and disease. Finally, we present a historical look at population health in Canada, providing a basic demographic picture of health and disease and how it has changed over time and examine how mortality and self-rated health are distributed across various population characteristics.

MOVING TO A POPULATION HEALTH PERSPECTIVE

From our discussion in Chapter 1, it is clear that health is a very difficult concept to define and to get much agreement on what it means. That does not make it unimportant. Health is a concept that consumes much of our time and energy. Health and disease are the subjects of many conversations. People will often talk about someone they know who just got diagnosed with cancer or who just had a heart attack or a stroke, or who was in a severe accident. People also talk about the activities they engage in that make them healthier, such as exercising or going swimming or for a massage. Most people think about health, illness, and disease as phenomena of the individual. While health is experienced at an individual level, it is also informative to move to examine health at an aggregate level across groups and populations.

Why would it be informative to talk about an individual-level issue at a population level? When we examine health at an individual level, it makes an implicit assumption that illness, disease, and health status are randomly distributed across the population. Everyone, regardless of background or status, has a relatively equal likelihood of suffering the same fate as everyone else. That is, there are no relationships between population characteristics and morbidity and mortality. Is this a valid assumption? Surely those whose jobs involve exposure to hazardous chemicals and materials or dangerous work environments would also be more likely to have health problems and injuries associated with the increased exposure. Those living near polluting factories or busy roadways are more exposed to noxious fumes that are linked to disease. People living in rural areas are more likely to be exposed to herbicides and pesticides used in the agricultural industry that have been shown to be associated with various forms of cancer. Those who cannot afford proper nutrition, what we call food insecurity, may be more prone to illnesses such as Type II diabetes. Who is more likely to be working in these jobs, living in these areas, and unable to afford proper nutrition? While these differences may be obvious, there are many patterns that exist that may not be quite so apparent. Examining patterns allows us to gain an understanding about who is at increased risk for various diseases. It also allows society to be better prepared, ensuring adequate health care resources.

Another reason to move from individual-level health to population-level health is our ability to better address health concerns. For example, Frieden (2010) developed and published the Health Impact Pyramid to describe the individual effort required for various public health initiatives and their overall effect on population health (see Figure 6.1). Regardless of whether the health outcome is an injury, a communicable disease (e.g., a sexually transmitted disease, STD), or a noncommunicable disease (e.g., cancer, heart disease), health interventions targeted lower down the pyramid will have a greater effect on overall health and require less individual efforts.

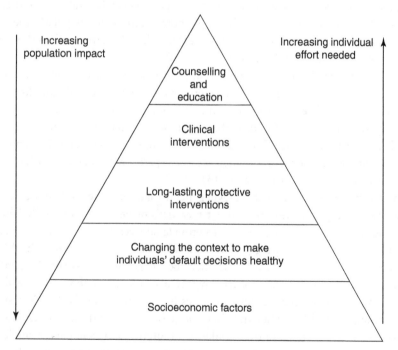

Figure 6.1 The Health Impact Pyramid

Source: Frieden, T. R. (2010). A framework for public health action: The health impact pyramid. *American Journal of Public Health, 100*(4), 590–595.

The novelty of this framework over previous public and population health frameworks is the bottom tier that accounts for socioeconomic factors, most importantly poverty (see Chapter 7).

Population Health Measures

Assessing health status at the individual level can take several forms, such as clinical examinations, diagnostic tests, and medical histories. Most often these occur within a health care setting in an interaction between a patient and a health professional. When we examine health and health status at a population level, it becomes more complex. How, then, do we promote health at the population level? What should we be focusing on? Moreover, if health is hard to define at the individual level, how do we measure the health of populations? Stephen Bezruchka (2010) argues that the population health approach should move beyond concepts used by us when we measure the health of individuals. He suggests that health can be measured at the cellular, individual, and population levels. To be healthy, cells need to have a constant supply of oxygen and glucose. Yet, if we are focusing solely on the health of individuals, we would refrain from suggesting to people that they constantly pump themselves with glucose and oxygen. To promote health at the individual level, we usually focus our efforts on promoting exercise and good nutrition as leading to a healthier lifestyle. Similarly, to promote health at the population level, we need to focus our efforts on developing a strategy that will address the needs of the population, not those of specific individuals (Bezruchka, 2010).

One of the principal benefits of population health measures is the ability to compare populations across space and time. This is often done to compare health and disease patterns between groups of people, such as men to women, province to province, or Canada to other countries. It is also useful to be able to follow a population over time to examine whether health patterns change. For example, the recent obesity epidemic in Canada and the United States is based on a drastic increase in the percentage of people with excessive body weight (Shields, 2006) (see Chapter 13).

Measures of health at a population level generally fall into three different categories, direct, indirect, and proxy measures. **Direct measures of health** are generally based on individual-level data that gets aggregated to provide an overall sense of the population. These could be based on reviewing patient medical charts or administrative health care data from provincial/territorial health insurance plans to get an estimate of the number of people with a specific diagnosis. Another way is to ask individuals about their health. In Chapter 2, we discussed recent survey initiatives by Statistics Canada that do just that: ask a whole range of health and health behaviour questions. From these, the responses are aggregated to provide a picture of the population of interest. An example is a single-item question asking, in relation to others your own age, how you would rate your health status on a scale from 1 to 5, 1 being excellent, 2—very good, 3—good, 4—fair, and 5—poor. Although some might argue against the merits of such a simplistic question, this question has been shown to correlate well with future physician evaluations, morbidity, and even mortality (Krause & Jay 1994; Thorslund & Norström, 1993). Another direct measure used in various Canadian surveys is the **Health Utility Index** (HUI). This is a multidimensional measure of health status, tapping eight domains: vision, hearing, speech, mobility, dexterity, cognition, emotion, and pain/discomfort (Roberge, Berthelot, & Wolfson, 1995). Other types of questions directly measuring health status query respondents about whether they have been told by a health care professional that they have a myriad of various diseases from heart disease to a mental illness. Many of these measures in various Canadian health surveys can be explored by the interested reader using <odesi>(http://www.odesi.ca) (refer to Box 2.2 in Chapter 2). However, this specific approach requires that persons are aware they have an illness.

Indirect measures of health are usually collected at the individual level as well but focus on markers and lifestyle behaviours that are connected to health outcomes. Health markers are factors that are linked to health outcomes but are not necessarily causal. For example smoking, obesity, and nutrition are not direct measures of a person's health. However, there is ample evidence that all of these are strongly linked to diseases such as cancer, heart disease, and diabetes. The number of people smoking today can provide some idea as to the potential burden of some cancers in the future. Again, much of this information is gleaned from various health surveys that can easily be accessed.

It is informative to use aggregated individual-level data to provide a snapshot of the population. The reverse is not necessarily so. Once data are aggregated, predictions about individuals are based on probability. You cannot infer that because someone smokes, he or she *will* get cancer, or because someone is obese that he or she *will* also have high blood pressure (hypertension). A direct inference from population-level statistics to specific individuals is labelled an **ecological fallacy**. Although someone who smokes is more likely to get cancer, you cannot infer that as an absolute, based on the link of smoking and cancer at the aggregated, population data level.

There are also metrics that are commonly used as proxy measures of health status. **Proxy measures of health** are usually population-level indirect measures likely to be associated with overall health status. Proxy measures of health are often used to compare across countries because it is easier to provide a common metric for more accurate comparisons. Many of the direct and indirect measures mentioned in this section are dependent upon the resources spent on collecting data, the cultural context of the meaning of some questions, and the cultural sensitivities of asking certain questions. Proxy measures are usually collected as part of the economic profile and vital statistics of countries, for example, the percentage of gross domestic product (GDP) spent on health care, or average life expectancy and number of practising physicians. A higher proportion spent on health care is assumed to be associated with a higher level of population health status. Average life expectancy (see the section that follows) is another proxy measure based on the assumption that a longer life expectancy is connected to better overall health status of the population. A final example is the number of physicians in a community, which assumes the more physicians in a population, the better the overall health status. Others argue, however, that the number of physicians only

Box 6.1

The Canadian Index of Well-Being

The Canadian Index of Well-Being Network is currently co-chaired by Roy Romanow and Monique Bégin. Roy Romanow is the former Premier of Saskatchewan and head of the Royal Commission on the Future of Health Care in Canada that produced the *Romanow Report*. Monique Bégin (see Researcher Profile in Chapter 3) was the Minister of Health who implemented the Canada Health Act in 1984.

The CIW moves beyond the usual measure of GDP (gross domestic product), a measure focused specifically on economic productivity of a country. The argument is that GDP tells us nothing about other important dimensions of the country such as the health of its people and environment. The CIW addresses this by considering eight dimensions to provide a single composite index (single value) to assess the overall quality of life of the citizens of a country. The specific dimensions are:

1. Living standards and income
2. Health of populations
3. Community vitality
4. Environment
5. Education
6. Time use
7. Civic engagement
8. Arts, culture, and recreation

The index provides a basis on which to compare changes within a specific country over time as well as differences across countries. In 2009, the first CWI report for Canada was released comparing Canadians and based on data from 2008 and 1994. Subsequent reports have been released every year to track the CWI of Canadians. The most recent report, for 2012, showed that Canada's GDP dropped by 8.3% but the CWI declined 24%. This indicates that impact of the 2008 economic crisis and subsequent recession had a much greater effect on the Canadian population beyond the economic state of the country.

Source: Canadian Index of Wellbeing. (2012). *How Are Canadians Really Doing? The 2012 CIW Report.* Waterloo, ON: Canadian Index of Wellbeing and University of Waterloo.

Note: The numbered dimensions are directly quoted from the Index.

predicts the cost of health care and not that of population health status. A promising new composite measure to assess population health and well-being is the Canadian Index of Well-Being (CIW) (see Box 6.1).

As we discussed in Chapter 2, no measure of health status is ideal and all have limitations. For example, for a variety of reasons, people may not be honest when asked about their health status, the presence of a specific disease, or their health and lifestyle behaviours. Someone may not be eager to indicate that he or she smokes, knowing that it is generally perceived as an unhealthy behaviour. Someone may also not be eager to reveal that he or she has AIDS or a mental illness, due to the stigmas associated with these diseases. Moreover, even asking someone his or her height and weight to try to assess whether he or she is obese is fraught with potential biases. Most people underestimate their weight but overestimate their height, biasing any population estimate toward more normal weight. To address some of these issues, Statistics Canada recently initiated the Canadian Health Measures Survey (CHMS) that collects direct measures of health, disease, and

Box 6.2

Canadian Health Measures Survey (CHMS)

In 2003, the Canadian government approved funding for the Canadian Health Measures Survey (CHMS) to complement current various survey initiatives, including the National Population Health Survey (NPHS), Canadian Community Health Survey (CCHS), and National Longitudinal Survey of Children and Youth (NLSCY) (see the research box in Chapter 2 on methodology for more detail on these surveys) (Statistics Canada, 2010a). Although the CHMS is a Statistics Canada initiative, the survey team works in collaboration with Health Canada and the Public Health Agency of Canada (PHAC). The intent of the national study was to establish baselines for many of today's health concerns and exposures as well as to gauge the prevalence of undiagnosed diseases among the population. The CHMS began in 2007 to collect direct physical health measures such as height, weight, blood pressure, physical fitness, and oral health. It also collected biological samples

to test for nutrition and to identify exposure to various contaminants, such as nicotine, lead, mercury, and VOCs (volatile organic compounds) as well as indicators of diseases such as hepatitis, diabetes, and kidney disease. The survey supplemented these direct measures with a questionnaire to gather data on socio-demographics and socioeconomic factors and other measures similar to the CCHS. Due to the complexity of collecting data, including bringing a tractor trailer–sized portable lab to collect specimens and take physical measures, the survey selects sites (various population areas) to sample a large number of people in a small area. For the first cycle of the CHMS, about 5600 Canadians between the ages of 6 and 79 at 15 sites across the country were sampled. Due to the sensitivity of the data, the CHMS is not publicly accessible, but is accessible with permission through Statistics Canada and its Research Data Centre (RDC) initiative.

exposure using blood and urine samples (see Box 6.2) (Statistics Canada, 2010a). For example, it can easily be determined if someone is a regular smoker by testing blood or urine samples for nicotine.

Even proxy measures can be problematic and can contradict one another, challenging their accuracy when comparing health statuses between countries. For example, in 2010, the United States spent 17.6% of GDP on health care compared with Canada that spent 11.4%. However, life expectancy in Canada in 2008 was 80.8 versus only 78.1 in the United States (OECD, 2012). So while the United States spent over 50% more on health care than Canada, overall life expectancy there was 2.7 fewer years. The limitations of health measures only emphasize the importance of having multiple measures to provide an overall understanding of population health.

EPIDEMIOLOGY

Examination of the patterns and spread of disease in populations is generally the work of epidemiologists. Epidemiology, quite literally, means the study of epidemics, focusing on the distribution and determinants of disease in an effort to identify how, why, and at what rate diseases spread through populations. The core focus is on groups of people as opposed to specific individuals (Kelsey, Whittemore, Evans, & Thompson, 1996). There are two primary goals of epidemiology. The first goal is to understand the rate at which a disease will spread through a population and the overall burden of the disease. A second and equally important goal is to identify the exposure that placed a person identified with the disease at risk. This is based on a model that considers three principal factors, including the person (host), the agent, and the environment (Kelsey et al., 1996). The **host** as a person is made up of various characteristics from genetic and biological to social and psychological, making that person more or less susceptible to any exposure. The **agent** is the carrier of the disease, such as a bacteria or virus or other infectious exposure. It can also be something non-infectious as in the case of asbestos. The agent is not necessarily the cause of the disease, as some people who are exposed may not contract the disease. The exposure to the agent only makes it more likely. The **environment** is the context, place, and time in which contact between host and agent occurs, making any transmission more likely to occur. When these three factors align, that is, someone who is more susceptible based on one or more characteristics is exposed to an agent due to the environment he or she is in, the likelihood of having a disease increases.

John Snow and the 1831 London Cholera Outbreak

Modern, population-based epidemiological inquiry has its historical root in the work of Sir John Snow (1815–1838). Snow investigated the 1831 cholera outbreak in the neighbourhood of Soho in London, England (Hempel, 2006; Vinten-Johansen et al., 2003). We now know cholera is an intestinal infection caused by a bacterium (*Vibrio cholera*) found in untreated drinking water. During Snow's time there was no way to see a bacterium, so people thought this disease was contracted through bad air, the *miasma* theory of disease.

Cholera has an extremely quick gestation period of one to five days producing diarrhea and vomiting leading to severe dehydration and a high risk of death without treatment. In previous outbreaks around England, thousands of people died. Snow mapped identified cases in Soho and found that they clustered around those who used one specific water pump located on Broad Street. He also noted two self-contained local facilities around this pump had much lower rates of illness. Specifically, only five of the 530 inmates at the Poland Street Workhouse (prison) that had its own water source contracted cholera. As well, there were no fatalities among the 70 workers at a Broad Street brewery who received a daily allowance of free beer. Using this as evidence, Snow petitioned local health officials to shut down the pump by physically removing the handle and, while they were skeptical, they complied. The severity of the cholera epidemic subsided.

The importance of Snow's approach was his method to identify the most likely cause of the outbreak through epidemiologic investigation. His identification of something in the water long predated the advent of modern microbiology by Louis Pasteur (1822–1895) that was made possible by the invention of the microscope. The observational methods used by Snow identified population patterns of the spread of the disease as well as the vector responsible for its spread, in this case, water from this specific pump. His techniques helped to establish the foundations for modern epidemiology and, more broadly, public health.

Statistical Fundamentals of Modern Epidemiology

The basis of modern epidemiological inquiry is the *rate* of a specific attribute (such as a disease, illness, injury, or death). The rate, a measure of frequency, is a ratio comparing the number of *cases* (persons with the specified attribute) to a specific *target population* over a specified time period. The mathematical basis divides the number of cases by the population and then multiplies this number by 10 to the power of a given number (10^n) to provide a rate given a specific number of persons.

$$\text{rate} = \frac{\text{number of cases in target population}}{\text{target population}} \times 10^n$$

The last part, multiplying it by a given power of 10, provides a number that is more meaningful. If the ratio is multiplied by 100 (or 10^2) it would be a percentage. For outcomes that are less prevalent in a population, it could be multiplied by 1000 (10^3), or 10 000 (10^4) or even 100 000 (10^5). For example, the smoking rate in Canada in 2010 was about 17%, that is, 17 persons per 100 smoked in 2010 (Canadian Cancer Society, 2012a). The rate of lung cancer in Canada in 2010 is 62 per 100 000 males and 49 per 100 000 females (Canadian Cancer Society, 2012b). If we were to express the rate of lung cancer as a percentage it would be 0.062% for males and 0.049% for females. Calculating the rate to reference a whole number makes the number more intuitive and easier to understand.

There are many types of rates to help understand and quantify the burden and spread of a disease in a population. Two important rates commonly used are the incidence rate and the prevalence rate. The **incidence rate** provides the number of new cases of a specific disease across a target population over a given period. This rate provides a sense of how fast a disease is spreading across a population. For example, an incidence rate provides health care practitioners with an understanding how fast a new infectious disease such as swine flu or SARS (severe acute respiratory syndrome) is spreading throughout a population. The **prevalence rate** provides an estimate of the total number of cases in a given population over a specific period of time that includes both new cases and existing cases but excludes cases (persons) who have recovered or died from the disease in that period. Prevalence provides a measure of the overall burden of a disease over a given period of time. This estimate can provide important information for health care systems in estimating expected service requirements and costs. Changes in the prevalence rate over time will provide an indication as to whether the disease burden is increasing or decreasing.

Both of these rates can be based on the entire population or can be adjusted to report on a specific subgroup of the population, commonly called an adjusted rate. This provides extra information such as how a disease may spread faster in one age group versus another age group. These are usually age-specific or **age-adjusted rates**; rates that would examine cases within an age range divided by the total number of people in that age range. For example, STDs (sexually transmitted diseases) would likely spread faster (have a higher incidence rate) among those in age groups that are both more sexually active with multiple partners and more likely to participate in unprotected sex. Adjusted rates can be broken down further to examine smaller groups such as adjusting for both age and sex or other higher risk groups. This more finely dissected information could greatly assist in focusing a public health intervention to target groups that are most at risk.

Epidemiological Study Designs

There are two principal study designs in epidemiology that attempt to identify exposures that cause disease: the cohort study design and the case-control study design. The **cohort study** is based on an exposure to the suspected risk factor. The design would entail recruiting a sample prior to or after a suspected exposure but prior to any disease outcome. An additional sample that has not had the exposure would also be recruited as the control group. The exposed and control groups are then followed over time and watched for the development of the disease. Cohort studies are very expensive and time-consuming to conduct because they require a large initial sample and that sample usually needs to be followed for an extended period of time for the disease to begin to appear. Moreover, the rarer the disease, the larger the sample required. However, this design provides very strong evidence for the causal linkage between exposure and outcome.

One of the most famous prospective cohort studies was the Whitehall Study in the United Kingdom (Marmot et al., 1984; 1987; 1991). The original Whitehall study followed civil servants for 10 years and found that a lower employment grade (as a measure of socio-economic status, SES) was related to higher specific-cause and all-cause mortality for both men and women. In fact, employment grade was a strong predictor after accounting for other commonly identified risk factors, including smoking, high cholesterol, and high blood pressure. The second Whitehall study, still ongoing, examined the effect of psycho-social factors on subsequent chronic health conditions and diseases, including heart disease. Preliminary findings show a gradient between lower employment grades and higher levels of work stress, chronic strains, and life events. Further analysis found that lower employment grades were linked to a number of biological and metabolic factors associated with onset of diabetes and heart disease, suggesting a link between psychosocial stress and later onset of disease (Brunner, 1997). The results and implications of the Whitehall study are discussed in the next chapter that examines the social determinants of health (see Chapter 7).

The **case-control study design** identifies people who already have the disease of interest (cases) and then examines whether they were previously exposed to the suspected risk factor. The samples are usually identified retrospectively, that is, after the disease state is known. Cases are identified and recruited into the study. These cases are matched to other persons who have similar characteristics but do not have the disease. Because the disease state is already known, case-control studies are less expensive and usually much quicker to complete than cohort studies. They are also much more economical when examining rare diseases.

Today, there are many sub-disciplines within epidemiology, including psychiatric epidemiology, social epidemiology, and disease-specific forms such as cancer epidemiology. Their common underlying premise is to examine how diseases are distributed across groups of people (i.e., populations) to identify the causes or precursors of the illness. In this text, we concern ourselves principally with social epidemiology. Mechanic (1978) described **social epidemiology** as providing "a framework that usefully integrates a description of disease distribution with a social science perspective on the process of disease occurrence and persistence" (p. 5). From this definition, social epidemiology examines risk factors ranging from the macro-level—such as poverty, education, and employment— the meso-level, including community and peer relationships—to the micro-level—such as family dynamics, individual lifestyle behaviours, and psychological factors. Many sociologists use a social epidemiological approach to examine health outcomes from physical to mental health (see Researcher Profile 6.1).

One of the principal criticisms of the epidemiological approach however, is that it focuses on negative outcomes (diseases) instead of positive outcomes (health). That is,

Researcher Profile 6.1

John Cairney

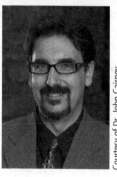

Courtesy of Dr. John Cairney

John Cairney is the McMaster Family Medicine Professor of Child Health Research, the Associate Director of Research in Family Medicine, and a Professor in the Departments of Psychiatry and Behavioural Neuroscience, Clinical Epidemiology and Biostatistics and Kinesiology. He is also an adjunct scientist for both the Institute for Clinical Evaluative Sciences (ICES) and the Centre for Addiction and Mental Health (CAMH).

Dr. Cairney, a sociologist by training, successfully incorporates epidemiological methods with the application of psychological and sociological theories to population health research. His work is multi-disciplinary, impacting the fields of population health, as well as behavioural sciences, epidemiology, exercise physiology, pediatrics, and sociology.

As one example of this, he is internationally recognized for his work examining the associations between childhood motor coordination problems (developmental coordination disorder or DCD), physical inactivity, and health-related fitness (obesity, physical fitness). He also examines associations between participation in recreational (leisure time) physical activity and mental health, both in relation to diagnosable disorders (e.g., bipolar disorder) and in relation to psychological distress and social stress using a population-level, social-epidemiological approach.

what are the factors and resources that keep people healthy? It is likely more than just the opposite of the factors that cause disease, but currently modern epidemiology seems unable to address this point. In the next section, we will examine various aspects of the distribution of the Canadian population to enable us to begin to understand the differential distribution of health and illness.

SOCIO-DEMOGRAPHIC CHANGES OF THE CANADIAN POPULATION

The Canadian population is a heterogeneous mixture of people with very different physical and social characteristics. When taking a population perspective to examine health, it is necessary to gain some insight as to how the population is distributed across various demographic characteristics. Population characteristics can be broken down into two types, ascribed and achieved. **Ascribed characteristics** are those factors that people generally have no control over, such as sex, age, race, and ethnicity. **Achieved characteristics** are those that people attain through various means, such as education. There are many ascribed and achieved characteristics that show considerable variation in Canada leading to great diversity in the population. In taking a population perspective in Canada to examine health, it is necessary first to attempt to gain some insight as to how the population is distributed across some of these various characteristics.

Age and the Aging of the Population

Canada, as of the 2011 census, had a total population of 33 476 688 million people (Table 6.1). The total population has doubled in just over 60 years. While that is a dramatic increase in a relatively short period, this overall total number does not tell the whole story. The population is increasing, but there are also dramatic shifts in the basic demographic profile of Canadians. First, the population is aging. What is meant by population aging? Population aging focuses on the differential distribution of age groups within an entire society. It examines changes over time of the mean and median age of the population and the proportions of people in various age categories such as children, adults, and older adults (generally defined as those aged 65 and above). An aging population means a higher number of persons aged 65 and older, the numerator, as a proportion of the total population, the denominator. So, not only does the number of persons in older age groups increase, it increases as a percentage of the whole population, relative to the percentage of people in young and middle age groups. In general, developed or high-income countries in Europe, North America, and Asia (notably Japan) have populations that are considered old or aged. If we examine the changing age distribution of Canada, we see that there is a decrease in the percentage of children (0 to 19 years) and an increase in the older cohorts. The cohort among those 65 and older has more than doubled from 1946 to 2011 (Table 6.1). The median age of the population has also increased by almost 13 years from 1946 to 2011.

Table 6.1 Total Population, Median Age and Age Distribution, Canada, 1946 to 2011

Year	Population (N)	Median age Years	0 to 19 %	20 to 64 %	65 and over %
1946	12 292 000	27.7	36.6	56.3	7.2
1966	20 014 880	25.4	42.1	50.2	7.7
1986	26 101 155	31.4	28.6	60.9	10.5
2006	32 623 490	38.8	24.0	62.8	13.2
2011	33 476 685	40.6	23.3	61.9	14.8

Sources: Statistics Canada. (2008) *Report on the demographic situation in Canada, 2005 and 2006,* 91-209-X, Ottawa: Statistics Canada.

Statistics Canada. (2012a). *Canada Year Book, 2012,* 11-402-X, Ottawa: Statistics Canada. Retrieved from www.statcan.gc.ca/pub/11-402-x/11-402-x2012000-eng.htm

The consequences of an older population are many, from economic to social to health. For example, the cost of some of the social programs for retirees such as the Canadian Pension Plan (CPP) and Old Age Security (OAS) is increasing while at the same time a smaller relative proportion of young people is moving into the workforce to support these programs. To address this labour deficit, the federal government recently increased the age at which someone can claim full CPP benefits from 65 to 67 years of age. This will force some people to work longer to get their full retirement benefits and will have a negative effect on employment opportunities for younger cohorts as they move into the workforce. The consequences of an aging population are discussed further in the chapter on aging (Chapter 9).

The aging of the population is not the whole story. When we examine this population increase more closely, it gets more complex. There are three factors that influence the growth and aging of a population, specifically births, deaths, and immigration. First, more people are living longer, which is another way of saying there are fewer deaths at younger ages. The average life expectancy of Canadians is continually increasing so more people are living longer. This would not have an effect on overall population aging unless it was increasing relative to the numbers of persons at the lower age groups.

Second, the fertility rate in Canada, as in other developed countries, has declined to a point where there are not enough births to maintain the current population. So in order to maintain the population and slow population aging, the government turns to immigration. It is hoped that letting more people who are of working age into the country will help offset increased longevity and falling fertility rates (Table 6.2). However, even with substantial increases in immigration rates, the mean age of the population continues to increase from 27.7 in 1946 to 40.6 years of age in 2011. Moreover, immigration brings with it a host of additional economic, social, cultural, and health consequences discussed briefly in the section that follows and also in greater detail in the next chapter.

Table 6.2 Components of Population Growth in Canada, 1986 to 2011

	1986	1996	2006	2011
Births	375 381	372 453	343 517	386 013
Deaths	184 224	212 880	228 079	252 561
Immigration	88 657	217 478	254 359	258 906
Emigration	50 595	48 396	38 551	52 456

Sources: Statistics Canada. (2008). *Report on the Demographic Situation in Canada, 2005 and 2006*, 91-209-X, Ottawa: Statistics Canada.

Statistics Canada. (2012). *Canada Year Book, 2012*, 11-402-X, Ottawa: Statistics Canada. Retrieved Feb 12, 2012, from www.statcan.gc.ca/pub/11-402-x/11-402-x2012000-eng.htm

Immigration and Emigration

Historically, most immigrants to Canada came from Europe. Before 1931, over 90% of all immigrants came from Europe; Asia made up about 3%. Since then, there has been a dramatic shift in immigration patterns. Over the past 30 years, the trend shows an increase in the percentage of immigrants coming from Asia and Africa (Statistics Canada, 2008b). Asia, including East Asian and South Asian countries, provided over 55% of all immigrants in 2007 (Table 6.3). The percentage of people immigrating to Canada from Europe decreased from 35 to 16%, less than half of what it was just 30 years previously. Moreover, even within Europe, the profile has changed over time. In the later part of the twentieth

Table 6.3 Percentage of Landed Immigrants to Canada by Region of Birth, 1981 to 2007

Region of Birth	1981	1986	1991	1996	2001	2006	2007
Asia	39.5	42.6	53.0	64.4	62.4	59.6	56.5
Europe	34.8	23.1	20.2	17.3	17.0	14.9	16.0
Africa	4.6	5.2	7.1	7.0	9.7	11.4	11.7
United States	6.8	6.1	2.3	2.2	2.1	3.5	3.7
Central America	1.2	6.3	5.9	1.5	1.3	1.7	2.2
Caribbean & Bermuda	6.8	8.9	5.6	4.2	3.4	2.7	3.4
South America	4.8	6.6	4.5	2.7	3.4	5.5	5.6
Oceania	1.4	0.8	1.0	0.6	0.6	0.5	0.6
Others	0.2	0.4	0.3	0.1	0.2	0.2	0.2
Total Numbers	128 642	99 353	232 803	226 073	250 638	251 643	236 759

Adapted from: Statistics Canada. (2008). *Report on the Demographics of Canada, 2005 to 2006*. Table A-4.1: Landed immigrants in Canada by country of birth, 1981 to 2007, (p. 60). Minister of Industry, Catalogue no. 91-209-X. Ottawa: Statistics Canada.

century, immigrants were mostly from Western European countries. In the first half of the twentieth century, when the Canadian government was encouraging rural settlement in the Prairies with the promise of free farm land, it included more immigrants from Russia, including Ukraine, and Eastern European countries such as Poland and Romania until World War II. People from those same countries that were behind the iron curtain of the Soviet Union (or communist USSR—Union of Soviet Socialist Republics) after World War II and before the fall of the Berlin Wall in 1989 comprise the majority of European immigrants today.

In 2007, the majority of immigrants came to Canada under the economic classification (55%). 28% were family reunifications, and 11% were refugees. The largest percentage of all immigrants, regardless of their classification, settled in Ontario (47%) with Quebec, British Columbia, and Alberta being the next largest recipients receiving 19.1%, 16.5%, and 8.8% respectively. The overwhelming majority of these immigrants settle in cities and suburbs and many settle near their own ethnic communities.

In addition to immigrants settling in Canada, there is also migration within the country, between provinces and within provinces. Migration is based, in part, on economic opportunities for employment and changes in the cost of living. Some cities and regions have seen large growth, principally because of the availability of employment. For example, between 2001 and 2006, Calgary and Edmonton have seen the largest in-migration of all census metropolitan areas (CMAs) in Canada. With respect to within-province migration, historically there has been a large move from rural areas to urban areas as families leave the farms and rural villages for employment opportunities in larger cities. More recently, however, there has been a reverse migration out of core urban communities into surrounding communities, a phenomenon called *urban expansion*. In fact, the surrounding communities of two of the largest cities in Canada, Toronto and Montreal, have seen a population decline from 2001 to 2006 while the surrounding peripheral communities (suburbs) have seen large population increases. Vancouver also saw overall population decreases but to both its core and surrounding communities. Part of this decline is due to the high cost of housing and property taxes in these cities that pushed many people to capitalize on selling houses and moving into surrounding communities. In the case of Vancouver, they moved even further away into communities several hours away, such as Kelowna.

Education and Employment

In addition to changes in various ascribed characteristics in Canada over time, there have also been changes over time in achieved statuses. One of these is the education level. From 1951 to 1975, the percentage of students attending grade school (kindergarten to grade 12) went from 82.9% to 98.9% (Statistics Canada, 1983). More telling, when we examine those in grade 9 and higher (14 to 17 years of age), the percentage went from 46.4% to 91.1%. Finally among those from 18 to 24 years of age in post-secondary school, the percentage went from 6% in 1951 to 19.5% in 1975. These changes in educational attainment align with urban expansion. Canada went from having almost half (48.1%) of its working-age population in agricultural pursuits in 1881 to 5.6% in 1971 (Statistics Canada, 1983). The reduction was very gradual, about a 5% decline of the total workforce each decade moving out of agriculture up until 1971. To compare with education, in 1951, the percentage in agricultural occupations was 15.9%. Today, agricultural occupations account for only 2.4% of the population. This change and its consequences are discussed further in the chapter on food (Chapter 13). With the reduction in the population employed in agricultural pursuits overlapping with the migration from rural to urban centres, there were concomitant increases in manufacturing, construction, transportation, finance, trade, and service employment. More recently, the manufacturing employment base has reduced as many of jobs shift overseas to places with lower labour costs.

The Constellation of Multiple Characteristics (Intersectionality)

Since we are concerned with how these various social-structural determinants influence sickness and disease, we must also consider that the structure of modern society is multiplex. Societies are not stratified hierarchically across a single factor. That is, people do not occupy separate, independent, socio-demographic categories. In Canada, for example, people are not only stratified by income, education, and occupation but also by gender, family structure, age, and ethnic status and race. Dimensions of social position cannot be conceptualized individually; they need to be considered as a constellation. For instance, the achieved characteristic of income is very much interconnected with sex. That is, historically, females earn about 70% of what males earn for similar jobs, a difference that continues to persist even today. This income difference across gender varies further by age with the differential being as close as 82% among those 18 to 24 but diverging to 64% among those 55 to 64 (Statistics Canada, 2001). There are several reasons proposed for this unequal income distribution by gender that vary across the different theoretical perspectives.

Another example of the interaction between statuses is the relationships between immigration, ethnicity, education, employment, and poverty. Table 6.4 shows the differences in unemployment rates comparing recent and long-term immigrants to Canada to those persons born in Canada, across educational levels. Regardless of education level, more recent immigrants have a much higher unemployment rate than longer-term immigrants or persons born in Canada. In fact, the greatest disparity across groups is among those most highly educated. It appears that education level makes little difference among new immigrants but education seems to become more important among immigrants who have been here for longer than five years. Moreover, if we examine poverty rates across immigrants from different regions, a further pattern emerges. Overall, visible ethnic minority groups generally from Africa, East and South Asia, and Latin America have persistently higher poverty rates than those from Europe and North America (Figure 6.2).

Table 6.4 Population Unemployment Rates among Those Aged 25 to 54 by Education and Immigrant Status in 2010

	All education levels (%)	No degree, certificate, or diploma (%)	High school graduate (%)	Post-secondary certificate or diploma (%)	University degree (%)
Born in Canada	6.1	12.9	7.1	5.6	3.5
Landed immigrants	9.5	14.9	10.1	8.9	8.6
Immigrants, landed 5 or less years earlier	14.7	18	16.2	14.3	14.4
Immigrants, landed more than 5 to 10 years earlier	9.5	16.1	11.9	9.1	8.2
Immigrants, landed more than 10 years earlier	8.1	14	8.9	7.7	6

Source: Statistics Canada. (2011). Population unemployment rates among those aged 25 to 54 by education and immigrant status in 2010. CANSIM Table 282-0106. Ottawa: Author.

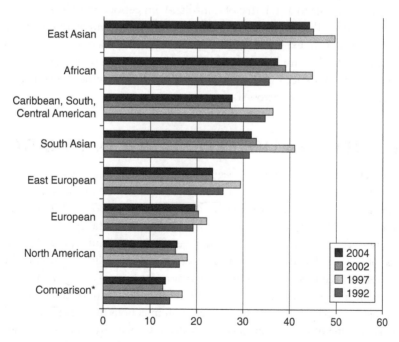

Figure 6.2 Low Income Rates among Immigrants in Canada Less than Ten Years by Region of Origin and Year

*Comparison group includes all Canadian-born plus immigrants living in Canada for more than 10 years.

Source: Picot, G., Hou, F., & Coulombe, S. (2007). *Chronic low income and low-income dynamics among recent immigrants* (p. 39). Catalogue no. 11F0019MIE—No. 294, Ottawa: Statistics Canada.

The idea of a constellation of social-statuses, or what some have termed **intersectionality**, is not new to the sociology of health (it is also discussed in Chapters 7 and 11). For example, some sociologists have proposed the *double* or *multiple-jeopardy hypothesis* to examine the health consequences of occupying two or more disadvantaged social positions (e.g., Ferraro & Farmer, 1996). Within the feminist perspective, others have talked about intersectionality as a way to identify systemic inequality based on multiple, intersecting statuses combining types of discrimination and oppression such as sexism, racism, ageism, and classism (e.g., Collins, 2000). In the area of health, much of this work has focused on age, gender, and social class. For example, McMullin (2000) examined the relationship between gender and social class and how the influence of social class determines differential access to resources. Women in lower socio-economic positions, unlike men, have a double disadvantage of living in both a capitalist and a patriarchal system. She argues that we must theorize about how all of these social structures influence personal circumstances simultaneously, rather than simply focusing on one aspect of social stratification.

Among immigrants, some have identified a phenomenon called the *healthy immigrant effect* (Kobayahsi & Prus, 2005). When immigrants come to Canada, they tend to be in better health compared with Canadian-born individuals; however, the health of immigrants declines over time to match that of Canadian-born persons and may even deteriorate further. Some explain this phenomenon by the discrimination and racism the immigrants face, while others tend to explain this deterioration in health as a result of adoption of the Canadian lifestyle (Kobayahsi & Prus, 2005). Therefore, to better understand how ascribed and achieved characteristics influence health, we need to examine the constellation of social-structural disadvantage across statuses.

MORTALITY AND LIFE EXPECTANCY IN CANADA

In the last section in this chapter, we begin to explore how some of these characteristics and the intersection of characteristics influence changes in mortality and life expectancy among Canadians. When we talk about health and health outcomes, the most concrete outcome is death. Mortality rates can vary from all-cause mortality (or the total death rate) to cause-specific mortality that examines specific diseases and injuries. In Canada, as in the rest of the developed world, there has been a marked reduction in mortality rates overall as well as a reduction in mortality due to more traditional causes such as infectious diseases, infant and perinatal mortality, and mortality due to nutritional problems. In 1882, the top 10 causes of death in Canada were all infectious diseases (Table 6.5). Over 100 years later, nine of the 10 top causes of death in Canada were chronic illnesses and injuries (both intentional and unintentional). This is referred to the **epidemiologic transition** wherein the majority of deaths of a specific country shift over time from acute, infectious diseases to chronic, degenerative diseases (see Box 6.3). The only infectious disease remaining in the top 10 was the category of influenza and pneumonia. These top 10 categories made up 76.4% of all deaths in 2009 in Canada (Statistics Canada, 2012, May 13).

Table 6.5 Top 10 Causes of Death in Canada 1882 and 2009

	1881*	2009**
1	Smallpox	Malignant neoplasms (cancer)
2	Typhus	Diseases of heart (heart disease)
3	Cholera	Cerebrovascular diseases (stroke)
4	Diphtheria	Chronic lower respiratory diseases
5	Dysentery	Accidents (unintentional injuries)
6	Measles	Diabetes mellitus (diabetes)
7	Tuberculosis	Alzheimer's disease
8	Typhoid	Influenza and pneumonia
9	Scarlet Fever	Intentional self-harm (suicide)
10	Meningitis	Nephritis, nephrotic syndrome, and nephrosis (kidney disease)

*Health Canada. (2001). *Canada Year Book. 1886.* Retrieved from www66.statcan. gc.ca/eng/acyb_c1886-eng.aspx?opt=/eng/1886/188601090095_p.95.pdf
**Statistics Canada. (2012b). Leading causes of deaths in Canada, 2009, CANSIM Table 102-0561. Ottawa: Statistics Canada.

The almost two-fold increase in the proportion of those 65 and older relative to the population is principally a result of the shift from infectious to chronic diseases. As our ability to fight infectious diseases results in fewer and fewer premature deaths, people live long enough to manifest chronic diseases. As a result, overall life expectancy

Box 6.3

The Epidemiologic Transition Theory

Initially postulated by Abdel Omran (1971), the epidemologic transition theory attempts to explain population dynamics and changing disease patterns and how these patterns interact with demographic, biological, sociological, economic and psychological factors. It is based on five propositions:

1. Mortality is a fundamental factor in population change;
2. The transition will include a long-term shift in disease patterns, gradually replacing deaths due to infections (e.g., cholera) with deaths due to degenerative diseases (e.g., cancer);
3. This transition will be most beneficial to the health and disease patterns for children and young women;
4. This transition will be closely associated with the socio-economic transition of the modernization of society;
5. There are three variations to this transition, including the classical (Western) model (e.g., Western Europe, United States, and Canada), the accelerated model (e.g., Japan), and the delayed model (i.e., most undeveloped and developing countries).

increases over time. We can examine these changes in life expectancy using tables that predict the total number of years of life left based on current age. The most common life-expectancy table predicts average number of years of life at birth. Another popular one is the number of expected years of life remaining at age 65. Differences in life expectancy are often examined across time, sex, provinces, and even countries. For example, the average life expectancy in Canada has increased from around 60 in 1931 to 71.3 in 1961 to 80.8 in 2008 (OECD, 2012). That is an increase of almost 20 years of life (almost 35%) in the span of only 80 years. If we separate it by sex, in 2008, females have a life expectancy at birth of 83.1 years compared to 78.5 for males. That is, females born in 2008 are expected to live almost five years longer on average than males. For those who have already survived to age 65 in 2008, the average expected number of remaining years is 21.6 for females and 18.5 for males (Statistics Canada, 2012b). So females who have made it to 65 in 2008 are expected to live on average to 86.6 (65 + 21.6) whereas males who have made it to age 65 in 2008 are expected to live on average to 83.5 (65 + 18.5).

Why would life expectancy be higher among those already 65? One reason is that life expectancy at birth accounts for all deaths through the course of life and many people simply do not make it to age 65 due to premature mortality, including possible infectious diseases, infant mortality, and accidents. Moreover, the gap between males and females is narrower among those already 65 simply because more males are likely to have died already, prior to age 65. This is due, in part, to injuries in their adolescent and young adult years, and due to diseases such as cardiovascular disease. If we examine the leading causes of death by sex, this becomes readily apparent (Table 6.6). Comparing males and females, more males than females die from cancer, heart disease, unintentional injuries (accidents) and intentional injuries (suicide), respiratory disease, and diabetes. Females are more likely to die from strokes, pneumonia, and Alzheimer's, diseases that are more closely associated with older age.

One of the most influential and controversial theses for understanding the dramatic increases in life expectancy and the shift from infectious diseases to chronic diseases is found in the work by McKeown (Colgrove, 2002). The McKeown thesis argued that increases in life expectancy from the 1700s to today are principally due to an increased standard of living that resulted in improved nutrition. McKeown discounted the effects of public health advances such as improvements in sanitation, public water supplies, vaccinations, and quarantine as well as any influence from advances in medical science and pharmaceuticals (Szreter, 2002). Although improvements in these other areas are certainly important historically, McKeown's work redirected the attention of the medical establishment beyond medicine and public health to acknowledge also the importance of more sociological factors, specifically increases in the standard of living among the masses. In keeping with this focus, the increasing gender gap in life expectancy favouring women is likely through reductions in family sizes and advancements in birth control. Fewer births reduce the exposure to risk of complications in pregnancy and childbirth, reducing premature deaths as a result.

Table 6.6 Ranking and Number of Deaths for the 10 Leading Causes of Death by Sex, Canada, 2009

Cause of death	Males Rank	Males Number	Males Percent	Females Rank	Females Number	Females Percent	Male-Female Ratio[1]
All causes of death	. . .	120 311	100.0	. . .	118 107	100.0	102
Malignant neoplasms (cancer)	1	37 452	31.1	1	33 673	28.5	111
Diseases of heart (heart disease)	2	25 950	21.6	2	23 321	19.7	111
Accidents (unintentional injuries)	3	6 045	5.0	6	4 205	3.6	144
Cerebrovascular diseases (stroke)	4	5 823	4.8	3	8 282	7.0	70
Chronic lower respiratory diseases	5	5 525	4.6	4	5 334	4.5	104
Diabetes mellitus (diabetes)	6	3 616	3.0	7	3 307	2.8	109
Intentional self-harm (suicide)	7	2 989	2.5	13	901	0.8	332
Influenza and pneumonia	8	2 694	2.2	8	3 132	2.7	86
Alzheimer's disease	9	1 932	1.6	5	4 349	3.7	44
Nephritis, nephrotic syndrome and nephrosis (kidney disease)	10	1 775	1.5	9	1 834	1.6	97
All other causes	. . .	26 510	22.0	. . .	29 769	25.2	89

. . . not applicable

[1] Number of males per 100 females.

Note: The order of the causes of death in this table is based on the ranking of the 10 leading causes for males.

Source: Statistics Canada. *Leading Causes of deaths in Canada, 2009*, CANSIM Table 102-0561.

**Statistics Canada. (2012b). Leading Causes of deaths in Canada, 2009, Catalogue no. 84-215-x2012001.

Finally, life expectancy is a relatively crude measure that accounts simply for longevity. However, life is potentially fraught with hardships that diminish quality of life, especially among the elderly. For example, females have a higher rate of Alzheimer's disease, a disease that is lengthy, progressive, and quite debilitating, negatively affecting quality of life (McIntosh et al., 2009). So even if overall life expectancy is longer among women, if they are living with a severe chronic illness, the quality of those extra years may be greatly diminished. One measure to account for quality of life in calculating life expectancy is **health-adjusted life expectancy (HALE)**. This measure takes into account living free of disease and disability that generally reduce quality of living, resulting in limited mobility or institutionalized living. The gap between life expectancy and health-adjusted life expectancy adjusts for the years that persons live with a disability or disease. For 2001, male life expectancy and HALE were 76.9 and 68.3 years respectively; female life expectancy and HALE were 82.0 and 70.8 respectively (Statistics Canada, 2006b). So although females live longer and are less likely to die prematurely from disease, they also live more years of their lives with a reduced quality of life.

In addition to sex, there are many additional factors that have an influence on mortality rates, life expectancy, and HALE that can also be assessed. Moreover, following the intersectionality framework already identified, various other factors combine to influence life expectancy and HALE. Table 6.7 illustrates the relationship between relative income level and both life expectancy and HALE for both males and females at age 25. There are three trends that we highlight in this table. First, as we would expect, females have a longer overall life expectancy and HALE compared to males across all income categories. Life expectancy also increases among higher income categories for both overall life expectancy and HALE regardless of being male or female.

Second, and more importantly, the increase among higher income categories is greater for HALE than for overall life expectancy. This suggests that not only are those in

Table 6.7 Remaining Life Expectancy and Health-Adjusted Life Expectancy at Age 25 by Income Decile and Sex, Canada, 1991–2001

Income Decile in 1991	Remaining Life Expectancy at Age 25		Remaining Health-Adjusted Life Expectancy (HALE) at Age 25	
	Male	Female	Male	Female
Decile 1 (lowest income decile)	48.6	56.5	37.0	42.9
Decile 2	49.5	57.0	40.0	45.6
Decile 3	51.1	58.2	43.0	48.4
Decile 4	52.1	59.1	43.7	49.3
Decile 5	52.9	59.4	46.4	49.7
Decile 6	53.2	59.8	46.5	51.2
Decile 7	53.8	59.9	47.4	50.7
Decile 8	54.4	60.1	48.4	51.8
Decile 9	54.8	60.6	49.0	52.2
Decile 10 (highest income decile)	56.0	61.0	51.1	52.4
Difference: Decile 10 minus Decile 1	**7.4**	**4.5**	**14.1**	**9.5**

Adapted from: McIntosh, C. N., Fines, P., Wilkins, R., & Wolfson. M.C. (2009). Income disparities in health-adjusted life expectancy for Canadian adults, 1991 to 2001. *Health Reports, 2009 20*(4), 55–64. 82-003-X

Note: The mortality data for this table come from the 1991–2001 Canadian Census follow-up mortality study. Data on health-related quality of life come from the 2000/2001 Canadian Community Health Survey (CCHS).

higher-income categories living longer, but they also have substantially more years of good health. Males at age 25 in the lowest income decile (lowest 10%) have an overall life expectancy of 48.6 additional years but only 37.0 years more once adjusted for health quality. In comparison, males at age 25 in the highest income decile have an overall life expectancy of 56.0 additional years and 51.1 years after adjusting for health quality, showing an increase in both life expectancy and HALE as one moves up the income gradient. The pattern among females is much the same. As well, the gap between overall life expectancy and HALE decreases for both males and females with higher income levels indicating that those with lower income will live a greater proportion of their lives with reduced quality of life.

Third, although both males and females benefit from higher income levels, males appear to benefit more in terms of both overall life expectancy and HALE compared to females as we move up the income gradient. The gap between overall life expectancy and HALE for males in the top income decile is 4.9 years compared to 8.6 years for females. In the lowest income decile the difference is 11.6 years for males and 13.6 years for females. These findings illustrate how the constellation of different statuses, for example both gender and income level, combine to influence mortality status and health more generally. We will explore this in much greater detail in the next chapter that investigates the social determinants of health and health inequities.

SUMMARY

In this chapter, we moved from examining health at an individual-focused level to a population-focused level. When we move to examine populations, it becomes more difficult to define and measure health and health status. These difficulties, however, have not discouraged scholars from continuing to explore the health status of population. Population health is too important to be dismissed simply because of difficulties in defining and measuring. When we move to examining health at a population level, we quickly realize that none of the available measures provide a complete picture of the health status of Canadians. If we use multiple measures, they can provide sufficient information to enable us to compare the health status of Canada to other countries as well as to examine differences in health status across groups within Canada. From this, we can readily see that Canada is composed of many groups across a broad array of ascribed and achieved characteristics. If we apply an epidemiological model that considers the host, agent, and environment, the importance of examining health status across groups becomes clear as these groups could vary greatly in their susceptibility and exposure.

The importance of this work on population health cannot be overstated as it not only serves to satisfy a scientific curiosity, but it also drives much of our national and provincial health policies and program initiatives and helps to prioritize the need for social action. As such, this work is far from just theoretical. From a sociological perspective, further examination of the distribution of disease needs to be examined with scrutiny as we explore the unequal distribution of health, illness, morbidity, and mortality in society. In the next chapter, we take a closer look at the social determinants of health and examine how our social environment shapes the health status and health inequities of the Canadian population.

Key Terms

Achieved characteristics—characteristics or statuses that people are able to attain and change to some degree through individual action such as education, marital status, occupation, and income

Age-adjusted rates—rates that would examine cases within an age range divided by the total number of people in that age range

Agent—the carrier of the disease such as a bacteria or virus or other infectious exposure

Ascribed characteristics—characteristics or statuses that people generally have no ability to change such as sex, race, and age

Case-control study—a study design that samples people based on having or not having the disease of interest and then retrospectively examining to see if there were differences in exposure across groups to explain the differential distribution of disease

Cohort study—a research study design where the sample is recruited based on the exposure to a risk factor and then followed to identify a future disease state

Direct measures of health—measures of actual health statuses such as disease states of an individual or population

Ecological fallacy—attributing characteristics of a population to an individual based on the aggregated, population-level data

Environment—in epidemiological terms, the context, place, and time where contact between host and agent occurs, making any transmission of disease more or less likely to occur

Epidemiologic transition—the shift in major causes of death of a specific country over time from acute, infectious diseases to chronic, degenerative diseases

Health-adjusted life expectancy (HALE)—a measure that estimates length of life free of disease and disability

Health Utility Index—a multidimensional measure of health status tapping eight domains, including vision, hearing, speech, mobility, dexterity, cognition, emotion, and pain/discomfort

Host—a person and the various characteristics (from genetic and biological to social and psychological) that make him or her more or less susceptible to any exposure

Incidence rate—provides the number of new cases of a specific disease across a target population over a given period

Indirect measures of health—markers and lifestyle behaviours that are not direct measures of health status themselves but are connected to health outcomes and disease states

Intersectionality—examination of the health consequences of occupying two or more disadvantaged social positions

Prevalence rate—provides an estimate of the total number of cases in a given population over a specific period of time that includes both new cases and existing cases but excludes those of have died from the disease during this period

Proxy measures of health—usually a population-level measure of some social or economic factor that gives some insight into the level of soundness and access to services of a population

Social epidemiology—"a framework that usefully integrates a description of disease distribution with a social science perspective on the process of disease occurrence and persistence." Mechanic (1978, p. 5)

Critical Thinking Questions

1. How do measures of health at a population level differ from measures at an individual level?
2. Why is population aging an important concern in relation to health care policy and programs?
3. What effect have the changing socio-demographic characteristics of the Canadian population had on changes in population health status and mortality?

Further Readings and Resources

McIntosh, T., Jeffery, B., and Muhajarine, N. (Eds.) (2010). *New directions in population health research in Canada*. Regina: CPRC Press.

Statistics Canada. (2008). *Report on the Demographic Situation in Canada, 2005–2006*. Catalogue no. 91-209-X Minister of Industry.

Canadian Institute of Health Information (CIHI)
www.cihi.ca

Data Library Initiative (DLI)
www.statcan.gc.ca/dli-ild/dli-idd-eng.htm

Health Canada
www.hc-sc.gc.ca/index-eng.php

<odesi> (Ontario Data Documentation, Extraction Service and Infrastructure Initiative)
www.odesi.ca

OECD Health Data, 2012
www.oecd.org/health

Statistics Canada
www.statcan.gc.ca

Chapter 7

Social Determinants and Inequities in Health

Chapter Outline

Learning Objectives

After studying this chapter, you will be able to:

1. Understand what is meant by the social determinants of health and health inequities;

2. Discuss the historical, Canadian, and international context of research and action in the social determinants of health;

3. Describe the health differentials across population groups stratified by income and class, sex and gender, and race and ethnicity, as well as the intersections across these social categories.

In this chapter, we build upon the content in Chapter 6 that described the overall population health trends and differences in Canada. With a solid grounding in the *social distribution* of health, we can now turn to the **social determinants of health**. We now examine the underlying reasons for variations in the distribution of health across social groups. A social determinants approach moves beyond individualist explanations to focus more broadly on underlying social structures as the *causes of the causes* of health, disease, and mortality. Specific sections will examine the impact of various social stratifications on health, including income and class, sex and gender, and race and ethnicity. Much of this discussion links back to the theoretical perspectives and concepts introduced in Chapter 1, but we also revisit and more fully expand upon the concept of *intersectionality* introduced in the last chapter.

SOCIAL DETERMINANTS OF HEALTH

The social determinants of health can be thought of as "how a variety of social factors such as education, income, gender, ethnicity, culture, work environment, social roles, and aging strongly influence the etiology, course, and outcome of disease" (Coburn, D'Arcy, & Torrance, 1998, p. 69). Abstractly, this description directs attention to some of the overlying social, structural, and environmental factors that influence people's health and disease. However, the potential processes involved in how these various factors interact and interconnect to influence the health and disease of individuals are complex. The following example from the Federal, Provincial and Territorial Advisory Committee on Population Health (1999) illustrates the potential complexities involved for a childhood injury and hospitalization:

Why is Jason in the hospital?
  Because he has a bad infection in his leg.
But why does he have an infection?
  Because he has a cut on his leg and it got infected.
But why does he have a cut on his leg?
  Because he was playing in the junk yard next to his apartment building and there was some sharp, jagged steel there that he fell on.
But why was he playing in a junk yard?
  Because his neighbourhood is kind of run down. A lot of kids play there and there is no one to supervise them.
But why does he live in that neighbourhood?
  Because his parents can't afford a nicer place to live.
But why can't his parents afford a nicer place to live?
  Because his Dad is unemployed and his Mom is sick.
But why is his Dad unemployed?
  Because he doesn't have much education and he can't find a job.
But why ...? (p. vii–vii)

From this example, it is clear that a variety of social factors surrounding people's lives and locations combine to have a complex, important role in influencing health and disease.

Some of these factors are situated at the individual and family level; others are situated within the community and the larger structural organization of society. These larger community and structural factors are far beyond the capacity of individuals to control. They are due instead to life circumstances. This perspective is not new; it has been clearly identified in some of the historical works on health and disease.

Historical Roots of the Social Determinants of Health

Although McKeown (1972, 1979), whose work was described in Chapter 6, was the first to use the term "determinants of health," the modern study of the social determinants of health has been argued to have taken its historical roots from the separate writings of Virchow and Engels during the mid-nineteenth century (Raphael, 2010). In 1848, German physician Rudolph Virchow (1848/2006) studied the so-called hunger typhus epidemic in Upper Silesia (Germany). As he described it:

> [T]here can now no longer be any doubt that such an epidemic dissemination of typhus had only been possible under the wretched conditions of life that poverty and lack of culture had created in Upper Silesia. If these conditions were removed, I am sure that epidemic typhus would not recur. (p. 2103)

Similarly, Freidrich Engels (1845/1987), in *The Condition of the Working Class in England*, wrote extensively about the social determinants of health highlighting the plight of the proletariat class in England. In Chapter 1, we highlighted a discussion by Engels about the strains that are placed upon the working poor that expose them to substandard living conditions. Continuing with this theme, he argues that:

> [S]ociety in England daily and hourly commits what the working-men's organs, with perfect correctness, characterise as social murder, that it has placed the workers under conditions in which they can neither retain health nor live long; that it undermines the vital force of these workers gradually, little by little, and so hurries them to the grave before their time. I have further to prove that society knows how injurious such conditions are to the health and the life of the workers, and yet does nothing to improve these conditions. (p. 64)

Not only did Engels and Virchow make the explicit link between living and working conditions and health, but also pointed out how political and economic structures that create inequalities are ultimately to blame (Raphael, 2010). From these historical roots, research on the social determinants of health has seen a resurgence in both Canada and internationally.

Canadian Antecedents

In their essay on the evolution of the social determinants of health in Canada, Glouberman and Millar (2003) describe how it involved two movements. The first movement focused on **health promotion**, which was first articulated by Hubert Laframboise and others in the federal department of Health and Welfare Canada in the 1974 Lalonde Report. (See Researcher Profile 7.1 on Hubert Laframboise) The second movement focused on **health inequity** that grew out of the work by Fraser Mustard and others associated with the Canadian Institute for Advanced Research (CIAR), a think tank funded by corporate and public sources.

Health Promotion Movement   The impetus for the Lalonde Report (1974), entitled *A New Perspective on the Health of Canadians*, was a response to three crises. First, with the advent of publicly funded health care, expenditures were rising rapidly. With both the 1957 Hospital Insurance and Diagnostic Services Act and the 1966 Medical Care Act ratified by all the provinces and territories, the full effect of the costs of universal health

Hubert Laframboise

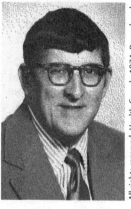

Mr. Hubert (Bert) Laframboise was the Assistant Deputy Minister of the Long Range Health Planning Branch of Health and Welfare Canada during the time that Marc Lalonde was federal Minister of Health (1971 to 1975). A sociologist by training, he was the (often uncredited) architect of the *Lalonde Report*. As noted in a detailed account of the making of the Lalonde Report, McKay (2000) writes:

> In the fall of 1972, Jo Hauser, one of the Policy Planning Consultants, brought the work of Thomas McKeown to the attention of the Director General. Taking an aggregate, long-term view of health, McKeown argued that the steady decline in mortality rates in England over the last century were entirely the result of changes in living standards, not the advancement of

medicine. In Laframboise's words, "his writings proved that the improvement of the health status of the people was far more a consequence of changes in lifestyle and the environment than it was a consequence of advances in medical science." This radical finding had a very strong influence on the work of the branch. (p. 7)

At the heart of the report was a de-emphasis of the importance of medical care and an emphasis on lifestyle and behaviour. McKay further describes:

> The very concept of lifestyle implied that behaviour was an area of self-determination that could be changed. This drew upon the liberal view of citizens as rational actors and the late 1960s idea of self-empowerment as the means for social change. Television was also recognised at this time as a powerful new tool for advertising products. In his correspondence, the DG, Bert Laframboise clearly shared the view that techniques of persuasion could be employed to modify behaviour. The Deputy Minister's files contained an article on social marketing sent from Laframboise to a long list of people. Using the power of T.V., social marketing was promoted as a new hope that could change the self-destructive health habits of Canadians. A contract for research into the ability to alter the behaviour of obese people through marketing was entered into in 1973. (page 9)

and acute care coverage was being felt. Second, there did not seem to be any matching increase in overall population health and life expectancy. This was not specific to the Canadian health care system; it was also highlighted in other countries with universal publicly funded health care systems, such as the National Health Service in Great Britain. Third, current medical interventions, while very effective in addressing acute and infectious diseases, were largely unsuccessful in addressing chronic conditions and diseases that were quickly becoming the leading causes of death in Canada.

To begin to better respond to these crises, the authors of the Lalonde Report proposed the concept of the **health field** that included four major components: human biology, health care systems, environment, and lifestyle. These four interrelated components were described in the report as follows:

> The **HUMAN BIOLOGY** element includes all those aspects of health, both physical and mental, which are developed within the human body as a consequence of the basic biology of man and the organic make-up of the individual.
>
> The **ENVIRONMENT** category includes all those matters related to health which are external to the human body and over which the individual has little or no control.
>
> The **LIFESTYLE** category, in the Health Field Concept, consists of the aggregation of decisions by individuals which affect their health and over which they more or less have control.
>
> The fourth category in the concept is **HEALTH CARE ORGANIZATION**, which consists of the quantity, quality, arrangement, nature and relationships of people and resources in the provision of health care. It includes medical practice, nursing, hospitals, nursing homes, medical drugs, public and community health care services, ambulances, dental treatment and other health services such as optometry, chiropractic and podiatry. This fourth element is what is generally defined as the health care system. (Lalonde Report, 1974, pp. 31–32)

Beyond introducing the health field concept, one of the key arguments in the report was that medical care was not the biggest determinant of health. That is, health care did not necessarily produce health at a broad population health level.

Some have argued that the health field concept and the consequent need for inter-sectoral collaboration and action needed to properly address the determinants of health were ideas that were ahead of their time (Glouberman & Millar, 2003). Indeed, this and other advances in the field of health promotion have resulted in more integrated policy action internationally than in Canada. Many, however, were concerned with the almost singular focus on health lifestyles.

Health lifestyles are ways of living that promote good health and longer life expectancy. They include both things that one *ought* to do and things that one *ought not* do. For example, the influential longitudinal Alameda County Study that examined the association between a number of behavioural and demographic risk factors and their influence on mortality found that pursuing a healthy lifestyle can enhance health and life expectancy. Based on this study, the researchers developed a list of good health practices that included (1) getting seven to eight hours of sleep each night, (2) eating breakfast regularly, (3) not snacking between meals, (4) controlling one's weight, (5) exercising, (6) limiting alcohol intake, and (7) never smoking (Kaplan et al., 1987) (see Chapter 10, Box 10.1).

Concomitant with the Lalonde Report was the ParticipACTION initiative, a federal program that began in the early 1970s funded initially by Health Canada. (For a complete history of the ParticipACTION initiative, see the University of Saskatchewan archives at: **www.usask.ca/archives/participaction/english/structure/timeline.html**.) It was an effort to use media to educate Canadians about healthy behaviour and promote individual lifestyle change. One of its most memorable ads came in 1973. It compared the health status of a 30-year-old Canadian with a 60-year-old Swede. The ParticipACTION project lasted until 2001 when it fell victim to budget cuts, only to be resurrected by the Conservative government in 2007.

Although the pursuit of a healthy lifestyle is an important determinant of health, the prominence of this approach both in the literature and in policy has been criticized on several levels. Health promotion advocates quickly recognized that an overemphasis on lifestyles in isolation from social and living conditions creates a "blaming the victim" mentality; you are sick because of what you do or do not do rather than where you live and work. Many materialist (Marxist), feminist, and environmentalist scholars and activists contend that healthy lifestyles are not freely determined by individual choice but are structurally conditioned and constrained by social position and location in the social organization of society (cf., Navarro, 1986). Additionally, the emphasis on lifestyles leads to a commodification of health (Waitzkin, 1983). Health becomes something you can purchase, like a pair of sneakers or a gym membership. It is argued that such a focus on the individual is consistent with the capitalist ideology wherein people either succeed or fail entirely as a result of their own efforts. In contrast to the emphasis on individual-focused, health lifestyles and behaviours, others suggest an alternate "to-do list" that has a much greater influence on health status. However, these factors are rarely, if ever, discussed (see Box 7.1).

These criticisms of the field of health lifestyles were reflected when health promotion policy directions were revisited a decade later in two seminal reports. The first was the federal/provincial/territorial report, entitled *Achieving Health for All: A Framework for Health Promotion* (Epp, 1986), that focused on how health inequities could be reduced through the strengthening of income security, employment, education, housing, business, agriculture, transportation, and social justice (Bryant, et al., 2011). The second report was *The Ottawa Charter for Health Promotion* (WHO, 1986) that resulted from the First International Conference on Health Promotion organized by the World Health Organization and held in Ottawa. These two documents articulated the principles of health promotion with the *Ottawa Charter* outlining five specific strategic frameworks for action that move far beyond individual-level factors:

1. Advocate for and build healthy public policies, because of how these policies shape how resources are dedicated and distributed at a societal level which, in turn, affect the determinants of health;

2. Create supportive environments and effective action by enhancing our knowledge base and building stronger alliances;

3. Strengthen communities and community-level action as these are the spaces, identities, interests, and concerns that people share;

4. Develop personal skills; and

5. Reorient health services to shift the emphasis from treating disease to improving health.

A Contrasting View of the Top 10 Tips for Better Health

The traditional ten tips for better health:

1. Don't smoke. If you can, stop. If you can't, cut down.
2. Follow a balanced diet with plenty of fruit and vegetables.
3. Keep physically active.
4. Manage stress by, for example, talking things through and making time to relax.
5. If you drink alcohol, do so in moderation.
6. Cover up in the sun, and protect children from sunburn.
7. Practice safer sex.
8. Take up cancer screening opportunities.
9. Be safe on the roads: follow the Highway Code.
10. Learn the First Aid ABCs: airways, breathing, circulation. (Donaldson, 1999)

The social determinants ten tips for better health:

1. Don't be poor. If you can, stop. If you can't, try not to be poor for long.
2. Don't have poor parents.
3. Own a car.
4. Don't work in a stressful, low-paid manual job.
5. Don't live in damp, low-quality housing.
6. Be able to afford to go on a foreign holiday and sunbathe.
7. Practise not losing your job and don't become unemployed.
8. Take up all benefits you are entitled to, if you are unemployed, retired, or sick, or disabled.
9. Don't live next to a busy major road or near a polluting factory.
10. Learn how to fill in the complex housing benefit/asylum application forms before you become homeless and destitute. (Gordon, 1999; personal communication)

Source: Adapted from Dennis Raphael, *Social Determinants of Health,* 2nd Edition (Toronto: Canadian Scholars' Press Inc., 2009). Reprinted by permission of Canadian Scholars' Press Inc./Women's Press.

The Ottawa Charter also focused attention on the necessary prerequisites for health—such as food, shelter, education, and peace—that address the structural aspects of society and the organization and distribution of both economic and social resources (Raphael, 2010).

An additional criticism or analysis of a focus on health lifestyles is derived from a post-structuralist concern with the regulation of the body. Turner (1996), for example, argued that the normative emphasis on healthy lifestyles has resulted in a series of bodily regimens. Moreover, lifestyle choices and consumer habits have developed into a primary source of social identity or that *you are what you consume* (Giddens, 1991). A focus on healthy lifestyles has also been deconstructed from a risk perspective (see Box 7.2) resulting in similar insights.

Health Inequalities Movement   Fraser Mustard, Robert Evans, Greg Stoddart, and their colleagues at the Canadian Institute for Advanced Research (CIAR), founded in 1982, were similarly influenced by the research and arguments made by Thomas McKeown

Managing Health in a Risk Society

As we discussed in Chapter 5, the concept of *risk society*, introduced by Beck (1992) and Giddens (1991), refers to the fact that individuals in our society are increasingly aware of the many risks that shape our existence and make us vulnerable to the dangers of living. This, in turn, shapes our response to these risks and changes our perceptions about the world around us to an unsafe and potentially hazardous place. While some of these risks stem from natural disasters, presumably out of people's control, other disasters, such as the dangers of nuclear war, an oil or toxic chemical spill, and many others, are the products of the human activity.

Some of the risks can be managed at the individual level while others become a source of concern for the provision of health care and health policy makers. Day after day, we hear about the management of *risk factors*—the factors that can contribute to emergence of disease and, therefore, should render closer attention by individuals and health care professionals. We know, for instance, that smoking is a risk factor for lung cancer, and that high blood pressure and cholesterol are risk factors for future heart disease, and eating candy is bad for your teeth. Although this information is often helpful to those of us who would really like to lead a healthier lifestyle, the information about new studies linking some of the behaviours to others is popping up every day and sometimes the messages contradict one another. For instance, despite much research done this field, there are still debates about the health benefits/dangers of having a glass of wine or a cup of coffee. According to Giddens (1991), however, the real problem lies not in the fact that medical research had not yet convincingly demonstrated the harm of consuming a glass of wine or a cup of coffee but in our preoccupation with the risks, and in our case, with health risks that really are out of individuals' control. Even those most devoted to managing a healthy lifestyle cannot keep up with the newly emerging debates, new findings, new studies, and new ideas about how to "avoid" risk. Hence, the quest for a healthier lifestyle, which is the hallmark of our health promotion policy, often seems an unachievable goal (this is further discussed in Chapter 12).

and by the Whitehall Study (see Box 7.4). The seminal work representing this perspective is *Why Are Some People Healthy and Others Not?* edited by Evans, Barer, and Marmor (1994). In this book they posed an argument that, although similar to the *Lalonde Report*—health care does not produce health—moved beyond individual lifestyle behaviours to focus on the underlying social structural environment. They examined the social and political reasons why the presumed close connection between health and health care persists, largely highlighting how professional self-interests (essentially medical dominance without actually naming it as such) is firmly implanted in the system (Link & Phelan, 1996).

Moving past the *Lalonde Report* and its focus on lifestyle, they identify a range of social and economic factors that have a powerful effect on both individual and population health in Canada. Drawing largely upon epidemiological research, they argue that the social and economic environments in which people live have a far stronger impact on health than both health care and individual health behaviours (Glouberman & Millar, 2003). One of the key areas of this group's concern was early childhood development. The group saw early development as being extremely important in regard to long-term health through education, employment, and the development of coping skills. This position aligns with the life course perspective, suggesting that the impact of early life events and transitions shapes the biographies of individuals and their subsequent life experiences (Pearlin, Schieman, Fazio, & Meersman, 2005).

Explaining this influence, Hertzman (2000) proposed to differentiate between factors that influence health: latent effects, pathway effects, and cumulative effects. **Latent effects** are the health implications of the biological and developmental experiences during the pre-natal period and early childhood years. For example, poor nutrition or in-utero exposure to second-hand tobacco smoke has developmental consequences that can have implications for health status in subsequent years (see Box 7.3). **Pathway effects** are the experiences that place an individual onto a specific life trajectory that exposes them to subsequent experiences, both negative and positive. For example, a prospective cohort study has shown that women who were victims of sexual assault as children and adolescents are placed on a life trajectory that make them more likely to be victims of sexual and physical assault as adults (Barnes et al., 2009). Other work has shown that children who experience significant adverse childhood events (ACEs) have more difficulties as adults in maintaining employment and intimate relationships and are more likely to engage in unhealthy behaviours (Felitti et al., 1998). Finally, **cumulative effects** are the sum of the overall experiences throughout life that combine and interact to influence the ongoing and long-term health of individuals.

Similar to the structuralist critique of the focus on health lifestyles, the health inequalities approach has also been the focus of various criticisms. First, there were concerns raised about the somewhat reductionist orientation of this model to socio-economic status. Critics argue that social reality is much more complex and multi-layered than assumed with this approach. That is, there are other critical resources to be considered, including knowledge, power, and social connections or social capital (Link & Phelan, 1996). Second, some critics argue that there is a lack of recognition of the fundamental causes of the differences in socio-economic status. As stated by Coburn et al., (2003):

> The CIAR model involves a clear if sometimes only implicit view of Canadian social structure. Society is viewed as a collection of interest groups in which some are more powerful than others but in which the state, informed by science, adjudicates among its own interests and those of the interests that make up society. Consequently, appeals for change are addressed almost entirely to policymakers. There is a heavy reliance on knowledge as a persuasive factor, but the complexities of what has been called "speaking truth to power" (i.e., the relationships between knowledge and power structures) are not addressed. (p. 393)

Finally, there is a concern that this approach is overly deterministic—that is,

> [W]hile population health research contributes to our understanding of the ways in which aspects of the social environment determine the health of populations, its models are unable to address the ways in which people, both individually and collectively, act to improve their health. (Coburn et al., 2003, p. 393)

Fundamental Causes of Disease   Many of the critiques of the *Lalonde Report* and the CIAR model can be framed within the fundamental-causes-of-disease framework. Within this framework, Link and Phelan (1995, 1996) and Phelan et al. (2010) make an important distinction between different kinds of risk factors in terms of spatial-temporal referents of distal and proximal. Refer back to the example of Jason at the beginning of this chapter. The proximal risk factors were playing in the junkyard while the distal risk factors were the father's unemployment and low education resulting in poverty. From this example, the distal risk factors refer to fundamental conditions that we might think of as "upstream" risk factors for disease. These fundamental conditions are based on structural and economic context that is determined by a person's social position, consistent with the CIAR model. However, it is not socio-economic status or poverty in isolation that is important. Instead, these fundamental causes differentially condition access to resources that allow individuals to protect themselves from proximal damaging elements in the social and physical environment (see Box 7.3). These resources are flexible and based on the given needs of a specific problem but can be thought of broadly as the knowledge, power, and means to control your own environment, making it more favourable and less harmful. It is the knowledge to make informed decisions and the capacity to successfully implement and act upon those decisions. It could include the ability to live in a more desirable neighbourhood, to send your children to a better school and involve them in extra-curricular sports and cultural activities, or to use your social connections to secure a job. It also includes behavioural decisions that flow from both knowledge and means. In Jason's example, it is both knowing the value of, and having the ability to afford, safe playground facilities and to have the resources to access appropriate and timely health care for the injury, regardless of the cost, before it became infected and required hospitalization.

Poverty or socio-economic status operates as a fundamental cause of disease by allowing people in higher socio-economic strata to use broadly serviceable resources, such as knowledge, money, and power, to avoid health risks and to minimize the consequences of disease once it occurs. Even when we develop the capacity to control and treat a disease, this capacity is unequally distributed, leading to differential morbidity and mortality rates. People of higher socio-economic status are more favourably situated to learn about the risks and to have the resources that allow them to engage in protective efforts to change their behaviours to avoid the risks and to seek treatment if necessary.

Another example is smoking and cancer. Only when information about the harmful consequences of cigarettes became widely known did the association between cigarette smoking and lower socio-economic status emerge. Prior to this, smoking was promoted through media and advertising as acceptable, luxurious, and a mark of affluence. When the evidence linking smoking to lung cancer and increased mortality became known, the prevalence of smoking and mortality rates fell much more quickly among those in higher socio-economic groups because they were better able to marshal their resources to take action (Singh, Miller, & Hankey, 2002). Other proximal lifestyle factors and health conditions such as diet, exercise, and obesity may be following a similar pattern.

Box 7.3

Poverty Affects Way Brain Works, Study Suggests

The Canadian Press

December 4, 2008 at 11:19 AM EST

VANCOUVER — A B.C. pediatrician has co-authored a new study that researchers believe shows that the brains of children from low-income backgrounds function differently from the brains of kids from high-income environments.

Tom Boyce, who serves as the B.C. Leadership Chair of Child Development at the University of British Columbia, said the study found certain deficits in the functioning of the prefrontal cortex in kids from low-income environments.

The prefrontal cortex is the region of the brain that is critical for problem solving and creativity.

"The conclusion was that something about the early environments of children growing up in less well-off families fundamentally affects the growth and development of that region of the brain," Dr. Boyce said.

"And that is concerning because we want all kids to have equal chances and it looks as though, because of this, that there may be some deficits in the development of the low-income kids."

In the study, 26 children, ages nine and 10, were chosen. Half came from low-income environments while the other half consisted of children from high-income backgrounds.

Each child's brain activity was measured on an electroencephalograph (EEG) while he or she watched triangles projected on a screen.

Each child was told that when a slightly skewed triangle appeared, he or she was to click a button.

Researchers found that children from low socioeconomic environments demonstrated a slower response to the unexpected stimuli.

The study was conducted at the University of California, Berkeley, where, in addition to his UBC duties, Dr. Boyce serves as professor emeritus of public health.

Robert Knight, director of University of California at Berkeley's Helen Wills Neuroscience Institute, and cognitive psychologist Mark Kishiyama also worked on the study, which was published in the Journal of Cognitive Neuroscience.

In a news release, Mr. Kishiyama described the response of low-income children in the study to the response of people who have had a portion of their frontal lobe destroyed by a stroke.

"These kids have no neural damage, no prenatal exposure to drugs and alcohol, no neurological damage," Mr. Kishiyama said. "Yet the prefrontal cortex is not functioning as effectively as it should be."

Dr. Knight suspects that with proper training, these brain differences can be eliminated.

"It's not a life sentence. We think that with proper intervention and training, you could get improvement in both behavioural and psychological indices," he said in a news release.

Dr. Boyce, who recognizes that such findings can lead to calls of class warfare, said that's a charge researchers tried hard to avoid.

"We believe that these are differences in the early experiences of kids growing up in low socioeconomic status families. It's not the fault of anybody. We're looking for things that can be done to make that better," he said.

When asked what parents can do to enhance their children's development, Dr. Boyce had a simple answer: Communicate.

"One of the differences that we do know about between low and high socioeconomic status families is that high socioeconomic status families just talk to their kids more," Dr. Boyce said. "Between birth and the third birthday, low socioeconomic status children hear 30 million fewer words than do kids growing up in middle and upper class families."

Source: [Entire Story] Poverty affects way brain works, study suggests. The Canadian Press. Reprinted by permission.

This view allows the possibility of dramatic changes in the association between socio-economic status and particular diseases as new information and intervention possibilities emerge. At the same time, these resources can be used flexibly to change proximal risk factors and their associated diseases. This alternative view predicts an enduring association between socio-economic status and disease overall regardless of the proximal, intervening risk factors. In the following sections, we focus on three specific aspects of the social determinants perspective, including income and class, sex and gender, and immigration.

INCOME AND CLASS DETERMINANTS OF HEALTH

Measuring Social Class

Typical sociology texts break down the social classes in Canada into three main groups—upper, middle, and working class groups. The upper class that makes up around 3 to 5% of Canadians are, in turn, made up of the upper-upper class, or *old money*, where the bulk of the wealth is inherited, and the lower-upper class, or the *nouveau riche*. Roughly half of the Canadian population falls into the middle class. The top half of this category, the upper-middle class, is typically made up of high earners in managerial and professional fields. The average-middle class group works in less prestigious white-collar or highly skilled blue-collar jobs (i.e., the trades). The next largest category is the working class that makes up a third of the population in Canada. They are largely employed in service jobs and lower-level, blue-collar jobs with less self-direction, control, and satisfaction and they have little accumulated wealth. Finally there is the lower class, or the poor, which makes up the remaining 15 to 20% of the population. Many of these individuals rely on social assistance whereas others are considered to be the "working poor" because their incomes are insufficient to cover necessities such as food, shelter, and clothing (Macionis & Gerber, 2010). Many of the working poor are becoming dependent on charities and community food banks to make ends meet and provide for their families. Increasingly, more working class and some average middle-class families are also utilizing these resources.

In the public health literature, however, there are three general approaches to the conceptualization of social class. The first equates social class with socio-economic status based on income, education, and occupation. A second conceptualization of social class is derived from a more Marxist tradition as a social group defined by its relationship to the economic mode of production (see Box 7.3). Finally, social class has also been conceptualized as a social group defined in relation to its possession and utilization of various forms of capital—economic, cultural, and social capital (Veenstra, 2007).

With respect to the first and most common conceptualization of socio-economic status, there have been a host of studies that have looked at health effects by different occupational level drawing either explicitly or implicitly on the following British Occupational Classification:

I. —Professional

II. —Intermediate

III. —Skilled non-manual and manual

IV. —Partly skilled

V. —Unskilled

The most influential of these studies are the Whitehall Studies in England led by Sir Michael Marmot introduced in Chapter 6. Basically, these studies not only reveal a difference in health among classes with higher occupational categories benefiting from better health, they reveal a **social gradient** where health status decreases incrementally as we move down the social ladder (see Box 7.4). They further find that the relationship between health and social status may be primarily a result of the social position itself and not just that it entails greater economic rewards and therefore purchasing power. Others have also proposed that health disparities are smaller when income differences within a society are narrower (cf., Wilkinson, 1996). This is what is referred to as **relative poverty**. Essentially, the relative aspect of poverty suggests that the greater the inequality of resources, the greater the inequality in health. This is in contrast to **absolute poverty** that is not having adequate financial resources to meet basic needs for shelter, nutritious food, clothing, and education.

Another means by which to measure class differences in health is by **neighbourhood income**. Using census data, neighbourhoods can be classified based on average household income level or by the percentage of households with income below the Statistics Canada defined low income cut-offs (LICO) to define poverty level. Based on the 2006 census, about 11.4% of all households were below the national poverty level

Box 7.4

The Whitehall Studies on Social Class and Health

The original Whitehall Study began in 1967 and was headed by Sir Michael Marmot (Marmot et al., 1978). It examined over 18 000 British male civil servants in London, initially over 10 years, comparing morbidity and mortality across different employment grades. What was found was an inverse relationship between employment grade and mortality across a range of diseases. Men in the lowest grade had a mortality rate three times higher than men in the highest grade. The effect was most prominent for heart disease. That is, those of higher occupational grades had lower mortality rates for coronary heart disease. They also found a positive relationship between occupational grade and height, of almost 5 centimetres (cf., Nettleton, 1995). In the second Whitehall study (Whitehall II) that included women (1991), the researchers found similar patterns.

They did not consider that the pronounced differences were caused by lifestyle and genetic makeup. Rather, the authors argued that *decision-making power* and *control* are important mediators of health inequalities. That is, although most believe that those at a higher occupational grade have more stressful lives as a result of their decision-making responsibility, what seems to be happening is that those lower on the chain of command are stressed due to having less control over their lives. This so-called *status syndrome* suggests that a lack of control over a person's work environment, work tasks and processes, and pace of work have consequences for differential morbidity and mortality rates.

For more information, please listen to the podcast of Sir Michael Marmot from the BBC program *The Life Scientific* first broadcast on November 1, 2011 (www.bbc.co.uk/programmes/b016ld4q).

while over 18% of all children lived in households that fell below the poverty level (Statistics Canada, 2006c).

When we examine variations in health at the neighbourhood level, we find that both men and women living in neighborhoods with higher income live longer while infants in poorer neighbourhoods are more likely to die (see Researcher Profile 7.2 of Richard Carpiano). Consistent with individual-level analyses, the mortality effects of neighbourhood are stronger for males whereas the morbidity effects are stronger for females. This is a common trend, as we will see when we examine sex/gender differences in health.

Statistics Canada has developed a measure of class based on **income adequacy** (Statistics Canada, 1980). Income adequacy is a measure that adjusts household income based on the number of people living in the household and where they live. Essentially,

Researcher Profile 7.2

Richard Carpiano

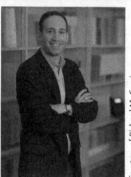

Courtesy of Richard M. Carpiano

Richard Carpiano is an Associate Professor in the Sociology Department at the University of British Columbia. His research centres on how social conditions contribute to the physical and mental health of adults, children, and the communities in which they live. He has also examined issues of social capital, social networks, theory-building in population health, social constructions of illness and risk, the measurement of community social environments, and the application of mixed methods to health research.

In his 2009 article "Concentrated affluence, concentrated disadvantage, and children's readiness for school: A population-based, multi-level investigation," Carpiano and his colleagues examine the relationship between neighbourhood concentration of affluence and disadvantage and the health and development of its residents (Carpiano et al., 2009). Their study population included 37 798 kindergarten children residing in 433 neighbourhoods throughout the province of British Columbia. Their findings suggest that increases in neighbourhood affluence are associated with increases in children's readiness for school. Particularly noteworthy is that the highest average child-level outcomes are not found in locations with the highest concentrations of affluence but rather in locations with relatively equal proportions of affluent and disadvantaged families. This finding lends further support to the social gradients thesis. Thus, concentrated affluence may have diminishing rates of return on contributing to enhanced child development, and children residing in mixed-income neighbourhoods may benefit both from the presence of affluent residents and from the presence of services and institutions aimed at assisting lower-income residents.

http://soci.ubc.ca/persons/richard-carpiano/

it rests on two assumptions: that a household of two is cheaper to maintain than is a larger household and that it is cheaper to live in rural and smaller urban communities. Statistics Canada calculates income adequacy, categorizing people into various groups based on household income and the low income cut-offs derived from the annual Survey of Labour and Income Dynamics (SLID), number of persons living in the household, and the size of the community. Income adequacy can be applied both at the family level and at the neighbourhood level by assigning LICOs that adjust for family size. Income adequacy has been shown to be a very useful measure to identify differences in health status and health outcomes.

Explanation of Class Differences

It is difficult to deny the strong associations between health and income, occupation, and social class. There have been a variety of explanations as to why these differences exist. The most robust analysis of the association between class and health is found in the British *Black Report* (1980) entitled *Inequalities in Health*. Commissioned by the Labour Government in 1978 to examine the persistent and widening class differences in health despite universality of access to health care services in the British National Health System (NHS), the commissioners examined four key explanations: (1) measurement artifact, (2) social selection, (3) cultural/behavioural differences, and (4) materialist causes (Blane, 1985).

The *measurement artifact* explanation posits that the relationship between social class and health is a result of the way that we measure class (discussed earlier in this chapter). When examining the evidence, the Commission came to the conclusion that the difficulties in measuring class actually serve to understate class differences in health. So the measurement artifact explanation could not explain away the association between class and health.

The second explanation, *social selection*, argues that the association between class and health is in the direction of health affecting social mobility and, as a consequence, social class. That is, those who are less healthy are less likely to achieve high income and socio-economic status. The commissioners found that this indeed does occur, particularly in the case of severe mental illness, such as schizophrenia, but that its overall effect was relatively minor. It could not explain the bulk of the association between class and health. (See Chapter 8 on mental illness for more complete discussion on this explanation).

The third and fourth explanations were considered to be the most pertinent. According to the *cultural/behavioural argument*, social class gradients in health are the result of social class differences in health and illness behaviours. That is, people in higher classes generally practise healthier lifestyles. There is indeed evidence to support this argument but, as we discussed, it is difficult to separate behaviour from its context. The evidence suggests that lifestyle behaviours are either intervening (proximal) variables or are constrained by the underlying structural influences on health. The commissioners were most convinced by the *materialist argument* that argues that class differences in health are the result of social structural differences between the classes. Although some have suggested that the evidence for this argument is more suggestive than conclusive, a counter argument is that there has been a failure to examine widespread, class-related causes of disease (e.g., poor housing) as well as a failure to examine summation and interaction of material factors. The following quote about the range of ways in which income and class affects health reveals the importance of taking a holistic approach:

> Income is a determinant of health in itself, but it is also a determinant of the quality of early life, education, employment and working conditions, and food security. Income also is a determinant of the quality of housing, the need for a social safety net, the experience of social exclusion, and the experience of unemployment and employment insecurity across the lifespan. (Raphael, 2010, p. 150)

Beyond this traditional materialism approach that focuses on the conditions of living are two additional perspectives. Raphael (2010) describes these as the *neo-materialist explanation* and the *psychosocial explanation*. In addition to the conditions of living as determinants of health, the neo-materialist perspective examines the social infrastructure. It focuses on why the material conditions of life have become so unequally distributed across the Canadian population. It essentially looks for the root causes of the causes of the causes (cf., Graham, 2004). The psychosocial perspective looks at how people compare themselves to each other, or how their relative position in the social hierarchy affects their health and well-being (Kawachi & Kennedy, 1997). These comparisons happen at both the individual and the communal levels. Perceived disparities at the individual level induce stress and other disease-producing effects. At the communal level, greater relative disparities reduce **social cohesion** among community members with consequent negative effects on health. This perspective enables us to dig more deeply into the mechanisms by which income and social class affects health.

The Manitoba *Mincome* Experiment

To further illustrate the link between social class and poverty on health, it is informative to examine a historical Canadian political experiment. From the late 1960s to the 1970s, the United States and Canada conducted field experiments to examine the effect of a guaranteed annual income (GAI) model to address income disparities and poverty. These experiments were initially implemented from a labour force perspective, to see if a GAI would create a disincentive to work (Hum & Simpson, 2001). Overall, the principal reduction in work effort was among adolescent males who stayed in school longer and mothers who extended maternity leaves, both of which could be perceived of as making longer-term investments in human capital (Forget, 2011). The North Carolina experiment showed higher elementary student test scores while the New Jersey experiment showed higher rates of school retention (Forget, 2011). These experiments also had implications for health and health inequality. Health was not generally considered in the United States experiments, but the Gary, Indiana, study did show reduced infant mortality rates.

The basic income experiment in Manitoba, co-funded by the newly elected New Democratic provincial government and the federal Liberal government under Pierre Trudeau between 1974 and 1979, called *Mincome*, was conducted in two parts. One part was in Winnipeg, modelled after the United States experiments. The second part occurred in Dauphin, Manitoba, using a saturation model in that the guaranteed minimum income project was universal, open to everyone in the town and area who fell below the poverty line (Hum & Simpson, 2001; Forget, 2011). This design allowed for examination of aggregate, community-level effects that could be compared with nearby rural towns that did not receive *Mincome*. All qualifying individuals and families in Dauphin were provided monthly cheques equivalent to $1200 per year indexed to inflation without the usual clawbacks for working while on welfare. (Note: the poverty cutoff in 1974 was $2100 per year compared to Statistics Canada 2008 poverty cutoff of $17 364 for an individual and $32 264 for a family of four respectively in a community fewer than 30 000 people.)

Interestingly, the *Mincome* study was ended abruptly as costs were higher than estimated and the prevailing political winds changed direction. The data were boxed and stored but not analyzed and a final report was never issued (Hum & Simpson, 2001). Thirty years later Evelyn Forget (2011), a health economist at the University of Manitoba, conducted an analysis of the Dauphin saturation study when the data were rediscovered in over 2000 boxes in an archive. She found that the *Mincome* experiment not only did not create a disincentive for recipients to work (except for a small number of previously poor, young mothers and teenagers), it had a range of unintended positive, longer-term population-level effects. First, the high school graduation rate increased in Dauphin, suggesting that poorer students did not have to leave school before graduating to find work to support their families. As identified in Chapter 6, educational attainment has a long-term positive impact on employability and health. Second, by linking the data to provincial Medicare health records, during the period of the *Mincome* experiment, visits to hospital dropped by 8.5% compared to other groups. There were also reduced hospital visits for work-related injuries and mental health problems. Finally, Dauphin residents also had a significant decline in physician visits compared to others. Forget (2011) concluded that the savings could be significant. Just using hospital visits, for example, an 8.5% decrease across Canada could potentially save about $4 billion annually.

SEX AND GENDER DETERMINANTS OF HEALTH

The literature on sex and gender differences in health usually distinguishes between *sex*, the biological differences between females and males, and *gender*, the socially constructed differences between men and women in our society. According to Lorber (2001), gender can be conceptualized as a social institution and a "process of creating distinguishable social statuses for the assignment of rights and responsibilities" (p. 26). As a *stratification* system, gender creates a social hierarchy in which men are more privileged than women of the same class or ethnic category, and as a *structure*, "gender divides work in the home and in economic production, legitimates those in authority, and organizes sexuality and emotional life" (Lorber, 2001, p. 27). This speaks to the differential in power relations, the relationship of men and women to the broader system of patriarchy, and gender-based inequality.

Gender can also be conceptualized as a *process* of "doing gender" (West & Zimmerman, 1987), creating differences between men and women in the course of social interactions. Gender is not only about these differences, but also about how the notions of masculinity and femininity are socially constructed and how individually we are socialized into these roles. As such, gender becomes a very powerful social construction that shapes not only our behaviours, but also the social conditions in which we live and experience our lives. However, most research focuses on sex to compare males and females as a proxy measure for these underlying social factors that influence differences far beyond any biological basis.

When we look at sex/gender differences in health, we can identify some interesting differences in the type of health problems experienced by men and women over the course of their lives, their utilization of health care services, and their health-related behaviours. It is essential to remember, however, that the majority of these differences cannot be explained away solely by the biological differences between males and females. Rather, gender differences in health demonstrate that, while gender is a social construct, it has strong influence on the health and well-being of the individuals.

Gender Differences and Morbidity and Mortality

Probably the most well-known adage accounting for the gender differences in health is that "women are sicker but men die quicker." Historically, women had a shorter average life expectancy than men primarily due to maternal death, poor nutrition, and the low status of women in society. While the overall life expectancy of both men and women has increased dramatically over the past century mainly due to improvements in public health, nutrition, and living conditions as well as advancements in medicine, gender differences have reversed, with women now outliving men by a number of years. Life expectancy for men and women born in the twentieth and twenty-first centuries shows that men, on average, live shorter lives than do women.

A longer lifespan for women does not mean that women will enjoy those extra years. Women do live longer, but they have more chronic illness and disability than men. When the rates of life expectancy are adjusted to account for the quality of life and living with a disability (e.g., health-adjusted life expectancy—HALE), women live only 2.3 more healthy years than men (68.9 for men and 71.2 for women) (see Table 6.7 in Chapter 6) (Statistics Canada, 2012d).

Gender differences are also evident in leading causes of death. Although the leading causes of death for both genders are cancer (ranked first) and heart disease (ranked second) (see Table 6.6 in Chapter 6), some of the notable differences are that men are more likely to die from accidents and unintentional injuries (5% of all deaths among men compared with 3.6% deaths among women). Another interesting finding is that suicide is ranked seventh on the list of leading causes of death for men (2.5% of all deaths) but does not make the top 10 causes of death among women, ranking thirteenth (0.8% of all deaths).

Gender differences persist not only in causes of death but also in the types of diseases that men and women experience over the course their lives. The morbidity patterns indicate that women are more likely to suffer from chronic diseases and mental disorders, especially depression (Denton, Walters, & Prus, 2004). Studies show that women are more likely to suffer from allergies, arthritis, rheumatism, asthma, high blood pressure, emphysema, and other non-fatal diseases that significantly decrease the quality of life and contribute to higher rates of disability among women (22.6% for women and 19.6% for men) (DesMeules, Turner, & Cho, 2003).

Finally, gender differences can be found in the patterns of hospitalization among men and women. When compared to men, women's hospitalization rates are approximately 20% higher, although more than half of women's overall hospitalization rates are due to pregnancy and childbirth (DesMeules et al., 2003). When pregnancy and childbirth are excluded from the analysis, women's hospitalization rates were actually lower than men's (DesMeules et al., 2003). Men are more likely to be hospitalized for circulatory and respiratory disease, as well as for injury and poisoning, whereas women are more likely to be admitted to the hospital due to cancer, mental disorders, and musculoskeletal diseases (DesMeules et al., 2003).

We have identified a number of health differences between males and females with respect to mortality rates and life expectancy, and morbidity and service utilization. At the start of this section, we discussed the difference between sex and gender, one based on biology and the other a social construct. Usually, it is inferred that the differences between men and women are biologically based. However, can biology fully explain the health differences among men and women? In the next section, we review a number of social explanations for these sex differences and discuss how gender impacts health and health-related behaviours.

Explanations for Sex and Gender Differences

As we mentioned in Chapter 1, sociological explanations for the phenomena of health and illness can be divided into two basic categories—the macro theories, dealing with a social organization of society, and the micro perspectives, examining the experiences of individuals in the context of social life. The contributions of feminist theories, which explore the impact of sex and gender on health and illness, cut across macro and micro theories. Some feminist explanations utilize macro perspectives and analyze gender as a social structure; others take a micro perspective looking at the impact of gender differences on everyday life. Although these explanations differ in their focus on the source of sex differences in health, they have one common feature—all of them have sought to understand how gender—a socially constructed category—creates the differences in morbidity, mortality, access to health care services, and experiences within health care system.

Gender Socialization and Gendered Experiences of Health and Illness

Gender socialization is a process that begins even before the birth of the child. When the expectant mother is choosing a pink or a blue blanket for her soon-to-be-born baby or choosing what colour to paint the nursery, she is assigning her unborn baby to a gender category. When guests at baby showers and birthdays bring gifts that are specific to boys or girls, they are reinforcing this gender categorization. Gendering is not only manifested in the selection of colours, clothing, and toys; it is also performed every day through many other actions, such as walking, sitting, standing, and interacting with others (Lorber, 1997; Lorber & Moore, 2002). Our assumptions about gender roles—or how we are supposed to behave as women or men—include a set of behaviours that are taught and rewarded as appropriate or inappropriate for each of us based on our sex. That is, females are assumed and expected to be caring, vulnerable, and emotional; men are assumed and expected to be strong, resilient, unemotional, and aggressive (Valverde, 1985). Paradoxically, while these gender norms are often explained by "nature" or biological differences, they often contradict biology. We know, for instance, that despite the portrayal of men as strong, male fetuses and male infants are more likely to die than female fetuses and infants. Moreover, there are some genetic-based diseases that are specific to males, such as hemophilia.

The gender norms related to masculinity and femininity also shape men's and women's responses to emerging health problems. It has been shown, for instance, that men are less likely to seek medical help than women, which can cause unnecessary deterioration in health conditions or progression of diseases due to the delay in seeking medical help (Lane & Cibula, 2000). Verbrugge and Wingard (1987) suggested that females' preventive actions might mean that their health problems do not become as severe as males. On the other hand, these differences in seeking medical help are not necessarily universal for *all* health conditions. Waldron (1995) found that patterns of sex differences for preventive behaviour are inconsistent, and that women delay just as long as men in seeking medical care for cancer and heart disease.

The impact of gender on medical diagnosis and reporting of medical problems is another aspect of social life that contributes to gender differences in health. The internalization of traditional norms of masculinity may influence men's readiness to talk about their disease with a doctor. This has been reported in instances when men are being diagnosed with the diseases that presumably can diminish their sense of masculinity, such as prostate cancer or erectile dysfunction (Chapple & Ziebland, 2002; Loe, 2004). On the other hand, popular cultural perceptions about women's overuse of health care services can become a reason for physicians to dismiss women's health concerns (Pederson & Raphael, 2006). As a result, physicians often interpret some women's health concerns as psychosocial in origin, and health care providers can often leave women undertreated (Pederson & Raphael, 2006).

Gender as a Mechanism for Stratification

It is important to realize that gender norms do not just "exist" in society. As we mentioned earlier, they also serve as a mechanism for stratification through oppression and the allocation of resources (Lorber, 2001). This oppression is sought to exert male dominance over women in our society (Connel, 1987). Although generally, this socially constructed hierarchy benefits men, it also causes men harm. What impact do gender norms have on men's health? Men are more likely than women to engage in risky behaviours (Thoits, 1995). These risks can be related to recreational activities, such as reckless driving or driving under the influence of drugs or alcohol, or engaging in violent or unsafe behaviours. Risk-taking is also related to working conditions because many more men are employed in jobs that have a high frequency of accidents and injuries, such as mining and construction, and they are more likely to willingly accept these risks. This increased risk-taking is evident in the statistics on mortality that show men as more likely to die as a result of an accident.

Women's work-related injuries are often "hidden" and under-reported as they are not usually lethal or acute. Women can be chronically exposed to occupational health hazards in their own homes or in the jobs that have over-representation of women but are not considered risky to their health (Pederson & Raphael, 2006), for example, ongoing exposure to harsh chemicals in cleaning products or chronic conditions due to repetitive strain or awkward lifting. Women also do most of the caring jobs in society, both paid and unpaid. Although this type of work can be very meaningful and important for women, it can also increase levels of stress and burnout, as well as cause deterioration in physical health (Denton et al., 2004).

The material and daily living conditions of men and women also have an impact on their health status (Pederson & Raphael, 2006). Women are more likely than men to live in poverty and to organize, provide for, and manage the care of people around them (Pederson & Raphael, 2006). Although provision of care makes women especially vulnerable to stress and burnout related to caregiving, it also allows women to build extensive social networks and feel connected to their families and communities (Connidis, 2010). Women have more social ties and more social support than do men, especially if we compare those men and women who are divorced or widowed (Connidis, 2010).

Although gender is a socially constructed category, it is evident that gender plays a central part in shaping men's and women's lives, their health, and their access to care. At the same time, because gender relations are deeply embedded in the everyday lives of individuals and the social organization of society, there are some unanswered questions about the complexity of the interactions between gender and health. For instance, when we compile statistics on morbidity and mortality, we do not necessarily rely on gender as a distinguishing factor—we look at males and females, the terms used to describe the biological differences, yet we make inferences about gender. While it is plausible that the majority of males adapt the norms of masculinity and the majority of females adopt the norms of femininity, the reliance on sex in the statistics on morbidity and mortality makes the theorizing about gender and health somewhat problematic (Lane & Cibula, 2000).

Another challenge in identifying the impact of gender on health is that gender cannot (and some scholars argue should not) be separated from other systems of oppression, such as class or racial differences (Crenshaw, 1995; Iyer, Sen, & Ostlin, 2008), a point that we revisit later in this chapter. What we do know is that gender matters

(Denton et al., 2004). What we do not know yet is exactly *how* gender matters, how it influences health, and what theoretical and methodological approaches would be most useful to illuminate the impact of gender as a social determinant of health.

RACE AND ETHNIC DETERMINANTS OF HEALTH

Another important cluster of characteristics that affect health are race, ethnicity, and minority status. Similar to the distinction made between sex and gender, there is an important distinction between **race**—typically considered to be a cluster of physical traits—and **ethnicity**—which denotes a more socially constructed, shared cultural heritage. **Minority status** adds a political and social-structural dimension because it refers to certain races and ethnicities of people who are socially stratified into subordinate positions within society (Macionis, Clarke, & Gerber, 1994). An even more contemporary term is **racialized**, which refers to the process by which certain characteristics are ascribed to people from certain "racial" categories, that is the reification of race (see Researcher Profile 7.3 of Gerry Veenstra). That is, certain racial groups are assigned a subordinate status based on negative perceptions based solely on physical characteristics. Li (2008) describes racialization succinctly: "[t]he social import of race has to do with society giving

Researcher Profile 7.3
Gerry Veenstra

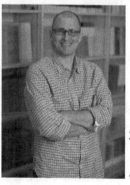

Courtesy of Gerry Veenstra

Gerry Veenstra is Professor in the Department of Sociology at the University of British Columbia in Vancouver, Canada. He is primarily interested in examining the health implications of social inequalities: by capitals and class, by "race" and ethnicity, and by intersections between gender, race, class, and sexual orientation. His ongoing research in the area of capital, class, and health relates to application of Pierre Bourdieu's theories and frameworks pertaining to fields, capitals, and habitus to health inequalities. His work on the nature of racial health inequalities in Canada does so by considering the distinctions between various aspects of people's suites of racial identities and explanatory factors such as socio-economic status and experiences of discrimination. As he states in his 2009 article in *Social Science & Medicine*, "Because processes of racialization are fundamentally processes of power and inequality, they likely have repercussions for health and well-being and, therefore, deserve attention from population health researchers, despite the difficulties inherent to operationalizing racialized identities in quantitative survey research" (Veenstra, 2009, p. 539).

significance to people according to selective phenotypic characteristics, and treating the resulting groupings as though they are naturally constituted in and of themselves" (p. 21).

Two key areas of research have dominated Canadian social science literature on racialized identity and health. The first deals with the health of Aboriginal Canadians whereas the second addresses the health status of immigrants to Canada.

Aboriginal Health

Aboriginal status can be broken down into First Nations, Inuit, and Métis populations. First Nations peoples are often further differentiated into those living on- or off-reserve. Epidemiologically, in terms of mortality rates, we find that Aboriginal Canadians on average have a lower life expectancy than other Canadians, by as much as seven years for both males and females. This is due largely to the high morbidity and mortality rates in their earlier years. Accidents, violence, and poisonings account for nearly one-third of all deaths among Aboriginals. Aboriginal Canadians are twice as likely as other Canadians to die from HIV/AIDS and four to nine times more likely to die from alcohol-related causes. Aboriginal groups experience diabetes at a rate three times high than other Canadians. They have higher rates of cirrhosis of the liver, tuberculosis, HIV, hepatitis C, high blood pressure, asthma, heart disease, sexually transmitted diseases, and aboriginal women have higher rates of cervical cancer (Health Canada, 2009, see Figure 7.1). Although the infant mortality rate has declined dramatically over the last few decades among Aboriginal groups in Canada, it is still double that of the Canadian population as a whole, and post-neonatal deaths are three times higher (Smylie, Fell, & Ohlsson, 2010).

Immigrant Health

The second key area of racial identity and health focuses on immigrants. Here we find a much different story, at least initially. That is, immigrants, on average, have lower standardized death rates and are healthier than non-immigrant Canadians. This is commonly referred to as the **healthy immigrant effect**. There are different explanations for a higher level of health among immigrants. One explanation is that Canada is highly selective of the immigrants it allows into the country. Those who are permitted to come to Canada generally tend to be in excellent health. The one exception would be refugees, who have poorer health status and a much higher risk of infectious diseases, particularly if a significant amount of time was spent in refugee camps (Health Canada, 2010). However, refugees make up a very small proportion of the total number of immigrants. Another possible explanation is a healthier diet and lifestyle that immigrants followed in their country of origin and continue to practise, at least temporarily, after immigrating to Canada.

With each passing year spent in Canada, however, this initial health advantage deteriorates as evidenced by their increasing rates of chronic diseases, such as diabetes and some cancers and their increasing mortality rates (Gushulak et al., 2011). This

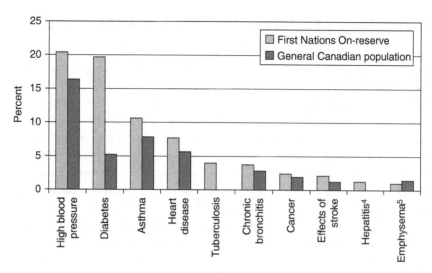

Figure 7.1 Age-Standardized Prevalence of Selected Health Conditions[1] among Adult First Nations On-reserve[2] (2002–03) and the General Canadian Population[3] (2003)

[1]The 2001 population for Canada was used as the standard population in the calculation of age-standardized rates.

[2]Includes respondents 18 years of age and older.

[3]The sampling frame of the CCHS excludes individuals living on Indian Reserves and on Crown Lands, institutional residents, full-time members of the Canadian Armed Forces, and residents of certain remote regions. (See References.) Includes respondents 20 years of age and older.

[4]Includes hepatitis types A, B, and C.

[5]For the general Canadian population in the CCHS, emphysema and chronic obstructive pulmonary disease (COPD) were asked in the same question. COPD includes chronic bronchitis and emphysema.

Notes:

a) RHS and CCHS data on prevalence of disease based on self-reporting of the respondent.

b) General Canadian population figures for tuberculosis and hepatitis are not available and are denoted as n/a.

Source: © All rights reserved. A Statistical Profile on the Health of First Nations in Canada: Self-rated Health and Selected Conditions. Health Canada, 2009. Reproduced with permission from the Minister of Health, 2014.

may be a result of acculturation to Canadian diet and lifestyle. Supporting this explanation is the fact that children of immigrants generally do not manifest the same healthy immigrant effect as they become acculturated more quickly into the Canadian lifestyle through school and other social interactions. There is also data to suggest that immigrants experience high levels of stress due both to migration and to ongoing difficulties integrating and succeeding economically in Canada. These stressors eventually erode their health resulting in higher rates of physical and mental health issues (see Chapter 8 on the stress process). Stressors associated with integration and economic success may vary across ethnic groups based on differential poverty rates (see Chapter 6, Figure 6.3).

Explanations for Racial and Ethnic Differences

It is generally agreed that biological differences among racialized and/or ethnic groups account for disparities in health. However, biological differences among groups tend not to be very strong and explain very little of the variance in health differences. Consistent with the previous discussions on class and gender differences, the two principal explanations for health variations are cultural/behavioural/lifestyle differences and the structural inequality of racism (whether overt or institutionalized) that result in unequal life chances and the interplay between these two sets of factors. For example, it is generally recognized that the health status of Aboriginal people is related to the broader social determinants of health. That is, their poor health status can be seen as reflecting the historical legacies of colonialism; racism; and the imposition of social, political, and cultural institutions (e.g., residential schools) that broke down the fabric of Canadian Aboriginal families and societies. For example, during the 1940s and 1950s, Aboriginal people in remote northern communities who were identified as severely malnourished were subjected not to nutritional supplements to address the problem but to nutritional experiments examining the effects of malnutrition on health. In collaboration with several government agencies, researchers examined approximately 1300 Aboriginals from various northern communities and six residential schools who were intentionally denied food and other medical and dental services to examine outcomes of malnutrition (Mosby, 2013). Although the long-term knowledge gleaned from these experiments is unclear, Mosby concludes that what is clear are the dehumanizing, paternalistic, and bureaucratic colonialist policies toward Aboriginal peoples by the government.

Even today, many Aboriginal people both on- and off-reserve continue to live in poor conditions and experience high levels of unemployment, poverty, and low educational attainment, all of which affect their health status. According to the Aboriginal People's Survey by Statistics Canada, a particularly pressing concern is lack of access to adequate housing that fosters the spread of diseases such as tuberculosis. It has been shown that the percentage of Aboriginal people living in overcrowded and substandard housing is five to six times higher on reserves and in the North compared with the Canadian population in general (Health Canada, 2009; Statistics Canada, 2007a).

Similarly, immigrant health has been described by Gushulak and colleagues (2011) as "a product of environmental, economic, genetic and socio-cultural factors related to when people migrated . . ., where and how they lived in their original home country, and how and why they migrated" (p. 952). These pre-migration factors interact with post-migration experiences to influence health. Changes and challenges posed by migration may include language and cultural barriers, changes in food, lifestyle and health habits, social exclusion, restricted admission to employment opportunities consistent with their qualifications, and limited access to health services. The coping strategies adopted by migrants to adapt to their new environments, such as creating links to social networks, are also relevant. For example, many international physicians immigrate to Canada but are unable to practise medicine here unless they complete their Canadian and province-specific certification. For immigrants from most countries, this can be costly and take years in additional courses and residency requirements with no guarantee of a licence at the end. Many just give up and take on other types of employment available through their social networks that are often far below their salary and status expectations.

INTERSECTIONALITY AND INTEGRATIVE MODELS OF THE SOCIAL DETERMINANTS OF HEALTH

Although we have considered class, gender, and racial differences in health separately, it is important to revisit our earlier discussion of **intersectionality** to make the case for an integrated view of these factors. That is, significant strides have been made in our methodological approaches and, by extension, in the literature understanding the social construction and intersection among class, gender, and racialized dimensions of health. In the case of immigrant health, for example, a growing body of research argues for a more nuanced approach that considers the intersection of migration status with other social indicators (e.g. age, gender, economic status) to understand which migrants are most vulnerable to health deterioration and the underlying reasons. This research suggests that immigrants who are older adults, women, with low-income, and members of racialized groups face a greater risk of health deterioration than other immigrants (Gushulak et al., 2011).

Intersectionality has remained a model focused on the combination and interaction of various social dimensions. As Hankivsky et al. (2011) articulate:

> [H]ealth is such a complex and multi-dimensional phenomenon, one determined and constituted in such great respect by the social, spatial, and temporal contexts in which people and communities exist. . . . Thus, it seems especially urgent—when theorizing and researching health—to apply analytical frameworks that account for and that take seriously the ways in which people's identities, the places they live, and those with whom they engage are constantly affected by power while also interlocking and overlapping in ever-dynamic, always relational, unbounded and unfixed ways. The framework of intersectionality offers excellent potential to do just this. (p. 1)

Although the transformational promise of intersectionality as a means to improve our understanding of the social determinants of health has been increasingly recognized, it has not made significant strides in transforming mainstream health research and policy (Hankivsky et al., 2011).

Moving even further toward a fully integrated, interdisciplinary model to explain health, additional ecological models have been proposed to include factors ranging from individual genetics and biology to the overarching social structure and environment. Two of the more well-known model depictions of the integrated nature of the various social determinants of health are featured in Figures 7.2 and 7.3. Each of these frameworks depicts the multi-layered understanding of the various intersecting influences of health.

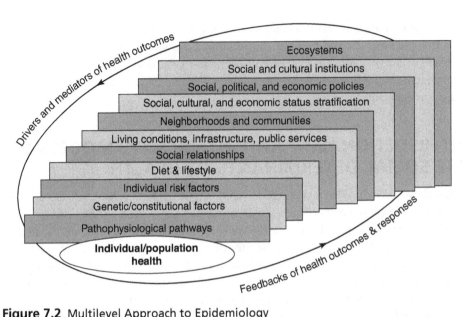

Figure 7.2 Multilevel Approach to Epidemiology

Note—This is a revised model from that originally proposed by Kaplan et al., 2000, p. 43, containing only seven levels.

Source: Reprinted with permission from Kaplan, G. A., Everson, S. A., & Lynch, J. W., The contribution of social and behavioral research to an understanding of the distribution of disease: a multilevel approach. Promoting health: Intervention strategies from social and behavioral research, 37-80. Copyright © 2000 by the National Academy of Sciences, Courtesy of the National Academies Press, Washington D.C.

The most proximate are biological and genetic factors and individual-level ascribed factors such as age, sex, and race. Moving outward from the biological and individual-level factors, the models take into account individual lifestyle and behavioural factors. These biological and individual-level factors are usually the easiest to investigate and are the ones most commonly identified as being associated with health during everyday discourse and in the media. Moving further outward, however, family and community factors are considered, and then the most distal factors, including socio-economic structural and environmental conditions.

As we have seen in the case of class differences in health, these more distal factors tend to be more difficult methodologically to link to health for a variety of reasons. The important point is not so much where the various factors are situated but that each of these factors is inseparably connected to each other in a complex and dynamic manner. That is, proximate factors are influenced, conditioned, and constrained by the more distal factors. Individual factors, including lifestyle choices, may vary across persons and groups, but they do so within the constraints of life chances imposed by the social-structural conditions in which people are required to live. For example, the living conditions of people of certain ethnic or racial group, age group, gender, and/or social class constrained their ability to make healthier choices in things such as nutrition and lifestyle.

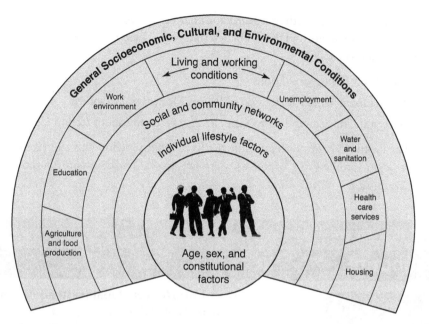

Figure 7.3 The Main Determinants of Health

Source: Dahlgren G, Whitehead M. (1991). Policies and Strategies to Promote Social Equity in Health. Stockholm, Sweden: Institute for Futures Studies. http://www.iffs.se/wp-content/uploads/2011/01/20080109110739filmZ8UVQv2wQFShMRF6cuT.pdf. Reprinted by permission of the Institute for Future Studies.

THE INTERNATIONAL CONTEXT OF THE SOCIAL DETERMINANTS OF HEALTH

A critically important activity focusing attention on the broader social determinants of health at the international level has been the WHO Commission on the Social Determinants of Health (WHO, 2008). Led by Sir Michael Marmot, the aim of the Commission was to focus on the "causes of the causes" of disease and premature death. These were described in the report as the social factors within which people live, grow, work, and age that, in turn, are shaped by social, political, and economic forces. The overarching theme of the Commission Report was that, "Social injustice is killing on a grand scale." As stated in the report:

> Social justice is a matter of life and death. It affects the way people live, their consequent chance of illness, and their risk of premature death. . . . Within countries there are dramatic differences in health that are closely linked with degrees of social disadvantage. Differences of this magnitude, within and between countries, simply should never happen. (p. 2)

The summary of the report, exemplified in its title, proposed a range of recommendations on how to "Close the Health Gap in a Generation." Taking the perspective that the underlying determinants of health inequities are interconnected as described above, they must be addressed through both integrated and comprehensive policies and programs that address both the proximate and the distal determinants. These recommendations focused on three principles of action:

1. Improve Daily Living Conditions
2. Tackle the Inequitable Distribution of Power, Money, and Resources
3. Measure and Understand the Problem and Assess the Impact of Action

Researcher Profile 7.4 introduces sociologist Ron Labonté who, with the Honourable Monique Bégin (profiled in Chapter 3), were important Canadian contributors to the WHO Commission.

Researcher Profile 7.4

Ronald Labonté

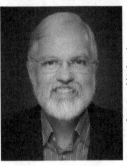

Courtesy of Dr. Ronald Labonté

(see **http://www.globalhealthequity.ca/content/ronald-labonte)**.

Ron has over 200 scientific publications and several hundred articles in popular media. His recent books include *Globalization and Health: Pathways, Evidence and Policy* (co-edited with Ted Schrecker, Corinne Packer and Vivien Runnels, Routledge. 2009); *Critical Public Health: A Reader* (co-edited with Judith Greene, Routledge. 2007); *Health Promotion: From Community Empowerment to Global Justice* (co-authored with Glenn Laverack, Palgrave Macmillan. 2007); *Health for Some: Death, Disease and Disparity in a Globalizing Era* (co-authored with Ted Schrecker and Amit Sen Gupta, Centre for Social Justice, 2005); *Fatal Indifference: The G8, Africa and Global Health* (co-authored with Ted Schrecker, David Sanders and Wilma Meeus, University of Cape Town Press/IDRC Books, 2004), and *Dying For Trade: How Globalization Can Be Bad for Our Health* (Centre for Social Justice. 2003).

Dr. Ronald Labonté, Canada Research Chair in Globalization and Health Equity, examines how globalization is affecting the health of a variety of groups in nations around the world. His research in health worker migration, medical tourism, global health systems reforms, global health diplomacy, and trade and human rights will help maximize health for all through a better understanding of how globalization creates health opportunities and risks.

For the WHO Commission on the Social Determinants of Health, Labonté coordinated the knowledge network hub on globalization from 2005 to 2007. This culminated in the report entitled, *Towards Health-Equitable Globalisation: Rights, Regulation and Redistribution* and 13 background critical evidence reviews

Prior to joining academia in 1999, Ron spent 10 years as international health promotion and public health consultant, and 15 years with provincial and local governments and NGOs in community health development.

SUMMARY

In this chapter, we have explored the underlying reasons for why the social distribution of health varies across groups through an examination of the concept of the social determinants of health and how this applies across the social cleavages of class, sex/gender, and race/ethnicity. We close with a story, as told by Irving Zola in an article by John McKinlay (1986), encouraging us to think more upstream about health:

> I am standing by the shore of a swiftly flowing river and hear the cry of a drowning man. I jump into the cold waters. I fight against the strong current and force my way to the struggling man. I hold on hard and gradually pull him to shore. I lay him out on the bank and revive him with artificial respiration. Just when he begins to breathe, I hear another cry for help. I jump into the cold waters. I fight against the strong current, and swim forcefully to the struggling woman. I grab hold and gradually pull her to shore. I lift her out onto the bank beside the man and work to revive her with artificial respiration. Just when she begins to breathe, I hear another cry for help. I jump into the cold waters. Fighting again against the strong current, I force my way to the struggling man. I am getting tired, so with great effort I eventually pull him to shore. I lay him out on the bank and try to revive him with artificial respiration. Just when he begins to breathe, I hear another cry for help. Near exhaustion, it occurs to me that I'm so busy jumping in, pulling them to shore, applying artificial respiration that I have no time to see who is upstream pushing them all in. . . . (p. 484)

Essentially this parable implies that dealing with more distal factors will indirectly address health status through changes in proximal, individual-level factors. We have seen this shift from the Health Promotion movement initially outlined in the *Lalonde Report* to the more recent Health Inequalities movement best illustrated in the Manitoba *Mincome experiment*. Although individual-level behavioural and lifestyle choices have a direct effect on health status, they are constrained within the social-structural context of peoples' lives. These social-structural contexts encompass a range of factors, including but not limited to social class, sex/gender, and race/ethnicity. We hope that such a focus on the *causes of the causes* of disease and health will prove emancipatory in that we will see that which has been socially constructed can be socially reconstructed into a system and society that better fosters health for all citizens.

Key Terms

Absolute poverty—not having adequate resources to meet basic needs for survival, including shelter, food, clothing, and education (contrast with relative poverty)

Cumulative effects—the sum of the overall experiences throughout life that combine and interact to influence long-term health and mortality

Ethnicity—a socially constructed, shared cultural heritage

Health field—a concept in the *Lalonde Report* identifying the four major components of health, including human biology, health care systems, environment, and lifestyle

Health inequity—refers to inequalities in health that are deemed unfair or that stem from some form of social or systemic injustice

Health lifestyles—ways of living that promote good health and longer life expectancy

Health promotion—strengthening the skills of individuals to encourage healthy behaviours and building the healthy social and physical environments to support these behaviours

Healthy immigrant effect—the consistent finding that new immigrants tend to be healthier and to have lower standardized death rates on average than non-immigrant Canadians

Income adequacy—a measure of income that is adjusted based on the number of people living in the household and the location and size of the community where they live

Intersectionality—an approach that encourages us to explicitly focus on multiple, intersecting statuses combining different layers of discrimination and oppression such as sexism, racism, ageism, and classism

Latent effects—health implications of the biological and developmental experiences during the prenatal and early childhood years

Minority status—a socially stratified political and social-structural dimension that categorizes certain racial and ethnic groups of people into subordinate positions in society

Neighbourhood income—grouping neighbourhoods on the basis of average household income or by the percentage of households with income below the poverty level

Pathway effects—experiences that place an individual onto a specific life trajectory that exposes them to subsequent experiences

Race—classification of people based on a cluster of physical traits such as skin colour

Racialized—attribution of social characteristics to people based on their race and physical attributes

Relative poverty—economic inequality that is socially and contextually defined either in terms of the location or society in which people live; how people perceive themselves as poor (or not) compared to others around them

Social cohesion—the feeling of shared social connections and the collective bonds and responsibilities

Social determinants of health—the social, political, and economic conditions of living and the way they are distributed among groups within a population leading to differences in population health status

Social gradient of health—refers to the sloping decline in population health status as we move down socio-economic and class positions

Critical Thinking Questions

1. What are the ways in which the social distribution of health is linked to the social determinants of health?

2. What are some of the proposed sociological mechanisms by which less hierarchical societies have fewer disparities and greater overall health status?

3. The literature on sex/gender and race/ethnicity reveals an interesting interplay between the biological and the social. Does the social determinants of health literature adequately address this balance? If not, how might it better acknowledge the role that biology plays?

Further Readings and Resources

Canadian Public Health Association. (1996). *Action statement for health promotion in Canada* Ottawa: Author. Available at www.cpha.ca/en/programs/policy/action.aspx

Glouberman, S. & Millar, J. (2003). Evolution of the determinants of health, health policy, and health information systems in Canada. *American Journal of Public Health, 93*(3), 388–392.

Hankivsky, O. (Ed.) (2011). *Health inequities in Canada: Intersectional frameworks and practices*. Vancouver, BC: UBC Press.

Navarro V. (2009). What we mean by social determinants of health. *Global Health Promotion, 16*(1), 5–16.

Mikkonen, J., & Raphael, D. (2010). *Social determinants of health: The Canadian facts*. Toronto: York University School of Health Policy and Management. Available at www.thecanadianfacts.org/

Rossiter. K., & Reeve, K. (2007). Board game on the social determinants of health. *The Last Straw* [board game]. www.TheLastStraw.ca

The Poverty Challenge
www.thepovertychallenge.org/

Chapter 8
Social Dimensions of Mental Illness

Chapter Outline

Learning Objectives

After studying this chapter, you should be able to:

1. Present a historical account of estimating rates of mental disorder, the current prevalence of mental disorder in Canada, and how it is distributed across various groups;

2. Compare and contrast social causation and social selection, two competing hypotheses to explain the differential distribution of mental illness;

3. Discuss various explanations of mental illness, including the stress process model as one potential model in the social causation framework that examines how social disadvantage and social stress may lead to increased risk of mental illness;

4. Present a historical account of the process of deinstitutionalization of the mentally ill in Canada and the United States.

Mental health and mental illness[1] (disorder) have long been examined by sociologists from various theoretical positions. Indeed, as far back as 1897, Emile Durkheim, considered one of the founding fathers of the discipline, turned his attention to social factors (conditions) of suicide. Since then, multiple volumes on topics examining such things as the prevalence of mental health problems and illness, the causes and consequences of mental health problems for individuals and society, and the issues surrounding health care services for those with mental health problems have been published. In this chapter, we provide a general overview of some of this work to provide the reader with a basic understanding of some of the social aspects of mental health and mental illness.

To begin, we should differentiate between mental health and mental illness. In previous chapters we devoted a great deal of space to differentiate health from illness. Mental health could refer to either good or poor health or one's mental state. The term **mental illness** is used to describe a psychiatric condition or diagnosis and is often used interchangeably with the term **mental disorder**. A mental disorder could be thought of as a mental abnormality in which a person exhibits strange or inappropriate behaviours. Disorders are recognized and defined by psychiatrists as meeting a specified number of symptoms that have been identified and agreed upon by the profession as standards for making a specific diagnosis. These diagnoses and the symptoms making up these diagnoses are listed in recognized professional volumes such as the *Diagnostic Statistical Manual*, Version 5 (DSM-V) of the American Psychiatric Association and the *International Statistical Classification of Diseases*, 10th Revision by the World Health Organization, 1992 (ICD-10). The diagnosing professional validates the clustering of certain behaviours and feelings indicating a psychiatric disorder, such as major depression, schizophrenia, or substance dependence. The diagnosis is often behaviourally based, unlike the case for other illnesses, such as heart disease or cancer that are physiologically or biologically based.

In this chapter we examine various aspects of mental illness from a social perspective. Initially we focus on the epidemiological rates of mental illness in Canada and the United States, including analysis of the distribution of illness across various groups. Then we look at competing explanations that may account for differential rates (i.e., differences between social groups) of mental disorder within society or that may explain the causes of mental illness. Finally, we briefly examine the historical process of deinstitutionalization in Canada and the United States, focusing specifically on the impact of this process on patients and the community at large.

---

[1]An earlier version of this chapter was published in Frankel, B. G., Speechley, M., & Wade T. J. (1996). *The Sociology of Health and Health Care: A Canadian Perspective*. Toronto: Copp Clark. This chapter was co-authored with John Cairney.

MENTAL ILLNESS IN CANADA
The Historical Development of Estimating Prevalence of Mental Disorder

Since psychiatric illness is recognized principally through behaviour instead of physiology, it is useful to look briefly at the epidemiological history of recognizing and estimating rates of disorder at the population level. Dohrenwend (1990) divided the history of psychiatric epidemiology into three periods or "generations." The first serious attempt to estimate the prevalence of mental disorder began between the turn of the twentieth century to World War II. It included 16 studies that relied mainly on informants and agency records to supply clinically relevant information. This approach estimated the prevalence of mental disorders in society to be about 3 to 4% based simply on "head counts" of the number of individuals residing in institutions (e.g., asylums, hospital wards).

The second generation of studies between World War II and the 1980s is marked by both the war and the development of the area of study known as **psychometrics**. Psychometrics is the science of systematic psychological measurement to examine such things as personality and IQ. Psychometrics expanded rapidly in the 1940s, and had a large influence on military conscription. After World War II, there was concern about "shell shock," or what we now call post-traumatic stress disorder (PTSD). Facilitating the rise in psychometrics, the military invested significantly in psychological testing of new recruits in the hopes of identifying and selecting out those who were psychologically vulnerable to traumas to reduce (it was hoped) the occurrence of PTSD. This resulted in large numbers of young men (and some women) being administered questionnaires measuring personality traits and psychological distress and impairment. These questionnaires identified large percentages of "healthy" people with symptoms of psychiatric disorder far beyond previous, first-generation estimates indicating that prevalence of mental disorder in the general population was much higher than expected based on estimates from the institutionalized.

Two of the most famous second-generation community studies were the Midtown Manhattan study conducted in New York City and the Sterling County Study in Nova Scotia. (Sterling County was a pseudonym to protect the identity of the actual county and its residents in Nova Scotia.) During this period, researchers began developing instruments to measure psychiatric disorder of the population. Instruments were based on psychiatric manuals such as the DSM-II (*Diagnostic and Statistical Manual of Mental Disorders*, 2nd Ed.) and the ICD 9 (*International Classification of Diagnoses*, version 9). Identification of disorder relied on directly administered semi-structured clinical interviews and standardized interview schedules such as the Psychiatric Status Schedule (PSS, Spitzer et al., 1970). These interviews, usually conducted by clinicians (psychologists and psychiatrists), reported a population prevalence of psychiatric disorder of about 20%. These instruments were generally effective at estimating **caseness** of disorder and had good inter-rater reliability but their accuracy in distinguishing among disorders was limited.

Caseness refers to the presence of a psychiatric illness generally with limited ability to identify the specific type of disorder.

The third generation marked a shift away from psychiatric clinical interviews to structured diagnostic interviews that lay-interviewers could conduct to replicate a psychiatric interview as closely as possible. Moreover, the interview schedules became increasingly refined to move beyond identifying caseness to differentiating among specific types of mental illness. These instruments were the precursors of today's interview schedules used to identify many different types of mental disorders. Some of the interview schedules developed included the Psychiatric Epidemiology Research Interview (PERI; Shrout, Dohrenwend, & Levav, 1986), and the Diagnostic Interview Schedule (DIS; Robins, Helzer, Croughan, & Ratcliffe, 1981).

The two main goals for these new diagnostic interviews were related to the accuracy of diagnosis (validity) and the replicability of diagnosis (reliability). Referring back to Chapter 2 on methodological tools, reliability can be divided into three types, including test-retest reliability, inter-rater reliability, and inter-item reliability (internal consistency). A structured diagnostic interview should be consistent in its specific diagnosis of an individual over time and across interviewers, and the items should be interrelated. Construct validity links the measurement or observation to its theoretical construct, in this case a specific psychiatric disorder. A specific aspect of construct validity is **criterion validity**, or how it compares when measured against a gold standard. In this case, the instrument is validated on the basis of how well it agrees with a clinician's diagnosis.

Examples of third-generation studies in Canada and the United States include the Epidemiological Catchment Area Study (ECA) by Robins et al. (1981), and the Edmonton Epidemiological Survey (Bland, Orn, & Newman, 1988a). The ECA was the largest community study to date, surveying over 20 000 people across five sites in the United States (Baltimore, Durham, Los Angeles, St. Louis, and New Haven) to identify incidence of illness as well as the lifetime and 12-month prevalence rates. Both the ECA and Edmonton studies used the Diagnostic Interview Schedule (DIS) and were remarkably consistent in their estimates of lifetime and 12-month prevalence rates of disorder. The ECA reported 32% overall lifetime prevalence rates of disorder and 20% one-year prevalence rates while the Edmonton study, interviewing a much smaller sample (3258 households), reported estimates of mental disorder of 33.8% lifetime and 21% one-year (Bland et al., 1988a) (Table 8.1). These findings show that approximately a third of the adult population has suffered from a mental disorder at least once in their lifetime. One fifth of the population either had a relapse or experienced their first episode within the previous year.

Others have identified a fourth and fifth generation of studies. The principal advancement in the fourth generation was the merging of rigorous measurement through the development of the Composite International Diagnostic Interview (CIDI) with national probability samples providing better estimates of the population prevalence of disorder. The CIDI was a collaborative effort by the World Health Organization (WHO) and the United States Alcohol, Drug Abuse and Mental Health Administration, based on ICD-10

Table 8.1 Prevalence of Specific Disorders (in percent) in the Edmonton Survey of Psychiatric Disorders

	Lifetime	One Year
Substance use disorders	20.6	9.1
Alcohol abuse/dependence	18.0	7.9
Drug abuse/dependence	6.9	2.6
Schizophrenia/schizophreniform	0.6	0.4
Schizophrenia	0.6	0.3
Schizophreniform	0.1	0.0
Affective disorders	10.2	6.8
Manic episode	0.6	0.2
Major depressive episode	8.6	4.6
Dysthymia	3.7	3.7
Anxiety/somatoform disorders	11.2	7.6
Phobia	8.9	6.2
Panic	1.2	0.7
Obsessive-compulsive	3.0	1.8
Somatization	0.0	0.0
Antisocial personality	3.7	2.4
Cognitive impairment	0.8	0.8

Source: Adapted from Bland, R.C., S.C. Newman, & H. Orn. (1988a). Period prevalence of psychiatric disorders in Edmonton. *Acta psychiatrica scandinavica, 77* (Suppl 338), p. 39.

and DSM-III, that could be completely administered by trained lay-interviewers, used in different languages for cross-cultural comparisons, and scored by computers to render diagnoses (Bland, 2010). The fifth generation focused specifically on children and adolescents (e.g., Streiner, Cairney, & Lesage, 2005). (See Box 8.1 on estimating child mental health and psychiatric disorder.)

The National Comorbidity Study (NCS), conducted between 1990 and 1992 in the United States, was the first study to use a national probability sample to assess the prevalence of major psychiatric disorders (Kessler et al., 1994). The most prevalent diagnoses of the NCS were major depression, alcohol dependence, and social phobia. It also examined **comorbidity**, the co-occurrence of more than one disorder. Among those with at least one disorder, 14% had three or more disorders accounting for half of all lifetime disorders. In Canada, the Ontario Mental Health Supplement (OMHS) of the Ontario Health Survey conducted between December, 1990, and April, 1991, also used the UM-CIDI (Offord, et al., 1996). It examined 8116 persons between the ages of 15 and 64 living in

Box 8.1

Measuring Child Mental Health in Canada

Streiner et al. (2005) suggest that the fifth generation in the history of psychiatric epidemiology focuses on identifying rates of disorder among children and adolescents. Children with emotional or behavioural problems place a heavy burden on their parents, perform more poorly in school, consume a large proportion of our health and social resources, and in the case of behavioural problems, are more likely to engage in delinquent behaviours. Canadian initiatives to assess child mental health have progressed significantly over the past decades.

The Ontario Child Health Study (OCHS) was one of the first population-level assessments of child mental health conducted by Offord and colleagues at McMaster in 1983 (Boyle et al., 1987; Offord et al., 1987). The Ontario government funded the study to examine child health and development and the health needs of children. Working with Statistics Canada, researchers sampled 3294 children aged 4 to 16 years in 1869 families. The survey measured various types of emotional and behavioural problems. Overall, they found that about one in five children suffer from some type of mental health problem. There were two follow-up studies in 1987 and 2001.

The Quebec Child Mental Health Study (QCHMS) was conducted in 1992 (Breton et al., 1999) under the mandate of the Ministry of Health and Social Services to assist in future child services planning in the province. The Quebec Family Allowance list was used to generate a representative provincial sample frame of children from 4 to 14 years of age resulting in a final survey sample of 2400 children. The study examined nine DSM-III-R disorders using the Diagnostic Interview Schedule for Children (DISC). Consistent with the OCHS, parent interviews resulted in a 19.9% overall prevalence rate of disorder among children.

The National Longitudinal Survey of Children and Youth (NLSCY) examined child health and development and life transitions. Based on the OCHS and QCHMS, the NLSCY began in 1994 with a large, nationally representative sample of Canadian children from newborn to age 11 (N=22 831) (Statistics Canada, 1997). The NLSCY had a much larger sample size, allowing for a more subtle examination of age-graded child characteristics. The children are followed every two years until age 25 to examine transitions into early adulthood. At every new wave of data collection, a new sample of birth to 2-year-olds is included to ensure the sample remains a good gauge of the current population. The NLSCY collects data from multiple sources, including the person most knowledgeable (PMK), who is typically the mother, the teacher, the principal of the school, and the children themselves, once they reach age 11 and older.

The NLSCY includes measures of antisocial tendencies for children 2 years of age or older, which allows for the examination of a younger population with symptoms of severe dispositional deficits (e.g., Wade, Pevalin, & Brannigan, 1999). The NLSCY also collects greater detail than previous surveys on the child and the child's environment, including family dynamics, parenting practices and problems, family dysfunction, and parental physical and mental health as well as several dimensions of scholastic performance, such as competence in reading, writing, and arithmetic.

Ontario. The findings of the OMHS were similar to previous studies in that males had higher levels of substance use disorders and antisocial behaviour while females had higher levels of affective and mood disorders. Finally, the researchers identified substantial levels of comorbidity with about 25% of those who reported having one disorder to have at least one additional disorder.

Current Estimates of Prevalence of Disorder

In 2002, Canada implemented the Canadian Community Health Survey, Cycle 1.2 Mental Health and Well-Being supplement (CCHS 1.2) (see Chapter 2 for a description of the health survey initiative by Statistics Canada and current national health surveys). The 2002 CCHS 1.2 was the first comprehensive attempt in Canada to examine the prevalence of multiple mental disorders and mental health service use using a national probability sample. (The 2012 Canadian Community Health Survey: Mental Health was not released in time for inclusion in this chapter.) The target population included people aged 15 years or older who lived in private dwellings (98% of the population). As a "community sample," it excluded specific populations, such as full-time members of the Armed Forces (surveyed separately), people living in health care and correctional facilities, on First Nation reserves, on government-owned land, in one of the three northern territories, and in remote regions.

The CCHS 1.2 was limited in the number of disorders compared to the OMHS and Edmonton study, including only major depression and mania (mood disorders); social phobia, panic disorder, and agoraphobia (anxiety disorders); and drug and alcohol dependence (Gravel & Beland, 2005). Questions were also asked to identify those likely to have an eating disorder, to be a problem gambler (gambling addiction), and those who had suicidal thoughts in the previous 12 months. Finally, the survey also included questions on mental health service use and barriers to accessing care. Table 8.2 presents the 12-month prevalence rates of disorder from the CCHS Cycle 1.2 Mental Health Supplement.

There are both consistencies and inconsistencies between the CCHS and earlier Canadian studies. Overall, the CCHS reported lower prevalence rates than the Edmonton study and the OMHS with the exception of a few specific disorders. The 12-month prevalence of any disorder (including substance disorders) was 10.6%, substantially lower than previous surveys. The lifetime prevalence of any anxiety or mood disorder (excluding substance dependence due to an error in the questionnaire) was around 20% of the population. The rates of comorbidity, as a proportion, were similar across the CCHS and OMHS with about 25% of those with one disorder manifesting at least one additional disorder. Gender and age differences were consistent across the studies with females reporting higher rates of mood and anxiety disorders and males reporting higher rates of substance use. Younger cohorts reported much higher 12-month rates of disorder.

One of the benefits of such a large sample in the CCHS was its ability to better examine links between mental illness and other social factors, including immigrant, socio-economic, and marital status (Table 8.3). Consistent with the healthy immigrant

Table 8.2 12-Month Prevalence of Psychiatric Disorder by Age and Sex, CCHS 2002

| | Age Groups | | | | | | | | Totals | | |
| | 15 to 24 | | 25 to 44 | | 45 to 64 | | 65 and over | | Sex | | Total |
Disorder	M	F	M	F	M	F	M	F	M	F	
Anxiety disorders (any)	4.3	8.8	4.2	6.9	3.3	4.8	1.2	1.8	3.5	5.7	4.7
Social phobia	3.3	6.1	3.1	3.8	2.2	2.8	0.8	0.9	2.6	3.4	3.0
Agoraphobia	0.4	1.3	0.3	1.5	0.4	1.0	0.4	0.4	0.4	1.1	0.3
Panic disorder	1.0	2.6	1.1	2.7	1.3	1.6	0.2	0.6	1.0	2.0	1.5
Affective disorders (any)	5.2	9.4	4.7	7.2	3.9	5.8	2.1	1.9	4.2	6.3	5.2
Major depressive episode	4.5	8.3	4.0	6.8	3.5	5.6	2.1	1.8	3.7	5.9	4.8
Manic disorder	1.3	2.3	1.3	1.1	0.7	0.6	-	-	1.0	1.0	1.0
Any Affective or Anxiety disorder	8.0	15.9	7.6	12.0	6.0	9.8	2.9	3.7	6.6	10.6	8.6
2 or more Affective and/or Anxiety disorders (Comorbid)	1.7	3.5	1.7	2.8	1.6	1.4	0.6	0.2	1.5	2.1	1.8
Substance use disorders (any)	11.6	5.5	5.1	1.8	1.7	0.4	0.1	-	4.5	1.7	3.1
Alcohol dependence	9.7	4.2	4.4	1.5	1.5	0.4	0.1	-	3.9	1.3	2.6
Illicit Drug dependence	3.5	1.8	1.1	0.5	0.2	-	-	-	1.1	0.5	0.8
Any Disorder or Substance Dependence	17.3	19.5	11.1	12.7	7.3	9.7	2.9	3.5	9.9	11.4	10.6
2 or More Disorders (Comorbidity)	4.3	5.1	3.4	3.5	2.5	1.7	1.1	0.3	3.0	2.7	2.8

Source: Based on Canadian Community Health Survey. (2002). Cycle 1.2, Derived Variable (DV) Specifications. *Public Use Microdata File.* Ottawa: Statistics Canada.

Table 8.3 12-Month Prevalence of Psychiatric Disorder by Length of Time since Immigration, Income Adequacy, and Marital Status, CCHS Cycle 1.2, 2002

Disorder	Time in Canada since Immigrating (yrs)			Income Adequacy					Marital Status			
	Not[1]	0–9	10+	Low	2	3	4	High	Married	C-L[2]	SDW[3]	Single
Anxiety disorders (any)	4.7	2.8	2.9	11.0	6.5	4.0	4.4	3.6	3.2	6.0	5.6	6.8
-Social phobia	3.0	1.6	1.6	5.9	3.4	2.3	2.8	2.5	1.9	4.1	3.1	4.7
-Agoraphobia	0.7	0.7	0.7	2.2	1.6	0.8	0.7	0.4	0.4	1.1	1.5	0.9
-Panic disorder	1.7	0.6	0.8	4.7	2.6	1.6	1.2	1.3	1.1	1.8	1.9	2.2
Affective disorders (any)	5.2	2.6	3.6	12.8	7.0	5.3	4.6	3.6	3.1	6.3	8.3	7.9
-Major depressive episode	4.8	2.5	3.4	11.8	6.6	5.0	4.2	3.3	2.9	5.7	7.8	7.4
-Manic disorder	0.9	0.4	0.5	2.7	0.9	0.9	0.9	0.5	0.5	1.2	1.2	1.5
Affective or Anxiety disorder (any)	8.7	4.7	5.6	20.0	11.8	8.0	7.9	6.4	5.7	10.3	12.3	12.2
2 or more Affective and/or Anxiety disorders (comorbid)	1.7	0.8	1.2	5.9	2.5	1.8	1.4	1.3	0.9	2.7	2.3	3.2
Substance use disorders (any)	2.4	0.3	0.8	4.8	2.8	1.8	1.9	2.0	1.0	3.6	2.0	5.3
-Alcohol dependence	2.0	0.2	0.7	3.5	1.8	1.5	1.7	1.8	0.9	3.1	1.8	4.5
-Illicit Drug dependence	0.5	2.0	0.1	1.5	1.2	0.4	0.3	0.3	0.2	0.7	0.4	1.4
Any Disorder or Substance Dependence	10.1	4.8	6.0	21.5	13.0	9.0	8.9	7.8	6.3	12.9	12.9	15.2
2 or More Disorders (Comorbidity)	2.7	1.3	1.7	7.7	3.9	2.8	2.1	2.0	1.4	4.1	3.2	5.1

[1]Not refers to 'not an immigrant'

[2]C-L refers to common-law couples

[3]SDW refers to separated, divorced, widowed

effect discussed in Chapter 7, the CCHS found that immigrants generally had lower rates of both affective disorders and substance dependence disorders. The overall rate of disorder was 4.8% for immigrants who had been here fewer than 10 years compared with 6.0% for immigrants who had been here longer and 10.1% for non-immigrants. The dissipation of this effect could be due to both acculturation and to the lower socio-economic status that many new immigrants must endure as their career aspirations are not met (for example, see Chapter 6, Table 6.4).

Other analyses using the CCHS 1.2 that specifically examine ethnicity and race found that people born in Africa, Asia, Europe, South and Central American, and the United States all reported lower rates of alcohol dependence, and, with the exception of Europe-born, lower rates of depression compared to Canadian-born (Ali, McDermott, & Gravel, 2004). These findings are consistent with earlier work examining the 1996 National Population Health Survey (NPHS) that found Asian and Black Canadians to have lower rates of depression than English Canadians (Wu, Noh, Kaspar, & Schimmele, 2003).

One of the most consistent and well-accepted findings in the field of psychiatric epidemiology is that lower socio-economic groups have higher rates of mental disorders (Eaton, 2000). The ECA study found that people who do not complete high school and people in unskilled occupations or were unemployed had higher rates of disorder (Robins, Locke, & Regier, 1991). Analysis of the CCHS 1.2 (Table 8.3) across **income adequacy**, a measure of household income that adjusts for the number of persons living in the household, showed a decreasing stepwise pattern in rates of disorder among successively higher income groups among all disorders with the one exception of alcohol dependence. Both the overall prevalence rate of any disorder and the prevalence of comorbid disorders declined from the lowest income adequacy group to the highest income adequacy group.

Finally, rates of mental disorder also varied by marital status. The Edmonton Study found that rates of disorder were highest among people who were divorced, widowed, or separated (46.5%), and among never-married or single persons (38.1%), compared to married persons (27.8%) (Bland et al., 1988). The CCHS data also found the married group to have the lowest overall prevalence rate of disorder (6.3%) (Table 8.3). Single persons had the highest overall prevalence (15.2%) while those living common-law and those separated, divorced, or widowed were in the middle (12.9% each). Across the non-married groups, the prevalence rates varied. For instance, those separated/divorced/widowed had the highest rates of affective disorders (8.3%) while singles had the highest rates of overall substance dependence (5.3%) and anxiety disorders (6.8%). Additional analyses examined marital status comparing married and single mothers and fathers examining the interaction between family status and gender (Wade, Veldhuzen, & Cairney, 2011). Overall, single-parent mothers and fathers had much higher rates than their married counterparts. As well, single mothers had the highest rate of both mood and anxiety disorders while single fathers had the highest rates of substance dependence disorders (Wade et al., 2011).

However, the distribution of psychiatric disorder across both SES and marital status are statistical associations. That is, we are unable to say, for example, whether marriage or the absence of marriage caused the disorder or whether the disorder inhibited a person's chances of finding a mate and getting married. This is a debate between social causation and social selection that will be discussed in the next section as we present some of the work that attempts to explain mental illness.

EXPLAINING MENTAL ILLNESS

There have been various theories postulated to explain mental illness. Historically, all involve some contribution of personal or psychological characteristics (e.g., personality), social factors (e.g., poverty, discrimination), and biological factors (e.g., genetics, infectious agents) as disease agents. Social factors continue to occupy a prominent place along suspected causes. Dating back to the nineteenth century, researchers have hypothesized a role for overcrowding in cities, poverty, social disorganization, discrimination, and other forms of stress associated with social disadvantage as risk factors for disorder. In the sections that follow, we provide an overview of some of the major theoretical issues that have confronted researchers interested in the social origins of mental distress and disorder. We conclude by reviewing a major sociological paradigm—the stress process—that has been used to understand how exposures to socially produced stressors shape mental health and illness.

Social Selection versus Social Causation

We have identified several social factors (e.g., gender, martial status, SES) that are associated to the prevalence of mental disorder and disease more generally (see Chapters 6 and 7). Indeed, we can say that the distribution of disorder across the population is socially stratified, with those in more advantaged social positions being less likely to have a mental disorder compared to those in more vulnerable, disadvantaged social positions. This is perhaps most notable in relation to SES. Individuals in lower income, education, and income groups have higher risk for psychiatric disorder. Inevitably this leads to an important question—was the disorder the cause or the consequence of a person's socio-demographic position? Obviously, it does not make sense to talk about a mental disorder causing *ascribed characteristics* such as a person's sex or ethnic origin; however, it is a pertinent question with respect to *achieved characteristics* such as marital status and SES. In the literature, this is framed in terms of social selection and social causation.

Social selection is generally discussed as the presence of a disorder creating a downward social mobility for the individual. An example of this could be that having a mental disorder leads to early school withdrawal that leads to a reduced chance of securing a well paying job resulting in lower overall income. **Social drift**, a type of social selection, refers to an intergenerational change in which successive generations will be continually downwardly mobile. This is where the troubles of one generation become compounded across subsequent generations, with each generation adversely affecting the next. An example here might be the negative social impact that is experienced by the children of a parent with a major mental disorder.

Social causation presents an alternative view that social position is a cause of mental disorder. It is based on three factors. First, individuals with low SES will experience a greater level of social stress, which increases the risk of disorder. Second, people in different social classes possess different resources with which to deal with stress. That is, people of higher SES would have more social resources with which to help offset the negative effects of stress. Third, inter-generationally, children born to parents of higher socio-economic status are less likely to be exposed to pre- and post-natal risks such as malnour-ishment and exposure to harmful chemicals (e.g., tobacco, alcohol, and industrial toxins) that predispose them to future problems. In this last example, we can think of the ways in which biological risks are themselves influenced (or conditioned) by social circumstances (Avison, 2010) (see Researcher Profile 8.1).

Historically, the debate between selection and causation focused on establishing or proving one over the other. However, accumulating evidence has shown that it is not an all-or-nothing game. Instead, it is a question of to what degree each influences the pro-cess (Eaton, 2000). The proportion of one over the other may differ for different ill-nesses. For example, the selection-drift hypothesis seems to be stronger for schizophrenia

---

Researcher Profile 8.1
William R. Avison

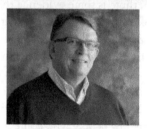

Source: Photography by Eric Gaston Simard

Dr. Avison's research focuses on how socio-economic disadvantage and associated types of social stressors affect the mental health of families and children. Within this focus, Dr. Avison led two large research studies—one examining single mothers and the other exam-ining unemployment—on how these disadvan-taged family statuses influence the health and well-being of family members. He has been

instrumental in the field and has published widely in international journals in sociology and psychiatry on the sociology of mental health.

Dr. Avison is past Chair of the Medical Sociology Section of the American Sociological Association (ASA), past Chair of the Sociology of Mental Health Section of the ASA, and of the Psychiatric Sociology Division of the Society for the Study of Social Problems. He is Editor of *Society & Mental Health*, the official journal of the ASA Section on the Sociology of Mental Health, a new journal that he was instrumen-tal in establishing. Dr. Avison was elected as a Fellow of the Canadian Academy of Health Sciences in 2012. He is the Chair of the Council for Canadian Child Health Research, representing all 17 Canadian academic health science centres with a focus on child and youth health.

than other disorders, in part because schizophrenia tends to have a much higher inherited component. Amato and Keith (1991), in a meta-analysis of child psychiatric disorder, found that children who had a schizophrenic parent had a probability of being diagnosed schizophrenic that was 12 times higher than the general population. Moreover, schizophrenia tends to occur early in life. Since the disorder affects a person's ability to form intimate attachments with others negatively affecting things like school completion and securing steady, desirable employment, it is easy to see how the illness can have a negative effect on things such as marital status, education attainment, occupational success, and income.

In analyzing a sample of 4914 young Israel-born adults of European and African descent, Dohrenwend et al. (1992) disaggregated the effects of selection and causation using ethnic status as a proxy for socio-economic status. As we noted previously, this is an interesting way to deal with the problem of what came first—social status or disorder. Ethnicity cannot be caused by mental disorder. However, in Israel, there are definite social consequences attached to ethnic status. These consequences are the result of social processes such as discrimination, not biological differences, creating an interesting "natural" experiment to disentangle selection from causation effects. Their results showed that both social selection and social causation processes operate. However, for certain disorders, the processes differ in relative importance. For example, schizophrenia tended to be much more socially selected whereas major depression for women and antisocial personality and substance abuse for men tended to be much more socially determined.

Generally, it does not make intuitive sense to consider schizophrenia as a disease that is caused by social factors. However, even while most of the evidence does show that it is much more influenced by social selection, there is some evidence that supports a causation argument. Link, Dohrenwend, and Skodal (1986) found evidence to suggest that a person's first occupation will be a major determinant for the onset of schizophrenia. Although people might have a predisposition toward the illness, there may be social processes that work as a catalyst. What is it about the first occupation that works as this catalyst? Link and colleagues predicted that it is the noisome characteristics of the job (e.g., heat, noise, hazards, fumes, cold, and so on) that may be important. Still, these jobs tend to be mainly blue collar and occupied by people who come from a lower SES, people who are predicted to have a higher rate of schizophrenia already. Therefore, they conclude that noisome work conditions may contribute to the onset of schizophrenia for someone who is already at high risk. A more contemporary example is the sharp increase in the incidence of schizophrenia seen in both first- and second-generation Caribbean immigrants to the United Kingdom (Jarvis, 2007). It is unlikely that this dramatic increase is attributable solely to biological factors and certainly it is the case that selection explanations on their own are inadequate to account for this phenomenon. As such, even in the case of schizophrenia, it would seem there is a role for social causation.

The support for social causation tends to be stronger for mental disorders such as depression. Depression has been investigated extensively in the context of social causation models such as the stress process model to be discussed. Generally, it tends to be more prevalent in women than men. It also tends to be greatly influenced by one's age. Mirowsky and Ross (1992) found that the association between depression and age is U-shaped; people at younger and older ages are much more likely to show symptoms than the middle-aged. The researchers suggest the lower levels of depressive symptomatology in middle age reflect gains in marriage, employment, and general economic well-being. If it were not for the loss of jobs, partners, and so on that accompany old age, they predict that the prevalence of depression would continue to decrease through old age. Contrary to this U-shaped relationship, Canadian data suggests that depression continued to decrease with age, rising again only slightly among the very old (Wade & Cairney, 1997). Further examination of this relationship showed that depression among younger cohorts was attributable to higher levels of social stress while depression among older cohorts was attributable to declines in both health status and social support (Wade & Cairney, 2000a).

While most research shows support for the social causation argument for depression, once again, it is not conclusive. Examining marital transitions, Wade and Pevalin (2004) found support for both social selection and causation processes. Those who exited marriage due to separation and divorce had a higher likelihood of depression two years prior and two years after the event compared to married people in a stable relationship (Wade & Pevalin, 2004). Alternatively, those no longer married because their spouses had died showed higher rates of depression the year of the event but their likelihood of depression was no different than those who were stably married in the years prior to or after the event. Further work examining mothers transitioning into and out of marriage found that the likelihood of depression among mothers who later separated or divorced was higher prior to the marital disruption than married mothers who remained married. Moreover, the rate of depression after the marital disruption remained high afterward. Single mothers who transitioned into marriage had higher rates of depression prior to the transition that remained high after marriage, contrary to what would be expected in a social causation framework (Wade & Cairney, 2000b).

Labelling Theory

Labelling theory is an off-shoot of social causation theory (see Chapters 11 and 12). Being labelled mentally ill or insane has profound effects on both a person's own self-identify and behaviour and how others perceive and behave toward the person bearing the label. The underlying premise of labelling theory is based on conceptualizing symptoms of mental illness as behaviour that does not conform to prevailing social norms or rules. These behaviours are classified as "residual deviance" in that they involve rule-breaking behaviours, often involving violation of taken-for-granted rules that govern normal social behaviours (Scheff, 1966, 1984). A classic example involves talking to yourself in public, which can be a symptom of psychosis connected to hallucinations. In North American society until recently it was considered deviant to talk to yourself (carry on a conversation with a person who is not there), especially in public settings. However, today with cell phones and wireless headsets, many people in public places look like they are talking to themselves, so it is becoming a more accepted behaviour.

Once someone is labelled as having a mental illness, it is extremely difficult to reverse. In a famous study, Rosenhan (1975) showed that the label of mental illness has an element of permanence. He trained eight people to be pseudo-patients and go to various psychiatric hospitals in five states. During the hospital interview, the pseudo-patients were told to say they were hearing voices (nothing specific, just nonsense words like "thud"). Every pseudo-patient was admitted to the psychiatric ward and diagnosed as mentally ill. Once admitted to the ward, they were instructed to act completely normal. The intent was to see how long it would take staff to realize that these pseudo-patients were not mentally ill. Rosenhan found that hospitalizations ranged from 7 to 52 days, averaging 19 days, before the "patient" was discharged. All were released with a diagnosis of schizophrenia in remission. Thus, while not currently showing any symptoms, once the label had been applied, others were quite reluctant to remove it.

Thomas Szasz (1967) takes labelling theory one step further to suggest that mental illness itself is a myth created by psychiatry and the label "mental illness" is "scientifically worthless and socially harmful" (Szasz, 1961, p. ix). Without considering the background of a disorder, the phenomenon of mental illness loses its meaning. Psychology is relativistic to the social forces that influence it; hence, psychology is dependent upon sociology. Certain behaviours may be entirely rational or understandable given the specific context in which they occur. However, psychiatrists have traditionally defined mental illness as separate and mutually exclusive of the social context consistent with the biomedical model. Szasz (1967) asserts that by defining certain behaviours as psychotic or mentally deranged, the psychiatrist essentially removes all blame from an individual for his or her actions. Whether the person is truly insane or just pretending, Szasz argues that the diagnosis will still be mental illness.

Perhaps understandably, the most vigorous critiques of labelling theory have come from those who work within the mental health field. If labelling theory is a bona fide explanation, how can we account for the high percentage of patients in hospitals who admit themselves voluntarily (Gove, 1982)? Furthermore, because of new drug therapies and treatment programs, patients usually do not remain in hospitals for long. This reduces the opportunity for the person to be socialized into the role of a deviant, as labelling theory suggests. Arguing against the issue of power in the labelling process, Gove (1982) also found that those in higher SES groups as well as people who occupy the powerful positions within a family are far more likely and much more quickly to be hospitalized than other family members.

Finally, if labelling were applicable, we would expect most of the patients to be embittered and hostile toward hospitals and institutions. Weinstein (1982) argues that labelling theorists who gave negative accounts of treatment and hospitals, such as Szasz (1967) and Goffman (1963), tended to exaggerate the negative aspects while neglecting the positive aspects. Weinstein showed that over 75% of all patients in institutions espoused positive attitudes toward treatment, staff, and the overall institution.

The Stress Process

Physiologist Hans Selye (1956) was the first to study the concept of stress as both a physiological and social phenomenon. He proposed a theory that focused upon the effects of external stimuli (electric shock) on the mental and physiological responses of an organism. This initial attempt at understanding stress created a wave of research in various disciplines, including psychology, epidemiology, and sociology, that focused on linking life stress with the onset of mental distress and disorder. Cassel (1974, 1976) studied the presence of environmental factors that might influence a person's vulnerability to mental distress and disease. Cobb (1976), in reviewing the research that links the concept of social support to psychological well-being, concluded that there was a strong relationship between social support and depression. Pearlin, Menaghan, Lieberman, and Mullen (1981) combined previous research on the components of stress and depressive symptomatology and hypothesized about the linkages between them in a social causation framework. They proposed the stress process as a means to combine prior work done on the specific domains of stress research in the sciences, most notably psychology and epidemiology, into a sociological framework from which to analyze the social causation processes.

The basic model presented by Pearlin et al. (1981) consisted of a stressor causing a subsequent health outcome (Figure 8.1). Operationalized, the stressor was a significant life event (LE), specifically recent loss of employment, and the health outcome was the onset of depressive symptoms. The basic model showed a very strong effect of stress on subsequent depression. The model increased in complexity by including additional stresses resulting from the life event, in this case the enduring economic strains that increased the total negative effect of job loss on depression. Finally, they examined whether certain protective mechanisms, specifically psychosocial resources and social support, could attenuate or offset the negative effects of the stressors on mental distress. Psychosocial resources included both self-esteem and perceived mastery. These resources reduced the

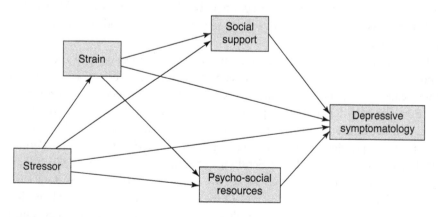

Figure 8.1 The Stress Process

total effect of job loss and the strains associated with job loss on depression. A person's social support network was also found to buffer the negative effects of a life event on mental distress.

Sources of Stress The stress process model provided a new way to study mental health by way of social processes and has guided many social researchers examining mental health. Subsequent research continued to manipulate and refine this model, gaining a better understanding of its dynamics. A **life events** approach, defined as negative or life-altering events occurring within the past year, has been a common approach in the literature. One way to measure life events is to present an inventory of possible events consisting of items that tap into an array of contexts. The following is a small selection of some of the questions used to measure life events that happened to you or a family member.

In the past 12 months:

1. Was there an abortion, miscarriage, or stillbirth?
2. Has anyone been fired or laid off?
3. Did anyone drop out of school?
4. Did someone close to you have a serious illness or accident?
5. Did you get married?

The respondents are given one point for each "yes" response that are summed to provide an individual's "life-events score." This technique has been very popular and has shown a very strong association with psychological distress. Turner and Avison (1992) moved beyond simple exposure to life events, which are the main factors leading to depressive symptomatology, to examining how a person managed an event and whether he or she successfully resolved it. They found that a resolved event did not have a negative effect on depressive symptomatology. Consistent with this, Brown and Harris (1989) argue that it is not sufficient to take into account the number of life events; it is necessary to take into consideration the context in which the stressor occurs. Sometimes one stressor, if it is severe enough, may be all that is necessary. Alternatively, a number of stressors that are not considered severe for that individual may not elicit any depressive symptoms.

Others have moved away from life events to examine other types of stressors such as **chronic strains**. Chronic strains have an enduring, eroding effect on psychological well-being because they persist over time. Wheaton (1994) concludes that chronic strains stem from the role demands that present long-term life difficulties distinct from life events that are discrete, time-limited events. Other forms of stressors have also been studied such as physical disabilities (Turner & Noh, 1988), daily hassles (Wheaton, 1994; Bolger, DeLongis, Kessler, & Schilling 1989; Kanner, Coyne, Schaefer, & Lazarus, 1981), and adverse childhood events (ACEs) (Felitti et al., 1998). Consistent with the original model presented by Pearlin et al. (1981), these alternative stressors have demonstrated strong effects on subsequent health outcomes. This shows the robust effects of stressors on the psychological stability of individuals.

Intervening Mechanisms of the Stress Process   In addition to sources of stress, the intervening mechanisms focused on various types of components that may buffer the negative effects of stress. Pearlin et al. (1981) looked specifically at self-esteem, mastery, and social support, which have continued to be the most common mediators studied. **Self-esteem** is a self-appraisal or emotional attitude of personal self-worth, while **mastery** is the sense of personal control over things that occur in your life. Some research has suggested that these mechanisms are key determinants as to whether someone will show symptoms of distress. In order to understand why some people demonstrate more symptoms than others, researchers examined vulnerability to stress or how different people may be differentially resilient or susceptible to stress (e.g., see Box 8.2 on gender differences).

The intervening mechanisms are proposed to operate in two different ways. First, as illustrated in Figure 8.1, the mechanisms are negatively influenced by exposure to stress in

---

Box 8.2

Gender Differences and Mental Illness

One of the most consistent findings across mental health surveys is the higher rate of depression among women. Even after adjusting for levels of stress, women remain twice as likely to manifest depression, prompting some researchers to conclude that females are more vulnerable to stress than males. That is, given exposure to similar levels of stress, women will be more likely to have an adverse reaction such as the onset of depression because they have fewer resources in which to withstand or buffer the effects of stress. This has been labelled the **vulnerability hypothesis** (sometimes referred to as the **buffering hypothesis**).

The vulnerability explanation ignores the fact that females may be more exposed to the stress experienced by others and explores how the size of one's social networks influences mental health. An alternative to this hypothesis is the **exposure hypothesis**. That is, higher levels of exposure to stress may make a person more likely to manifest depression. While much research has found that the quality and quantity of social networks may assist in reducing the effect of stress on depressive

symptomatology, it can also be a source of stress itself (Haines & Hurlburt 1992; Revenson et al., 1991). Women's risk of exposure to stress would be greater because they are more affected by the stress of others.

Another possible explanation for this gender difference is the singular focus on depressive symptomatology as the principal outcome in most stress research (Aneshensel, Rutter, & Lachenbruch, 1991). If we consider other health outcomes we may come to a different conclusion. Focusing on depression alone as the main outcome of stress may falsely classify people who manifest different symptoms as not affected by stress. While women are about twice as likely to manifest depression, males have a much higher likelihood of alcohol and drug abuse. By examining a broad array of outcomes, both health and behavioural, that result from stressful experiences, we see very similar patterns across genders suggesting that observed gender differences may not be due to vulnerability or exposure but may be due instead to a limited focus on potential outcomes (Wade, 2001).

a direct fashion. The exposure diminishes personal coping resources and social support, which precipitates a direct increase in psychological distress. Think of resources as a type of bank account that contains a finite amount where both deposits and withdrawals can be made. During times of stress, people tap these resources. As they are used to a greater and greater extent, the account balance decreases, resulting in fewer available resources. The second manner in which intervening mechanisms operate is through moderating the negative effects of stress. That is, those with higher levels of resources are able to better withstand exposure to stress. Given two individuals exposed to a similar stressful event, the one with greater social support, self-esteem, and mastery would be less vulnerable and better able to withstand its negative impact.

Although the stress process model has provided a better understanding of how stress can influence mental health, in doing so, the social-structural aspects that predispose people to certain life trajectories that may prove more stressful than other life trajectories has been neglected (Phelan, Link, & Tehranifar 2010; Pearlin, 1989). Sociology, ideally, focuses upon the consequences of underlying social structures and institutions for individuals in their daily lives. Instead of concentrating on the stress process as operating in a social vacuum, void of outside influence, a new direction has began to focus on the sociological aspects of mental health that are affected by underlying structural conditions (such as SES), people's shared values, and the social roles that people occupy the and consequences attached to these roles (Phelan et al., 2010). The importance of examining these underlying factors is evident in the differential prevalence rates of disorder across groups as already shown.

MENTAL ILLNESS AND DEINSTITUTIONALIZATION

In the seventeenth and eighteenth centuries, medieval asylums across Europe evolved into a special type of institution that incarcerated the mentally and physically ill from both the community and other types of deviants, specifically criminals (see also Chapter 5, specifically Box 5.1). Weinstein (1990) suggested that the underlying basis for this gradual shifting of patients from institutions that housed criminals was not necessarily based on humanitarian ideals but rather the intent was to prevent the spread of "madness" to others.

By the late eighteenth century, Weinstein (1990) noted, however, humanitarian ideals consistent with the Enlightenment began to play a role in the treatment of the mentally ill. This era brought about new therapeutic techniques for dealing with the institutionalized. The new treatments—dubbed the "moral treatment approach"— were humanitarian innovations aimed at therapeutic goals (Wright, Mortran, & Gouglas, 2003). The change in attitude toward the mentally ill initiated the rise of mental institutions that persisted for almost two hundred years, well into the mid-twentieth century. During this period there was also a gradual shift from private to public facilities, giving the state more control over care of the mentally ill. With this control also came state responsibility, both financial and moral. In Canada, the first asylums for the mentally ill (lunatic asylums) were established in Quebec, Ontario, and the Prairies during 1845 to 1857 (Fierlbeck, 2011, p. 198). The asylums were a more humane alternative to the poorhouses where the mentally ill had previously been held. In the asylums, it was believed, people with mental health problems could learn to have order and peace in their lives by doing simple tasks (such as gardening) and getting along with others (patients and orderlies). The popularity of asylums grew toward the end of the nineteenth century, and during the years from 1845 to 1902 the spending on the mental hospitals exceeded spending on medical hospitals and prisons combined (Wright et al., 2003).

The 1950s marked the peak in the numbers of psychiatric patients under the institution-based psychiatric treatment model in Canada and the United States. Up to this point, these hospitals contained people suffering from a variety of disabilities who today would be defined under alternative categories, such as developmental delays, and neurological conditions, such as dementia. From 1960 to 1976, the number of beds in psychiatric institutions across Canada decreased by over two-thirds (47 633 to 15 011) coinciding with the shift to psychiatric care in medical hospitals as psychiatric beds in hospitals increased from 844 to 5836 (Goering, Wasylenki, & Durbin, 2000).

The shift from mental institutions to hospital psychiatric units and community care was based on several factors. First, the increasing cost of keeping large numbers of people in institutions, often for life, was a substantial and ongoing financial obligation for governments. Second, overcrowding and dwindling funding for psychiatric institutions over time meant that asylums had moved from their original intention of moral treatment to warehousing large numbers of people who could be more appropriately and less expensively cared for elsewhere (Mulvale, Abelson, & Goering 2007). For example, older patients who suffered from senility resulting from old age were shifted to more appropriate institutions for their specific needs. Third, an understanding of the biological elements of mental disorders led to the discovery of new psychoactive and antidepressant drugs and other therapeutic treatments, assisting psychiatry in being recognized as a bona fide medical discipline. Around the world, these discoveries seemed to offer the promise of community-based treatment with short-term hospital-ization when required rather than the long-term institutionalization of patients (Kirby & Keon, 2004). Fourth, in Canada, the shift coincided with the introduction of federal cost-sharing for publicly financed hospital insurance through the Hospital Insurance and Diagnostic Services Act (HIDS, see Chapter 3), and later for physician services through the Medical Care Act. Because psychiatric hospitals were excluded from HIDS funding (Greenland, Griffin, & Hoffman, 2001) that matched federal funding at a 50–50 level with provinces for the construction of new hospitals, provinces and territories had significant financial incentives to expand mental health care within general hospitals through psychiatry units and to establish community care in outpatient clinics affiliated with the general hospitals (Mulvale et al., 2007). As a result, psychiatric units in hospitals increasingly gained recognition and acceptance (Greenland et al., 2001). However, there were far fewer beds available in hospitals compared with institutions for inpatient treatment of mental illness. This increased the need for community-based and hospital outpatient care coupled with short-term, acute inpatient care when required.

Patient Rights and Critical Voices

With this shift toward deinstitutionalization, the issue of patients' rights become much more apparent. Freddolino (1990) noted that until the 1960s, patients were generally void of individual rights in institutional settings. What went on in these institutions was largely out of sight and out of mind of the general population. From the 1960s onward however, patients and other vulnerable populations in the community began to demand the right to refuse treatment, the right to the least restrictive treatment alternative, and other rights directed toward daily living, such as the right to privacy. Similarly, family members began to demand the right to treatment on behalf of their loved ones. The right of individuals to be incarcerated against their will was also questioned for all but the most severe cases.

Until the early 1950s, hospitals were seen as the solution for the problem of mental illness. In reality, there were few effective treatments and attempts to address the severe problems experienced by the mentally ill. Weinstein (1990) argues that by the late 1950s and 1960s, the psychiatric hospital itself was perceived as a social problem. Sociologists such as Goffman (1963) began to criticize the psychiatric hospital as the main driving force maintaining mental illness. Goffman provided a rich account of life in such institutions, describing the control and de-humanizing effect it had on patients. Consistent with the core tenets of sociology, this work stressed the important of context in the lives of patients, and how the "place" shaped the experiences and subjective identities of those who lived there. This wave of critical literature from the academic community furthered the justification for deinstitutionalization. Movies such as *One Flew Over the Cookoo's Nest* in 1975 dramatized psychiatric hospitals as harmful to patient rights as well as their health and well-being.

Some argue (as already noted), however, that this critical research forgot to consider the patient's viewpoint (Weinstein, 1990). Sociologists such as Goffman criticized the system from the perspective of a person who was from the outside, neglecting the perspective of the patient who was directly involved. Weinstein (1990) argues that more than 30 studies espouse positive attitudes by the majority of the patients toward the institution and staff. He argues that this critical research may have ignored the historic function of the mental institution. Patients suffering from mental disorders were there because of an opportunity to improve their condition at a time when there were few alternatives.

Community Psychiatric Services

With the push toward deinstitutionalization, outpatient care, and community services came the realization that patients were inadequately prepared for life outside the hospital. Even in an ideal community that was willing to accept them and had the services in place to support them, this transition was difficult. Community-based services, such as housing and outpatient treatment and rehabilitation, were inadequate to deal with the large influx of inpatients, some of whom had not lived in the community for decades (Wasylenki, 2001; Wegner, 1990). Although the underlying motive was to reduce the enormous cost of inpatient care for the mentally ill, some of these savings gained through hospital closures were supposed to be reinvested into creating a community-level infrastructure to ease the transition for the patient and community. Wegner (1990) argues, however, that government intention to do this was little more than rhetoric. Once on the outside, many patients were forced to live on the street. Many others were imprisoned, shifting the expense from one government ministry to another but still failing to address the needs of patients. (It is interesting that, in some respect, we had come full circle. Removing the mentally ill from criminal institutions was the original impetus in earlier centuries to develop mental asylums.)

> The patient has been taught to be self-centered, dependent, over-medicated, under-stimulated and most of all, placid. The first thing many patients did was to slice a vein or jump out a window to win a ticket back to the only home they had known. Eventually, however, most had to face the fact that the door had slammed behind them. (Capponi, 1985, 8)

And yet other patients found their community experience positive. This was more likely if they had a well-established and accepting personal social support network outside, including family, friends, and formal services (Capponi, 1985).

Concurrently with the International Year of Disabled Persons in 1981, the attitude of governments toward former psychiatric patients began to change. During the 1980s both the community and governments began to address issues surrounding deinstitutionalization, providing required care to citizens who had been released without support from psychiatric hospitals. Governments and communities came to realize that former patients deserved the same respect as other citizens. People living with mental illness have the same needs as others—the need for "a home, a job, a friend"—the slogan of mental health consumer/survivor advocacy groups. People with mental illness have the same need for self-actualization and should be given every advantage to pursue these goals and the assistance required to succeed in satisfying these needs (Plamondon, 1985). Each person should be supported on his or her journey of recovery to define a meaningful life for him or herself (Mental Health Commission of Canada [MHCC], 2009; MHCC, 2012).

Although the vast majority of former residents of psychiatric hospitals have been released and most of the institutions in Canada have been closed, a few remain open and continue to treat the most complex patients, often on an outpatient or short-term inpatient basis. People come in to the institution when they need assistance and leave as soon as it is feasible. Psychiatric hospitals still maintain a small number of long-term residents, many of whom are held involuntarily under a psychiatric certificate because it is believed that their release would pose a threat to themselves or the community.

Box 8.3

Phases of Deinstitutionalization

Wasylenki (2001) talks about three phases of the shift to deinstitutionalization. The first phase was the release of long-term patients into the communities with an expectation that they would receive necessary services there. Moreover, reintegration into the community was expected to help to lessen the stigma of mental health. Unfortunately, this policy was based not on scientific evidence but instead was done for political and economic reasons and there was little preparation for either the patients or communities to ensure services were available.

The second phase was characterized by conflict between various stakeholders. Conflicts arose between community service providers and hospital providers, between consumers (patients) and family organizations, and between patients and their family organizations and the various professions. Consumers organized and were increasingly successful in gaining government support for services such as housing, income, and community integration that were seen as equally important as treatment needs focused on by many professional organizations. Family organizations focused on and lobbied for more research and treatment and for greater resources for families to assist them with their caregiving.

The third phase was marked by an evidence-based approach and an emphasis on best practice models. There was greater cohesion among all groups to work together to address the coordination of social, community, and health services. There have also been revisions to legislation to address the needs of consumers and their families as well as new approaches to treatment, such as Assertive Community Treatment (ACT) and Community Treatment Orders, as effective and high-quality community-based treatment alternatives to involuntary hospitalization.

SUMMARY

Mental illness is perhaps the area of health that has been most studied by sociologists and other social scientists. It provides an excellent opportunity for researchers to examine not only the sociology *in* medicine but the sociology *of* medicine. For example, through the labelling of behaviours as deviant, we socially construct illnesses that may or may not have an identifiable biological basis.

Because many are without any biological basis does not mean mental illnesses are unimportant or less serious than other illnesses. Only recently have we become more aware of both the human and health care costs of mental illness as we become better able to identify its prevalence and distribution across the population as well as its precursors and consequences. While usually not directly linked to death with some notable exceptions such as suicide, mental illnesses are strongly related to the onset, management, and successful treatment of a host of other chronic health conditions and diseases, including diabetes, cancer, cardiovascular disease, and asthma as well as a number of health conditions and risky behaviours such as obesity, high blood pressure, physical inactivity, smoking, excessive alcohol use, and insufficient sleep (Chapman, Perry, & Strine, 2005). Mental illnesses, including depression, alcohol and substance use, schizophrenia, and dementias, have also been identified as some of the most significant illnesses reducing overall adjusted life expectancy due to living with a disability. With regards to depression specifically, it has been identified by the Global Burden of Diseases project sponsored by the World Health Organization as the leading cause of Years Lost to Disability (YLD) for both males and females for high- as well as medium- and low-income countries (Mathers, Lopez, & Murray, 2006). A recent report published in Ontario, *Opening Eyes, Opening Minds*, is the first Canadian study to estimate the burden of mental illness in the population (Ratnasingham et al., 2012). The study concluded that the burden of mental illness in Ontario was 1.5 times greater than all cancers combined, and more than 7 times greater than all infectious diseases. This is because mental illnesses tend to strike relatively early in a person's life course, meaning that people live with these illness for decades.

Recently in Canada, mental illness has received much greater interest from health professionals and health policy makers as an important factor in the health and well-being of our population. The 2006 Kirby Report on mental health, *Out of the Shadows at Last*, was the first comprehensive look at the mental health status health care services in Canada aiming to address the mental health needs of the population. The report made 118 recommendations on how to improve the current situation in mental health and called for a national, coordinated strategy to address the needs of Canadians (Standing Committee on Social Affairs, Science and Technology, 2006). As part of recommendations of the report, in 2007 the federal government established the Mental Health Commission of Canada. The goals of the commission are (1) to develop a national mental health strategy, (2) to share the knowledge across provincial jurisdictions, and (3) to promote public campaigns that will fight the stigma attached to mental illness. In 2012, the Commission published the very first Canadian mental health strategy along with 109 recommendations on improving the mental health of Canadians (MHCC, 2012). These recommendations focus not only on health policy makers but also on business, social services, and citizens with the goal of transforming how we understand mental health, mental illness, recovery, and well-being as well as expanding mental health promotion and prevention efforts and the nature of services and supports delivered to support people with mental illness in their recovery journeys (MHCC, 2012).

Key Terms

Buffering hypothesis (vulnerability hypothesis)—given exposure to similar levels of stress, one group will be at a greater risk of manifesting a negative outcome due to a fewer resources

Caseness—the ability to identify the presence of psychiatric illness generally but the inability to differentiate between specific types of psychiatric disorders

Chronic strain—a stressor that persists over time having an enduring and eroding effect on psychological well-being

Comorbidity—co-occurrence of diseases or disorders, often used to identify persons with two or more psychiatric disorders

Criterion validity—the comparison of the constructed instrument to a gold standard

Exposure hypothesis—the greater the exposure to stress, the greater the likelihood of manifesting an adverse outcome

Income adequacy—a measure of household income adjusted for the number of persons living in the household

Labelling theory—whereby mental illness is considered to be attributable to the social processes of defining and learning based on the meaning we attached to people's behaviours that deviate from socially accepted norms

Life event—usually defined as a negative or life-altering event that occurred within the past year

Mastery—a sense of personal control over the things that occur in a person's life

Mental disorder (or mental illness)—a mental abnormality from normal development that may be exhibited by non-typical or inappropriate behaviours and defined by psychiatrists as meeting a specified number of symptoms that have been identified and agreed upon by the psychiatric profession as standards for making a specific diagnosis

Psychometrics—the science of measurement, usually but not exclusively related to subjective phenomena such as IQ or personality

Self-esteem—a self-appraisal or emotional assessment of personal self-worth

Social causation—the view that social position or social disadvantage or events are the cause of mental disorder

Social drift—an intergenerational change whereby successive generations will be continually downwardly mobile and socially disadvantaged as a result of mental disorder

Social selection—the presence of a mental disorder creating a downward mobility and social disadvantage within the same generation

Critical Thinking Questions

1. Thinking about the historical development of the identification, measurement, and classification of mental illness, what are some possible next phases in this process?

2. Discuss how both the social causation and social selection hypotheses complement each other in understanding the development of mental illness.

3. What are some of the factors that continue to be important for the success of the ongoing process of deinstitutionalization and community integration?

Further Readings and Resources

Cairney, J., & Streiner, D. L. (Eds.) (2010). *Mental disorder in Canada: An epidemiological perspective*. Toronto: University of Toronto Press.

Government of Canada. Minister of Public Works and Government Services Canada. (2006). *The human face of mental health and mental illness in Canada*. Ottawa: Government of Canada, Cat. No. HP5-19/2006E

Mental Health Commission of Canada. (2012). *Changing directions, changing lives: The mental health strategy for Canada*. Calgary, AB: Author. www.mentalhealthcommission.ca/english/pages/default.aspx

Rae-Grant, Q. (Ed.) (2001). *Psychiatry in Canada: 50 years*. Ottawa: Canadian Psychiatric Association.

Canadian Mental Health Association
www.cmha.ca/

Canadian Psychiatric Association
www.cpa-apc.org/index.php

Centre for Addiction and Mental Health
www.camh.ca/en/hospital/Pages/home.aspx

Mood Disorders Society of Canada
www.mooddisorderscanada.ca

Chapter 9

Social Dimensions of Aging, Health, and Care

Chapter Outline

Learning Objectives

After studying this chapter, you should be able to:

1. Explain aging as a social process from a range of theoretical approaches;

2. Look at aging as a lifelong, healthy process of development and not as something that necessarily requires medical intervention;

3. Understand what is meant by population aging, and its implications;

4. Compare and contrast the types of formal and informal care for older adults, including long-term care, home care, residential care, and aging at home strategies;

5. Explain the facets of end-of-life care, including palliative care, and better understand various perspectives on the controversial issue of assisted suicide.

Most people think of aging as something to do with the transition into and the occupancy of roles having to do with old age.[1] But aging takes an entire lifetime. Aging involves physical, social, and emotional growth and changes across the course of a life, and everyone ages at the same rate—one year at a time. Although aging is a fact of life for everyone regardless of whether they are young or old, this chapter focuses principally on issues surrounding aging during the later stages of life. This has been an area of great interest among social scientists examining health, illness, and health care.

In this chapter, we discuss several issues surrounding health and aging, beginning with an overview of some of the theoretical approaches to understand the process of aging. We then move to show how aging, usually more narrowly defined as a disease or illness within the biomedical paradigm, can be thought of within a broader healthy aging perspective. We then shift our focus to the most prominent societal concerns with the aging of the population in Canada in relation to the experiences of health and illness and the provision of health care services. This includes both formal and informal caregiving (formal and informal care providers) and alternative ways for providing care, including end-of-life care.

AGING AS A DISEASE OR A LIFE PROCESS

Aging is a natural process as the body and mind develops, grows, matures, and then slowly deteriorates. In the literature on health and health care, aging is often defined as an illness or disease requiring medical intervention that has important consequences for health and other care services. Just as we describe the overall process of medicalization in Chapter 12, there is a similar process of the **medicalization of aging** has happened simultaneously with that of other natural occurrences, such as childbirth. "Stop the aging process!" or "how to look younger than you are" are slogans touted by numerous ad campaigns that market products from face cream to hair transplants to exercise equipment. As Larkin (2011, p. 30) describes, "This focus on medicalization and anti-aging contributes to the idea that aging is something wrong to be feared…and to be treated with pills and potions." The common message from society is that aging is something that is undesirable, something to avoid at all costs, and something that can be prevented or cured.

This conceptualization of aging has several social implications for older adults and their caregivers, including quality of life, dignity and self-worth, and stigma and discrimination. Some have labelled this as **cultural gerontophobia**, or a societal fear of the aged

---

[1]This chapter was co-authored with Margaret Denton.

and aging in our youth-obsessed culture. We contrast this perspective with a different conceptualization of aging—that of **healthy aging**, that is, aging as a natural process in the course of life as something to look forward to and embrace. Before we begin to outline the stages in healthy aging, it is important to describe the broader theoretical perspectives that inform a discussion of aging as a social process.

THEORETICAL APPROACHES TO THE STUDY OF AGING

The field of *social gerontology* focuses on aging as a *social* process. Although aging is clearly a physiological process, many aspects of aging fall into the social realm. A number of theoretical approaches explain the social processes associated with aging. In what follows, we summarize some of the most dominant views on aging.

Classical Gerontological Theories

Early, classical gerontological theories focused primarily on the adaptation to aging and the role of social structures in easing off the transition to old age (Hatch, 2000). Aligned within a functionalist perspective, *disengagement theory* saw aging as a process of withdrawal from social life and social roles. According to this theory, social institutions allow individuals to gradually withdraw from certain aspects of social life so as to prepare themselves for their ultimate withdrawal from society—death. To ease off the impact of this withdrawal on the individual and on society, older persons cease to continue to perform their usual social roles and begin to lose interest in pursuing active social interaction. For instance, people retire and no longer contribute to economic life of society. This gradual withdrawal is beneficial because reduces the bond between an individual and the social world and prepares older people (and society) to accept their aging and death (Hatch, 2000). Aging, according to this perspective, is not a positive experience—it is associated with withdrawal and decay.

Contrary to this perspective, *activity theory* sees successful aging as an active engagement in the social life. Activity theory assumes that when people are socially engaged, they maintain a positive self-concept, and this positive view contributes to a better adaptation to aging. To experience successful aging, older people must be actively engaged in social life, and if they are no longer capable of pursing their old roles (e.g., that of a full-time employee), they can shift and take on new roles (e.g., that of a volunteer). Building on these assumptions, *continuity theory* argues that we should understand aging as a process that is tied to our lives. We build our relationships and form personal identities our whole lives, and when we age, our roles and statuses change in accordance with our previous life experiences but they do not simply disappear without a trace (Hatch, 2000).

Although these classical theories of social gerontology have different and even opposing views on aging process, they have a common link—they all view aging as a process of adaptation of the individual to society. This view is consistent with the structural functionalist perspective that envisions the social world based on equilibrium. Critical and conflict theorists, however, challenge this position. Their emphasis on inequalities that are embedded in the organization of social life is evident in their conceptualization of aging.

Critical Perspectives on Aging

Although we often take for granted the social regulations that society establishes in relation to age, we should also acknowledge that these regulations are socially constructed and create a system of inequality based on age. Most of us are probably grateful for the laws prohibiting seven-year-olds from driving cars or buying alcohol, but these laws can also be seen as oppressive—they deny some rights to some people based on their age. Moreover, while some age discrimination is legalized and widely supported in society, other instances of age discrimination are less formal and less justifiable. Older people, for instance, may be denied career opportunities based on their biological age or may receive less passionate care from their health care providers.

Ageism—or discrimination of people based on their age—is embedded in our society, at both the structural level and the level of social interaction. Critical perspectives on aging draw our attention to age-based inequalities and focus on political, economic, and cultural relations that shape the experiences of aging. The *political economy perspective*, for instance, examines the impact of the political and economic organization of society on people's experiences of aging. Scholars working from this theoretical framework analyze the allocation of resources, such as retirement funds and pensions (Minkler & Estes, 1991), or the intersection of age with other forms of social inequality (e.g., based on race, gender, class). People working from this perspective are also often critical of the negative portrayals of aging bodies that contribute to the development of the profitable anti-aging industry marketing everything from cosmetic surgery to anti-wrinkle creams (Bengtson, Burgess, & Parrot, 1997).

Given that the majority of aging individuals are women, and that gender is embedded in the structures of social inequalities, feminist scholars explore the link between age and gender, seeking to understand the role of society in the process of aging and the experiences of older adults from the prism of gendered organization of life. *Critical gerontology*, a relatively new approach in studies of aging, supports this position, but it also emphasizes the importance of social action and empowerment. This position argues that the diversity of older people and our critical approach to the social structures shaping the experiences of aging should move beyond theoretical knowledge to empowerment of older people to create social change that addresses ageism (Bengtson et al., 1997).

Life-Course Perspective

While these earlier and later developments in social gerontology are shaping the theoretical debates in the field of aging, they do not fully incorporate the view of aging as a *process* that starts at birth and lasts throughout the life course. Using micro-perspectives (e.g. activity theory) or macro-approaches (such as a political economy approach), researchers tend to study aging as a "snapshot" in time. The life-course perspective provides a wider view on aging, incorporating micro and macro approaches in its theoretical framework.

The life-course perspective provides an interdisciplinary approach, bringing together the theoretical assumptions from a variety of disciplines, including sociology, psychology, history, family, and health studies (Hatch, 2000). This perspective focuses on aging as a process that unfolds throughout the life cycle from birth (Connidis, 2010). Macro factors such as major political, economic, or ideological changes shape the experiences of individuals and can influence the transitions and timing of major life events (Putney & Bengtson, 2005). The ultimate goal of this perspective is to understand the process of aging and to incorporate the impact of previous life experiences and social structure on human agency.

Although the life-course approach has gained widespread popularity across disciplines, a number of underlying principles form the core of the perspective (Bengtson et al., 1997). These principles include the importance of history and personal biography, the sequence and timing of personal **transitions** that are coupled with choices and constraints, and the interdependence of linked lives. Bengtson et al. (1997) proposed that the goals of the life-course perspective are to explain:

1. the dynamics, context, and the process of aging;

2. age-related transitions and life trajectories;

3. the role of cultural context and social structure locations on the experiences of the individuals; and

4. the impact of time, historical period, and cohort effect on the lives of the individuals.

Using these tenets and objectives, scholars have commonly inquired into cohort effects on attitudes, perceptions, experiences, and actions (Hatch, 2000; Putney & Bengtson, 2005; Shenk, Kuwahara, & Zablotsky, 2004).

The life-course perspective gained tremendous popularity in social sciences in the past few years. Although some scholars critique this perspective for being too broad in its scope, it allows us to see aging as a process that occurs throughout a person's life. This is the approach that we take in this chapter.

HEALTHY AGING

While much of the discussion on aging and health focuses on illness, disease, and death, aging is about much more than that. Getting old certainly signals the end of some experiences, activities, and opportunities, but it can also open the door for others to take their place that may be just as rewarding and exciting.

The broader concept of aging refers to the entire life course beginning at birth and continuing until death. As such, **aging**—or the gaining of experience, reaching developmental milestones, growing emotionally, and changing physically—happens as long as one continues to live. To understand healthy aging later in life, it is useful to have some sense of healthy aging while young. A look back at childhood theories of healthy aging allow us to see more clearly the social, political, and physical aspects of healthy aging of adults into old age.

Healthy Aging in Childhood

Healthy aging in childhood is generally presented as reaching developmental achievements. A number of theorists have proposed theories of development. Piaget (1932, 1952) proposed the theory of *cognitive development*, identifying developmental milestones as children progress through childhood and into adolescence. His theory proposed that children evaluate their world through four stages. The first stage, the *sensory-motor stage* occurring between birth and age 2, is where children move from merely responding to stimuli around them to actually manipulating things and become active participants in their environment. During this stage, children are **egocentric**, meaning they are unable to perceive the needs, wants, and desires of anyone else. In the *pre-operations stage* (between 2 and 7 years old), the child moves away from egocentrism developing a firm sense of what they perceive as right and wrong that they expect others to share with them. The third and fourth stages move from *concrete operations* in older childhood to *formal operations* in adolescence. The child develops the ability to deal in a logical fashion, to generalize, and to deal with abstract concepts. For example, sarcasm is difficult for children to grasp until they move into the formal operations stage and are able to understand more latent and tangential meanings.

George Herbert Mead (1934), one of the fathers of symbolic interactionism, examined child development and differentiated between young children and older children in their ability to play versus their ability to participate in games. Play, according to Mead, allowed children to take the role of another, as in cops and robbers, superheroes, or playing "doctor." The child would be able to take on concrete adult roles. This developed a sense of subject and object as the child develops a sense of self. Through participation in games, the child is able to generalize to many objects and comprehend how objects and roles relate to each other. To participate in the game of baseball, Mead's favourite example, a child needs to be able to not only play her position; she also needs to understand the other positions on the field in order to successfully anticipate actions of others. This is central to personality development, the ability to function and know a person's specific role and the roles of others in groups. Play and games developed the two central components of self, what Mead called the "I" and the "me." The "I" is the active and subjective part of the self as in "I did this." The "me" is the passive and object part of the self as in "this happened to me." These dual aspects of self are reflexive and allow a person to be both subject and object. The development of this reflexivity is the essence of the ability to develop relationships through life. In Chapter 11 we described the importance of this distinction through the illness experience.

Perhaps the most famous works historically on childhood development and aging are those of Sigmund Freud and Erik Erikson. Freud (1905) proposed the Psychosexual Stages of Development, which included five developmental stages: oral, anal, phallic, latency, and genital. Each developmental stage contained a physical, psychological, and adult character-type theme that the child had to achieve in order to move to the next phase and ensure a psycho-social-sexually healthy adult. Failure to resolve problems at one stage would leave the child disadvantaged as an adult, regressing to that stage in the face of stress.

Eric Erikson (1950, 1959, 1968, & Erikson, 1987), a protégé of Freud, modified the original five-stage theory describing child development, and, more important for our purposes, expanded it to include three additional stages of development during adult life. In Erikson's formulation of the "eight stages of man," he left behind Freud's psychosexual orientation, taking a more psychosocial focus. He postulated that healthy psychological development was obtained through social interaction and relationships as a person successfully or unsuccessfully navigated the crises of opposing forces involved in each stage. According to his theory, a child or adult could underdevelop or overdevelop a trait through a specific crisis or attain a healthy ratio necessary for success. For example, during the first stage, the development of *trust versus mistrust* that coincided with Freud's oral stage, a child must develop a healthy level of trust in others but not too much to be gullible and not too little to be mistrustful of everything. A proper ratio will result in a sense that things will be okay. The next four childhood stages included *autonomy versus shame and doubt, initiative versus guilt, industry versus inferiority*, and *identity versus role confusion* (see Table 9.1).

Table 9.1 Stages of Development as Outlined by Various Theorists and Researchers

Age	Piaget (1932, 1952)	Freud (1905)	Erikson (1950, 1968, & Erikson, 1987)	Vaillant (2002)
0–1½	Sensory-Motor	Oral	Trust vs. Mistrust	
1½–3½	Pre-Operations	Anal	Autonomy vs. Shame	
3½–6		Phallic	Initiative vs. Guilt	
6–Puberty	Concrete Operations	Latency	Industry vs. Inferiority	
Post Puberty and Adolescence	Formal Operations	Genital	Identify vs. Role Confusion	
~20s			Intimacy vs. Isolation	Identity
~30s				Intimacy
~40s			Generativity vs. Stagnation	Career Consolidation
~50s				Generativity
~60s			Integrity vs. Despair	Keeper of Meaning
~70s+				Integrity

Healthy Aging in Adulthood

At this point, Erikson moved beyond Freud to describe further developmental stages in adulthood. Erikson identified three stages roughly equating to early, middle, and late adulthood, during which the adult develops further psychosocial skills through crises. The sixth stage, *intimacy versus isolation*, is where young adults learn to love and be intimate with a significant other. This is the bonding of one to a special "other" in reciprocal, mutually beneficial, committed relationships. While this principally reflects the primary relationship, it also applies to close friends and work colleagues. Failure to achieve this could result in social isolation. Or, in the other extreme, it could result in promiscuity and shallowness of relationships wherein there are no intimate bonds or meaningful affiliations. Both outcomes result in isolation from emotions and intimacy.

The middle adulthood stage focused on the clash of *generativity versus stagnation*. Generativity was a giving back to others, mentoring younger persons, or a giving back to society—a "pay it forward" mentality. In this stage, people put their time into raising their children or helping in the community. In this sense, it is the generational reproduction of values and culture, a passing down of these things from one generation to the next. Failure to find the right balance in this stage could result in either a lack of care, rejection of values and culture, or an overextension of the self.

Erikson's final stage occurred in old age involving the crisis of *integrity versus despair*. This is where people reflect back on their lives to assess their lifetime achievements and legacy. Questions surrounding the meaning of life and one's purpose in life arise in this "taking stock." Positive self-reflection to these questions results in a comforting wisdom, an integrity that we are content, happy, and ready for our eventual demise. Failure at this stage results in either discontent and struggle to find meaning and purpose, while reliving the failures of your life or, it could go to the other extreme as a dogmatism. In this sense, it is an absence of reflection that carries a sense of having been right all along, in an almost "intransigent adolescent frame of mind" of knowing everything and unwilling to consider challenges to your views.

Recent work by Vaillant (2002) on healthy aging, building on Erikson's work, describes six developmental *tasks* as opposed to stages, emphasizing that they are not necessarily linear. These tasks include identity, intimacy, career consolidation, generativity, keeper of meaning, and integrity. While not completely accurate, you can think of these tasks as moving across the decades of adult life as people become septuagenarians (in their seventies) and octogenarians (in their eighties). The two tasks that differ from Erikson's work are career consolidation and keeper of meaning. *Career consolidation* infers contentment with a person's central adult roles regardless of any financial compensation. The key is perceived value that reinforces a commitment to succeed in the role or occupation instead of just enduring it. *Keeper of meaning* moves beyond generativity and mentorship to preserving the culture and institutions for society more generally.

Consistent with Erikson, the final task of *integrity* is the feeling that the journey was worth it and your life has made a contribution. The alternative is *despair*, where you are left seeking a purpose for your life, reflecting back with negative feelings about past experiences and past failures (real or perceived) and your pending demise.

Interestingly, this concept of healthy aging also aligns well with Antonovsky's (1979, 1987) model of **salutogensis**, a term coined in direct response to the pathogenic focus on disease and illness to redirect attention away from disease and toward health. Within this salutogenic framework was the concept of **sense of coherence** that provided people with a sense that the world was a predictable, understandable, and meaningful place. Sense of coherence aligns with later stages of development, specifically integrity and generativity. A recent analysis of the longitudinal National Population Health Survey (NPHS) examined how various factors predict change in health status among middle-aged groups and seniors (Martel, Bélanger, Berthelot, & Carrière, 2005). Whereas for those between 45 and 65, the central factors were lower chronic social stress and higher income, among those 65 and older, the important factors were a higher sense of coherence and greater leisure time and physical activity. In both groups, higher education was related to staying healthy.

Health and Illness in Old Age

In addition to social-psychological changes, healthy aging also entails living and coping with deterioration of the physical body and the onset of multiple chronic conditions. As Figure 9.1 outlines, the proportion of the population with one or more chronic conditions increases with age to the point where an additional 30% of Canadians over 80 reports living with four or more diseases compared with the cohort aged 45 to 64. The most prevalent chronic conditions reported by seniors were arthritis and rheumatism, affecting 44% of seniors in 2009. Nevertheless, many seniors (44%) still perceive their health to be in excellent or very good condition (Public Health Agency of Canada [PHAC], 2010).

As a consequence of physical deterioration, a particularly important health concern among seniors is falls. Indeed, the most common cause of injury among seniors in Canada is falling. It is estimated that a third of seniors are likely to fall at least once each year. Falls are especially common among seniors suffering from cognitive impairment. Those who live alone or who are housebound due to chronic health conditions are at greater risk for falls. Both the increased likelihood of a fall and the severity of the consequences of that fall are linked to the condition of osteoporosis, characterized by low bone mass and thinned and weakened bones, a condition that is more prevalent among women than men (29% vs. 6% of those age 65 and older) (PHAC, 2010).

Another critical issue facing older Canadians is dementia, including Alzheimer's disease. In 2008, an estimated 400 000 senior Canadians were living with dementia, with rates being higher among women than men. Based on current prevalence rates, it has been estimated that the number will more than double within 30 years based on the aging of the population (PHAC, 2010).

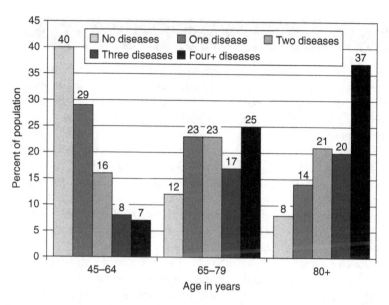

Figure 9.1 Proportion of Population with One or More Chronic Diseases,* by Selected Age Groups, Canada, 2009

*Diseases include angina, asthma, arthritis or rheumatism, osteoporosis, high blood pressure, bronchitis, emphysema, chronic obstructive pulmonary disease, diabetes, heart disease, cancer, effects of a stroke, Crohn's disease, colitis, Alzheimer's disease, Parkinson's disease, cataracts, glaucoma, thyroid condition, mood disorder, and anxiety disorder.

Source: Public Health Agency of Canada [PHAC]. (2010). *The Chief Public Health Officer's Report on the State of Public Health in Canada 2010.* Retrieved from www.phac-aspc.gc.ca/cphorsphc-respcacsp/2010/fr-rc/cphorsphc-respcacsp-06-eng.php

So both individually and at a sociocultural level, there is a tension between the recognition of aging as a natural and positive process to be embraced versus an approach where aging is thought of as a condition or an illness to be resisted through medical or behavioural means. Box 9.1 outlines two case studies that problematize the resistance of aging or at least societal norms of an aging population.

Box 9.1

Two Case Studies Problematizing the Resistance of Aging

Case Study 1: Sexy Seniors

Sociologist Barbara Marshall of Trent University, problematizes the increasing sexualization of seniors in her (Marshall, 2010) essay, "Science, medicine and virility surveillance: 'sexy seniors' in the pharmaceutical imagination." She argues that while sex has historically been seen primarily as the prerogative of the young, more recently the emphasis has been on

(continued)

Box 9.1 (*Continued*)

the maintenance of active sexuality as a marker of successful aging. She describes a new cultural consensus that appears to have emerged that not only emphasizes the importance of continued sexual activity across the lifespan, but links sexual function with overall health and encourages increased self-surveillance of, and medical attention to, late-life sexuality. Drawing on historical accounts, clinical research, popular science reporting, and health promotion literature, she explores several key shifts in models of sexual aging, culminating in the contemporary model of gender, sexuality, and aging that has made aging populations a key market for biotechnologies aimed at enhancing sexual function. Two central concepts frame her analysis: "virility surveillance," where age-related changes in sexual function are taken as indicative of decline, and the "pharmaceutical imagination," where sexual life courses are reconstructed as the effects of drugs revise standards of sexual function. After consideration of how narratives emerging from qualitative research with older adults challenge the narrow depiction of sexual functionality promoted by pharmaculture, she calls for continued critical inquiry into the biomedical construction of sex and age.

Case Study #2 Disciplining Old Age

Sociologist Stephen Katz, also from Trent University, critiques the way in which old age has been increasingly "disciplined" or reified in his 1996 book *Disciplining Old Age: The Formation of Gerontological Knowledge*. Using the work of Foucault, Katz inverts the usual trajectory of gerontological history to illustrate the ways in which gerontology, as a discipline, constructed the subject of old age. As he says about the Foucauldian approach, "Rather than looking at the history of gerontology to discover how knowledge disclosed the problems of old age, we can look at how the subjectification of old age made gerontological knowledge possible" (Katz, 1996, p. 11, as cited in Hirshbein, 1998). Katz uses specific examples to explore the disciplining of old age. He traces the medicalization of the aging body from premodern times to the present, and the creation of an elderly population through institutions, pensions, and social surveys. He examines the medical and popular texts that created a science of old age, and the disciplinary activities of gerontological organizations. Although Katz emphasizes the construction of subjects by disciplines, he does not imply that these subjects have no agency. Instead, he argues that, "elderly persons, constructed as bodily, individual, and demographic subjects, also become agents who strategically mobilize political action" (Katz, 1996, p. 26, as cited in Hirshbein, 1998). Throughout his book, Katz questions traditional assumptions about gerontology, particularly the heroic history of the discipline as the acquisition of knowledge to assist older people. Katz does acknowledge, however, that despite his critical reading of gerontological knowledge, "gerontologists have bettered life in old age" (Katz, 1996, p. 135, as cited in Hirshbein, 1998).

POPULATION AGING AND CHANGING CANADIAN DEMOGRAPHICS AMONG THE ELDERLY

Population aging has been discussed in detail in Chapter 6. The age group most commonly defined as old, those aged 65 and over, is the fastest-growing age group in Canada, almost doubling in the past 50 years. Moreover, as this cohort increases in size and the population continues to age, old age has been further differentiated into the "young-old," the "middle-old," and the "old-old." According to the 2011 Census, Canada's population aged

65 and over stands at 4.3 million (13.7% of the total population) of whom 1.2 million are 80 and over (3.7%). The 2011 Census reports 4.945 million people aged 65 or older or 14.8% of the total population (Statistics Canada, 2012c). This is an increase of 14.1% from the 2006 census. Unfortunately, at the time of writing, information was not available from the 2011 census on the breakdown of age groups within the elderly but it is readily apparent that the numbers are increasing. The aging of the population is expected to continue over the next three decades with those 65 and over expected to reach 9.8 million by 2036, doubling to 25.5% of the population (Statistics Canada, 2007b). Recently, the Canadian government has even started keeping track of the number of **centenarians** (those who are 100 years old or more). In 1996, there were 3100 people at least 100 years old with female centenarians outnumbering male centenarians by about 5 to 1. This number grew to 3600 in 2001 and to 4100 in 2006 to 5825 in 2011. To put this age in perspective, today's centenarians were alive during World War I and alive prior to Canadian women having the right to vote.

The aging of the Canadian population will continue to have a pronounced effect on many facets of Canadian life. For example, economically, the percentage of persons receiving government pensions is growing while there are fewer people as a proportion in the workforce to fund those pensions. This is one of the reasons for the recent federal move to shift the official retirement age from 65 to 67 to defer pension payments.

Population aging influences population health, which translates into additional pressure on our health care system. Some argue that it will have repercussions for the care of older adults and for the growing workforce providing this care (Home Care Sector Study Corporation, 2003a; Carrière, 2006). When we discuss the health needs of an aging population, it is important to move from discussing the "elderly" as a homogeneous group to differentiating them into groups. Differences in age translate into differences in use of health care services and health care costs. The average dollars spent annually on health care for those who are 80 or older is $18 160 compared to $10 742 spent for people whose age is 65 to 79 (Canadian Institute for Health Information [CIHI], 2010). Moreover, as medical science and technology advances and people live even longer, there will be more time to manifest additional illnesses and conditions and more time to live with them, which will continue to drive health care costs among the elderly (Canadian Health Services Research Foundation [CHSRF], 2011). Some have labelled this phenomenon as **apocalyptic demography**. According to Gee (2002), this is an ideology that perceives old age as a burden on the assets of society as resources get allocated to deal with the sick, elderly populations at the expense of younger, healthier cohorts. Gee and other Canadian medical sociologists, such as Herb Northcott (see Researcher Profile 9.1), argue that this is a myth. They suggest that rather than blaming the aging population for rising health care costs, we should focus our attention on the reorganization of currently existing services. Even Canadian health economist Robert Evans disagrees, arguing that only 0.8% of the increase in Medicare costs is attributable to the aging of the population. The majority is attributable to the private components of the system such as prescription drugs, dental care, and home care (Evans, 2010 further detailed in Chapter 3 on the history of Canadian Health Care). Others such as the CSHRF also challenge this myth:

Herbert Northcott

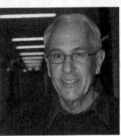

Donna Fong/Herbert Northcott

Herbert Northcott, a Professor of Sociology at the University of Alberta, has been working to debunk the inaccurate and negative pictures of the impact seniors have on society. "The population aging trend is about the increase in the percentage of the population that are seniors." The problem with the public dialogue around this trend is that it's all too easy to misconstrue, leading to talk of an "impending demographic crisis." Northcott goes as far as to say that, if there is a crisis, it's being constructed, and it's almost "apocalyptic" in tone. "We talk about it as a challenge, a problem,

a crisis—apocalyptic demography leading to eventual and inevitable economic and social disasters, including pension shortfalls and a health-care system collapse as a suddenly seniors-top-heavy population sucks the public purse dry with their pension and health care needs—this is simply not going to be true."

The Winnipeg-raised author of *Aging in Alberta* and *Changing Residence: The Geographic Mobility of Elderly Canadians* points out that these demographic trends unfold very slowly, sometimes over the course of decades, giving us plenty of time to prepare. "When we surveyed a representative sample of adults, we found that they believed seniors would constitute a crisis—a belief that has no justification. People heard it articulated so much that they believe it. When I reviewed all the local needs assessment surveys I found that most seniors are healthy, happy and living independently. It's simply a myth that most seniors constitute a burden," explains Northcott.

Source: Adapted from Kosowan, G. (2001). Population aging prof breaks down myths. Available at: www.archives. expressnews.ualberta.ca/article/2001/07/234.html

The good news is that problems expected to arise from population aging can be managed with smart changes to care delivery for the elderly. It's the other issues—such as the growing cost of healthcare services and the increased costs arising from technological innovation—that are causing expenditures to escalate. These are the cost drivers that require our foremost attention. (CHSRF, 2011)

HEALTH CARE FOR OLDER ADULTS

Lower[2] fertility rates that have accompanied population aging and shifting work patterns, particularly among women, has resulted in a general trend moving elder care away from the family to the formal care system. The increase in chronic and, indeed, multiple (co-morbid) chronic health conditions and diseases with age requires more

---

[2]This section is a revised version of the chapter written by Margaret Denton (2009) for the report, *The Role of Immigrant Care Workers in an Aging Society: The Canadian Context & Experience.*

care. However, the structure of the health care system in Canada historically is largely organized around the treatment of acute, curative care rather than chronic disease management. The **insured services** covered by Medicare are governed by the five principles of the Canada Health Act (universality, accessibility, portability, comprehensiveness, and public administration) include primary medical care and acute care, which are price-regulated and protected from user fees and extra billing. **Extended health services**, including residential long-term care, home care, adult residential care, and ambulatory health services, are not. As a result, the fragmented, privatized system of health care for older adults has a broad range of consequences for the various forms of long-term care.

Long-Term Care in Canada

Context and Definitions Long-term care (LTC) is an umbrella concept used in Canada to describe a complex system of care for persons who are at significant risk because of having progressive and/or chronic conditions, and who require services to meet their long-term functional needs. (Continuing care has been used interchangeably with long-term care as a service concept, organizing framework, or division of government. For example, some provinces use continuing care to describe the overall system and use the term "long-term care" to describe facility care.) According to Chan & Kenny (2001), the

> four essential features of long-term care in Canada are that (1) the care will be long-term; (2) it is an integrated program of care across various service components, that is, a service continuum; (3) it is a complex service delivery system, not a type of service; and (4) the efficiency and effectiveness of the system are based not only on the efficiency and effectiveness of each component, but also on the way that the service delivery system is structured. (p. 87)

The main components of long-term care service delivery systems in Canada are institutional care in LTC facilities and home care/community-based services. LTC services are not fully insured in any jurisdiction. The balance among these components and the range of services within each component vary from province to province, within an overall national framework that sets guidelines for access to care. Each province has developed its own terms and conditions under which services are provided (Canadian Health Care Association, 2004). This has resulted in differences in provincial policies, organization, availability, delivery, costs, eligibility requirements, coverage limits, covered services, and public investment of non-insured home care health services. Further, there are no commonly accepted terminology, standards, or comprehensive data for home care (MacAdam, 2004). Similarly, this has led to provincial differences in accountability, system design, funding, policies and regulations, facility ownership, costs to residents, residency requirements, and minimum comfort allowances for institutional care (Canadian Health Care Association, 2004; Berta, Laporte, Zarnett, Valdmanis, & Anderson, 2006).

Long-Term Care Expenditures in Canada   Health care expenditures in Canada have been rising in absolute terms as well as per capita and as a percentage of GDP (CIHI, 2005). In 2003, total health expenditures in Canada were $123 billion and were forecast to reach $142 billion in 2005 (CIHR, 2005). Health expenditures on long-term care, however, were only a fraction of total expenditures in 2003, totalling 9.3% or $11.4 billion on nursing homes and other residential care facilities (CIHR, 2005) and 4.0% or $3.4 billion on home care (CIHI, 2007b).

Although the provinces have rapidly increased funding for home and long-term care, it has not kept up with demand. In Canada, home care expenditures have increased by 204% in the decades since 1991 and by 209% in other health institutions, which include nursing homes and residential care facilities. Nursing homes and other forms of residential care still absorb 80% of the total long-term health care budget; however, the growth in expenditures for home care have been increasing at a faster rate than the budgets for residential care (MacAdam, 2004). The LTC institutional share of the health care pie has risen to 10.3% in 2006, or $15.5 billion (CIHI, 2008). In response to increasing costs, many home care programs have implemented cost containment mechanisms, such as restricting the number of hours of care, the number of visits or services, changing eligibility criteria, and training family members on how to provide care. There has also been a trend to using unregulated home care providers, such as personal support workers or health care aides, to perform many of the tasks done previously by nurses (Sharkey, Larsen, & Mildon, 2003).

Residential Care Facilities for Older Adults in Canada

Defining long-term residential care in Canada
The two main types of residential care services are *chronic care hospitals* or chronic care units within hospitals, and *long-term care facilities* that provide multiple levels of care that cover clients at intermediate and extended-care levels (Chan & Kenny, 2001). Chronic care hospitals or units provide care to persons who, because of chronic illness and marked functional disability, require long-term institutional care but do not require all of the resources of an acute, psychiatric, or rehabilitation hospital. Professional nursing staff provide 24-hour coverage and physician and other health and social specialities are on-call. Long-term residential care facilities (also called nursing homes or homes for the aged) provide a protective and supportive environment to clients who can no longer live at home. Residents receive assistance with the activities of daily living, 24-hour surveillance, assisted meal service, and professional nursing care and/or supervision, including supervision over medication (Chan & Kenny, 2001).

The term *residential care facilities* refers to facilities with four beds or more that are funded and licensed or approved by provincial/territorial departments of health or social services. Apartments or other facilities (e.g., assisted living or retirement homes) not providing any level of care are not included in this definition (Statistics Canada, 2007c).

According to a 2005/2006 survey of residential care facilities in Canada, there are 2086 homes for older adults serving 196 242 residents. Payment for resident-days in homes for the aged come primarily from provincial health insurance plans, although about 13% comes from other sources such as self pay (Statistics Canada, 2007c, p. 42). The amount coming from other sources varies by province from a low of 0% in Québec, to 14% in British Columbia, 17% in Ontario, 21% in New Brunswick, and 33% in Prince Edward Island (Statistics Canada, 2007c, pp. 43–47). There are also sizable differences in per capita expenditures on homes for those aged 65 and over by province. British Columbia ($1874) and Ontario ($2475) had the lowest per capita expenditures while Saskatchewan ($3348) and Manitoba ($3287) had the highest with the other provinces and territories falling somewhere between (Statistics Canada, 2007c, p. 11).

Ownership of Long-Term Residential Facilities in Canada   Homes for older adults fall into three broad categories of ownership: private (proprietary), government (federal, provincial, and municipal), and not-for-profit (lay- and religious-operated facilities). Private-sector homes constitute 54% of the ownership with not-for-profit (24%) and government (22%) making up the rest (Statistics Canada, 2007c, p. 13). Government-owned facilities house more people than the not-for-profit or for-profit sector homes (Berta et. al., 2006). Regional variations exist, with government-owned LTC facilities more likely to be in Alberta, the Prairies, and Ontario, while for-profits dominate Eastern Canada and for-profits and not-for-profits co-dominate in British Columbia (Berta et al., 2006).

Utilization   According to the 2001 Census, close to 7 to 8% of all seniors are institutionalized in Canada and the percentage increases with age, with 35% of all seniors 85 and over living in institutions (Cranswick, 2005). Although the overall proportion of seniors residing in LTC facilities has been declining for men and women and all age groups, nursing home residents are more likely to be women, living without a spouse, and on low incomes (Trottier et al., 2006). Other factors strongly associated with living in a LTC facility include a recent hospital admission; having one or more problems with the activities of daily living; having a severe disability; and having a debilitating chronic condition, such as Alzheimer's disease, urinary incontinence, or the effect of a stroke.

Who Works in Residential Care Facilities?   Residential care facilities include a wide variety of care workers. According to the 2005–2006 survey of residential care facilities in Canada, 158 732 workers were employed in the 2086 homes for the aged. Nearly half (48%) of these care workers were part-time employees. There is a paucity of research on care workers in long-term care facilitates. There is research on the nursing workforce, but data on nurses working in long-term care facilities are rarely examined separately. We do know that compared to acute-care hospitals, the long-term care sector had the lowest ratio of nurses to patients. The long-term care sector identified difficulties recruiting new graduates at their sites, noting that new graduates were more interested in working in acute care. Other factors contributing to nursing shortages in LTC included the lack of full-time positions, workload demands, difficult clients, and isolation/rural challenges. Caseloads can be so heavy that it often falls upon nurses to direct care and delegate functions of care to be carried out by aides. This is of particular concern because the acuity of clients and the complexity of their care have been increasing in recent years (O'Brien-Pallas et. al., 2004).

Home Care in Canada

Defining Home Care in Canada Home care is defined as the ". . . array of services which enable consumers incapacitated in whole or in part to remain in their own homes, often with the effect of preventing, delaying or substituting for long-term services" (Home Care Sector Corporation, 2003a, p. 3). Although each province has organized home care differently, there are some common features: entry to all home care services is by way of provincially designated public agency and eligibility is based on need as determined by a provincially uniform assessment process (MacAdam, 2004). Currently, all provinces provide three types of home care—post-acute care, supportive care for the chronically disabled, and end-of-life care—within one umbrella program. Professional services (nursing, rehabilitation, and case management), pharmaceuticals and medical equipment/supplies, support for essential personal care needs, and assessment and case management are offered at no cost to clients (MacAdam, 2004) (see Table 9.2).

Table 9.2 A Comparison of Workers in Residential v. Home Care Sectors

Types of Direct Care Workers in Residential Care Facilities*	Types of Paid Care Workers in the Home Care Sector**
	Home Support Workers (also called personal care attendants/workers) deliver the basics: a washed floor, a clean bathroom, a stocked fridge, a hot meal, laundered clothes and linens, and a safe bath.
Registered Nurses may include the Director of Nursing, the Assistant Director of Nursing, supervisors, and general duty nursing staff who qualify as registered nurses.	**Registered Nurses** provide a continuum of nursing services designed to support consumers of all ages to remain in their homes during an acute, chronic, or terminal illness.
Registered qualified nursing assistants/licensed practical nurses are persons authorized to function as nursing assistants according to appropriate provincial legislation.	**Licensed/Registered Practical Nurses** working as members of the interdisciplinary team, use the nursing process and nursing concepts to provide care to a diverse population of consumers, and their caregivers, within the community setting.

Physiotherapists are responsible for the maintenance and improvement of the functional capacity of a resident through procedures including exercise, massage, and manipulation.

Occupational therapists are responsible for the maintenance and improvement of the functional capacity of the resident through the practice of activities of daily living and the development of vocational and manual skills.

Other therapists would include speech therapists, behaviour therapists, group therapists, etc.

Physiotherapists enable consumers to remain in their home by working to improve the mobility and functional independence of consumers in the home environment.

Occupational therapists enable the client to participate in daily activities (i.e., bathing, functional mobility, meal preparation, shopping) and support the role of family and caregivers.

Case managers establish client eligibility for home care programs; assess the client's health, functional, and social status; and establish the supportive service plan to assist consumers and their families to regain optimum health status or provide the required care, services, and supports to ensure the client, caregivers, and/or the community are supported through complex disease issues and end-of-life care.

Activity/recreation staff includes any staff involved in setting up or maintaining a program of social activities, recreation, and hobbies for the residents.

Other direct care staff—nursing aides, health care aides, dieticians, counsellors, orderlies, social workers, graduate nurses, chaplains, etc.

Other home care occupations include social workers, dieticians, respiratory therapists, speech/language pathologists, physicians, and psychologists.

* *Sources:* Statistics Canada: Residential Care Facilities Survey. (2010c). Guide: Instructions and Definitions. Retrieved from www23.statcan.gc.ca/imdb-bmdi/document/3210_D1_T1_V15-eng.pdf

**Canadian Home Care Association. (2003a). *Canadian Home Care Human Resources Study, Final Report* (p. 11). Retrieved from www.cdnhomecare.ca/media.php?mid=1030.

Models of Home Care Delivery

There are two basic models of public home care delivery: a *provider model* in which services are arranged for and provided through staff hired by home care agencies, and a *self-managed home care model* in which clients are given cash or service vouchers to manage and arrange for all aspects of service provision, including hiring, tasks provided, and quality of care (MacAdam, 2004). All provinces and territories offer the provider model, but only eight offer both models (Québec, British Columbia, Alberta, Ontario, Manitoba, New Brunswick, Newfoundland, and the Northwest Territories). If people are not eligible for publicly funded home care, they are able to purchase home health services privately. It is estimated that about 20% of total home care expenditures are paid for privately (MacAdam, 2004, p. 395).

Utilization   Data from the 2003 Canadian Community Health Survey indicates that the rate of publicly funded home care users is 25 per 1000 population or 1.2 million Canadians, aged 18 and over (CIHI, 2007a). The proportion receiving home care increases with age: 6% of those aged 65 to 74, 15% of those aged 75 to 84, and 32% of those aged 85 and over. Women were more likely than men to receive formal home care. Those most likely to receive home care lived alone, had been admitted to a hospital in the past year, had one or more chronic conditions, and reported social assistance as their main source of income. The most frequent types of care provided included housework, followed by nursing care, personal care, and meal preparation (Carrière, 2006). In 2003–2004, provincial and territorial government spending on home care averaged $105 per person. Of this, $57 was spent on home health care, including professional and nursing care; and $60 for home support, such as personal care, housework, meals, shopping, and respite care (CIHI, 2007c).

Human Resource Issues in Home Care   There are a variety of health workers providing home care services. The Canadian Home Care Human Resources Study (CHCHRS) (Home Care Sector Study Corporation, 2003b) reported that in 2002 there were 9241 registered nurses (RNs), 2854 licensed practical nurses (LPNs), and 32 300 home support/personal care workers (PCWs) working in home care in Canada. There were differences in the percentage of occupational groups working for different sectors. Government home care programs were more likely to employ people working in professional occupations, such as therapists and RNs, but fewer LPNs. The not-for-profit sector had a disproportionate share of LPNs, whereas the for-profit sector employed a higher proportion of home support workers (Home Care Sector Study Corporation, 2003a). Home care work is predominately a female occupation and the majority of home care workers are over 40 (Home Care Sector Study Corporation, 2003b).

Working conditions in home care are typically poor across Canada, no matter what model of service organization and delivery is employed (Aronson, Denton, & Zeytinoglu, 2004). Home care work is characterized by low levels of pay, few fringe benefits, job insecurity, and lack of career and training opportunities (Home Care Sector Study Corporation, 2003a). Many workers are employed part time or work casual hours (i.e., paid either by the hour or by the visit and hours are not guaranteed) (Canadian Association of Retired Persons [CARP], 2001) and workers are expected to work weekends and evenings. Job-specific factors, such as high travel costs, occupational health and safety issues in clients' homes, heavy client loads, limited time to care for clients, and increasing acuity of sickness in patients are additional difficulties experienced by home care workers

(CARP, 2001). Difficulties experienced in providing care in home settings include unsanitary conditions in houses, lack of cooperation from consumers and informal care givers, physical or verbal abuse, sexual harassment, and racial discrimination (Home Care Sector Study Corporation, 2003b). Other factors that contribute to job dissatisfaction are low wages and professional isolation, high levels of stress or burnout, lack of recognition, and work-place injuries or disabilities (Denton, Zeytinoglu, Davies, & Lian, 2002). As a result, the recruitment and retention of home care workers has been challenging. Canadian medical sociologist Margaret Denton has undertaken a great deal of work on the home and long-term care workforce (Denton, Zeytinoglu, & Davies, 2003) (see Researcher Profile 9.2).

Informal Care and Aging at Home

In addition to formal care provided by a range of health care providers described in the previous sections, a great deal of informal care is provided in the home by family members (see Figure 9.2). Because women usually assume most of the responsibilities for the

---

Researcher Profile 9.2
Margaret Denton

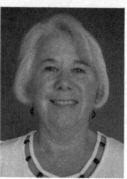

Courtesy of Margaret Denton

Margaret Denton is a Professor of Sociology and Health, Aging, and Society at McMaster University, Hamilton, Ontario. Her areas of research expertise include women's health; heath services research (home health care); age-friendly cities; age inequality; and work, retirement, and pensions. A case study of the home care sector in a mid-sized city in Ontario undertaken by Denton with colleagues Denton, Zeytinoglu, Davies, & Hunter (2006) reveals that, in a five-year period between spring 1996 and spring 2001, of the 620 visiting home care workers employed by the three non-profit agencies in 1996, 320, or 52%, had left the agency. During that time, the turnover rate for nurses was 54% and for PSWs 50%. In a related study of the association between casualized employment and turnover intention in home care for older adults, Zeytinoglu, Denton, Davies, & Plenderleith (2009) found that controlling for variety of other factors, "casual hours and perceived employment insecurity and labour market insecurity are positively and on-call work is negatively associated with home care workers' turnover intention (p. 258)." Commenting on these results, researchers conclude that such findings represent evidence on the impact that casualized employment strategies have on home care workers' turnover intention.

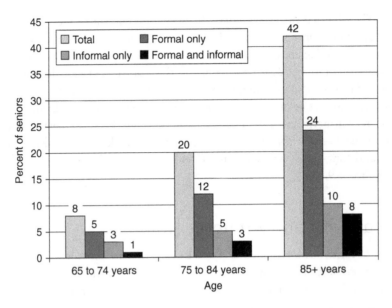

Figure 9.2 Percentage of Seniors Who Received Home Care in the Past Year, Canada, 2003

health of family members, the most likely informal care providers are women (a wife, daughter, daughter-in-law, or niece). Although there are positive elements of being a care provider, it has also been found that there is a resulting social isolation and lack of "downtime" that may arise from caregiving responsibilities that can result in caregivers experiencing poorer physical and emotional health (PHAC, 2010) (see Researcher Profile 9.3). Sociologist Susan Reverby (1987) has described this situation as causing the **caring dilemma** wherein (most often) women feel obliged to provide care within a society that at the same time does not allow women the means by which to determine how that care is to be provided.

Palliative and End-of-Life Care

We include this topic in a chapter on the social dimensions of aging, recognizing that, in the literature, there has been a general disconnect between the scholarship on aging and dying. As Clark and Seymour (1999) describe in their book *Reflections on Palliative Care: Sociological and Policy Perspectives* that both biology and culture and their intersection affect the process of death and dying. They propose the term **deathways** as the ways in which society structures and constrains the pathway to death or the trajectory of dying, and how this often neglects the experience and response to

Anne Martin Matthews

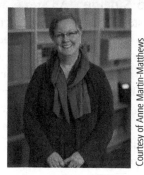

Courtesy of Anne Martin-Matthews

Anne Martin-Matthews, Professor of Sociology at the University of British Columbia, has recently completed two terms (2004–2011) as the Scientific Director of the Institute of Aging, one of 13 national Institutes of the Canadian Institutes of Health Research. Under her leadership, the CIHR Institute of Aging led the development of the Canadian Longitudinal Study on Aging (CLSA), a 20-year study of 50 000 Canadians aged 45 to 85,

launched in 2009. The Institute of Aging has also developed strategic initiatives on Cognitive Impairment in Aging, on Mobility in Aging, and on Health Services and Systems for an Aging Population. Her publications include over 140 articles on health and social care, aging and social support, work–family balance, and rural aging; and two books, including *Aging and Caring at the Intersection of Work and Home Life: Blurring the Boundaries*. As noted by Papanikolaou (2008), this latter book

> aims to capture and conceptualize the complexity of informal care to older people at the intersection of work and life in different 'care work' contexts. It explores the flowing boundaries of caregiving across different care-giving societies . . . [through] contributions from 25 experienced academics looking at different aspects of the junctions between the private and public life, between professional and non-professional responsibilities, and between paid and non-paid work. (p. 44)

human suffering. Ameliorating this disconnect would enable the link between dying and caring, and ultimately bereavement, which is an important experience in a person's life course. We are, as a society, not very good at palliative and end-of-life care, and this may reflect our general aversion to dealing with the topic of death and our cultural gerontophobia.

The cultural and ethnic diversity of the Canadian population raises an additional set of concerns about the services provided to the aged and to palliative care patients. Canadians come from diverse ethnic and cultural backgrounds and different groups have different needs. While Western culture places strong emphasis on informed consent and the right of patients to "know the truth" about their health conditions, in some cultures (Chinese, Japanese, Korean, Ethiopian) family members are expected to protect the patient by "shielding the truth" about his or her condition (Turner, 2002). Some Canadians may feel discussing end-of-life care gives them the ability to express their wishes and to make sure that they are met, whereas others may view talking about death as a "bad omen" (Turner, 2002).

Due to fiscal constraints and lack of available long-term care facilities, older people might be "forced" into accepting a place in long-term care or residential facility where they may be completely isolated from their religious or cultural group. Our population is aging but it is also becoming more diverse, which will have immense repercussions on how to provide and organize care.

Patient Control over Dying and Assisted Suicide An area of increasing concern among sociological scholars, health professionals, ethicists, and lay persons is patient control over dying, which can lead to the charged issue of assisted suicide. Although decisions concerning how, when, and where patients should die have traditionally been the exclusive domain of health professionals, patients and their families are demanding increasing control over these decisions. This reflects a broader consumer orientation among health care users. Nevertheless, there is evidence to suggest that health care professionals maintain control over decisions even in the presence of patients' **advanced directives** or living wills (Kelner, Bourgeault, Hébert, & Dunn 1993). Health professionals often feel a tension between both their personal beliefs and sense of clinical autonomy, and their desire to heed their patients' wishes. One of the means by which some health professionals addressed this tension is through passive means, such as walking very slowly (informally referred to as a "slow code") to resuscitate a patient (Kelner & Bourgeault, 1993).

SUMMARY

In this chapter, we examined the tensions among viewing aging through the lens of various theories, and the view of aging as a medicalized transition to the life course perspective that emphasizes healthy aging. We have provided details about the aging Canadian population and showed some ways in which care has been structured and may need to be restructured to meet the changing needs of this population.

Specifically, we have provided evidence to detail how Canada's universal, publicly funded health care system has not been designed to accommodate a national approach to long-term care of older adults. Community-based home care and institutional LTC are not publicly insured services under the Canada Health Act and each province has developed its own terms and conditions under which these services are provided. As a result, an important problem facing the Canadian long-term care system is the regional disparities in the types of services and level of care available to seniors, including access to home and facility-based care. Beyond these issues, we have highlighted how in both the formal and informal care sector that most primary care providers for older people are women and they are disproportionately affected by the structure and organization of care both as care providers and recipients. At issue is the future supply of workers to this care sector. We concluded with an examination of end-of-life care with a focus on the growing interest and concern with older adults' control over their own dying. In all, the social dimensions of aging, health, and health care are dynamic and in a continuing state of flux.

Key Terms

Advanced directive—an advanced specification of the types of medical procedures one would or would not want to undergo if one became mentally incompetent or unable to communicate one's wishes

Ageism—discrimination on the basis of age

Aging—the natural process of gaining experience, reaching developmental milestones, emotionally growing, and physically changing as one increases in age

Apocalyptic demography—an ideology that perceives old age as a burden on the assets of society as resources get allocated to deal with sick, elderly populations at the expense of younger, healthier cohorts

Caring dilemma—the tension caused by being obliged to provide care without the right to determine how that care is to be provided

Centenarian—a person who is 100 years old or more

Cultural gerontophobia—a social and or cultural fear of aging that is often exhibited with an obsession with maintaining a young appearance or demeanour in a youth-obsessed culture

Deathways—the ways in which society structures and constrains the pathway to death or the trajectory of dying

Egocentric—a focus on the needs, wants, and desires of the self, disregarding others

Extended health services—include residential long-term care, home care, adult residential care, and ambulatory health services not covered under the principles of the Canada Health Act (universality, accessibility, public administration, portability, comprehensiveness) and restrictions on user fees and extra billing

Healthy aging—a process of positive development and progression through life

Insured services—include primary medical care and acute care covered by the five principles of the Canada Health Act

Medicalization of aging—the process by which the natural process of aging is reconceptualized as a disease that is to be addressed by a range of medical (principally pharmaceutical) interventions

Salutogensis—a term coined by Antonovsky in direct response to the pathogenic focus on disease and illness to redirect attention away from disease and toward health

Sense of coherence—a perception that the world makes sense; that it is a predictable, lucid, and meaningful place

Transitions—from a life-course perspective, are conceptualized as shifts in social identity that can be triggered by major life events (e.g. birth of a child, marriage, etc.)

Critical Thinking Questions

1. What are the pros and cons of medicalization as applied to the topic of aging?
2. What are the health care implications of the various conceptualizations of aging?
3. What factors need to be considered when balancing the care needs of older adults and their desire for independence, and how does this influence health care policy and service delivery?

Further Readings and Resources

The Canadian Association of Retired Persons: A new vision of aging in Canada. www.carp.ca/

Martel, L., Bélanger, A., Berthelot, J.-M., Carrière, Y. (2005). Healthy Aging. In *Healthy today, healthy tomorrow? Findings from the National Population Health Survey*. Statistics Canada Catalogue no. 82-618-MWE2005004. Ottawa: Statistics Canada.

Public Health Agency of Canada. (2010). *The chief public health officer's report on the state of public health in Canada 2010*. Available at www.phac-aspc.gc.ca/cphorsphc-respcacsp/2010/fr-rc/cphorsphc-respcacsp-06-eng.php

Chapter 10
Self Care and Health Care Behaviour

Chapter Outline

- **Learning Objectives**
- **Models of Health Behaviours and Health Care Utilization**
  - *The Health Belief Model*
  - *Social Cognitive Model*
  - *Stages of Change Theory*
- **Health Beliefs and Health Practices**
- **Sociological Approaches to the Study of Illness and Health Behaviour**

- **Interacting with the Formal Health Care System**
- **Complementary and Alternative Medicine**
  - *Definitions*
  - *Who Uses Complementary and Alternative Medicine and Why?*
- **Globalization and Medical Tourism**
  - *Where Are People Travelling and Why?*

Learning Objectives

After studying this chapter, you should be able to:

1. Apply the various explanations and theories that try to predict health care utilization to health care seeking behaviour;

2. Understand the context of lay health beliefs and practices and how gender and culture can influence these phenomena;

3. Describe the process by which how people come to interact with the various elements of the formal and informal health care system;

4. Reflect on the evolution of the role of people from patients to consumers in a global health environment.

Imagine that you are not feeling well. At what point do you decide to seek help? And what kind of help do you decide to seek? Do you first care for yourself with a range of home or over-the-counter remedies? At what point do you decide to seek professional care? Do you consult your family members or friends before making an appointment? Do you go to see a family physician, a nurse practitioner, or an alternative health care practitioner, such as a homeopathic specialist or a naturopath? The decisions that people make about care and seeking medical help are strongly rooted in social perceptions about health and illness. These perceptions are shaped by the social context within which individuals experience health problems. For instance, you may decide not to seek medical help if you are experiencing mild symptoms of a cold but you would likely change your mind if you were to develop a high fever. Pre-existing chronic health conditions, health status, age, gender, ethnicity, and interactions with others all play a role in forming decisions about seeking professional care. Your decision can also be influenced by the design and the structure of our health care system and your relationship with your health care provider. Do you think you would make a different decision about seeking medical help if your doctor could make a home visit? If you could see your doctor without booking an appointment, would you be more likely to go? If you had to pay a fee for a visit, would this affect your decision? If complementary and alternative medicine were free, would you be more likely to consider this type of care?

In this chapter you will learn about health beliefs and their impact on health practices, health care seeking behaviour, and health care utilization. We will discuss gender and cultural differences that affect health beliefs and practices. We will also discuss various conceptual models that are used to understand health care utilization among individuals. Examining formal care, we will look at provider–patient interactions in the formal care setting (e.g. physician–patient interaction) and understand the impact of the social status and health status of patients on these interactions. We will discuss how power of knowledge shapes medical encounters and analyze the shift toward **consumerism** in provider–patient communication and interactions. The last part of the chapter will focus on complementary and alternative medicine (CAM) and alternative methods of seeking help and consuming health services.

MODELS OF HEALTH BEHAVIOURS AND HEALTH CARE UTILIZATION

Understanding patterns of health behaviour and health care utilization are of critical importance to sociologists and health policy analysts. If we know why people choose to seek medical help and what paths they take in utilizing the health care system, we can design more effective public health campaigns, better redistribute health care system resources, and improve the health outcomes of the population. Psychologists, sociologists, and public health analysts have developed a number of conceptual models that help to predict health care utilization. These models, as Redding and colleagues (2000) suggest, should be viewed as "a roadmap of the health behaviour territory" (p. 181). They do not necessarily predict the behaviour of individuals seeking medical help, but they can be guiding tools to identify important social, structural, and psychological factors that play roles in health care utilization behaviour. In what follows, we describe three of these models and demonstrate their strengths and weaknesses in explaining health behaviours.

The Health Belief Model

The Health Belief Model analyzes people's health beliefs to determine the actions that they take to preserve their health (Rosenstock, 1974). It involves four specific factors (see Figure 10.1). *Perceived susceptibility* refers to an individual's perception of being at risk of developing a particular problem or condition. The *perceived seriousness* of the problem or condition refers to the individual's belief about the potential impact that this condition can have on her or his health. Both of these perceptions can be categorized together as an assessment of the threat that a condition has on a person's health. Considering the effectiveness of health protective behaviours, individuals assess the *perceived benefits* and *barriers* associated with preventive health actions that together make up the expectations of outcome. Based on the perceived threat of a condition and the potential outcome of intervention, individuals decide whether or not to take an action and to modify their behaviour. This last action step is also based on the individual's perceived ability to carry out the recommended action.

The Health Belief Model has undergone a number of modifications since its emergence in the early 1970s (Armstrong, 2000) but it remains influential in health research and health policy. Testing the usefulness of this theory on our own experiences, we may consider our decision making about receiving flu shots or other vaccinations. For example, you might ask yourself if, during the recent H1N1 flu epidemic, you considered receiving the flu vaccine and how you went about rationalizing your choice of actions considering the perceived susceptibility and the seriousness of the disease, the benefits of receiving the flu shot, and the costs associated with getting the vaccination (e.g., waiting times, going to the clinic, side effects, and so on).

Although the Health Belief Model has been influential, it has received its share of criticism. Despite the later incorporation of social factors into the model (such as level of social support), some argue that it still lacks a recognition of the social and economic context for the individual actors (Calnan, 1987). The major criticism of this model is its assumption that people's *behaviours* are rational and reflective of their *beliefs*. Evidently,

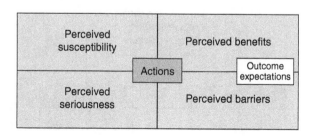

Figure 10.1 The Health Belief Model

it is very common for people to behave in ways that contradict their beliefs about risks, health, or illness. For example, most if not all people who smoke cigarettes know about the health risks involved but choose to continue this behaviour.

Social Cognitive Model

The Social Cognitive Model analyzes people's health beliefs through the triadic relationship among cognitive and personal characteristics, behaviour, and the environment. Taking its roots in social psychology, this model seeks to connect personal behaviours with social and environmental factors impacting the behaviours of individuals. These three factors influence each other and build a model of health behaviour (see Figure 10.2). According to this model, health behaviours do not exist in a social vacuum but are learned and influenced through social interactions and environmental factors. Similarly, behaviours can be influenced by environmental factors and personal beliefs.

To understand how health behaviour can be modified, we revisit smoking. Why do some people, despite knowing the dangers of tobacco, continue to smoke? Social cognitive theory provides a number of explanations for this phenomenon. First, individuals vary in perceptions about their *self-efficacy*, or the confidence that they can change their behaviour. If they tried to quit before and failed, it may prevent them from trying again. Similarly to the ideas presented in the Health Belief Model, some individuals may perceive the outcome of quitting as less beneficial than avoiding the challenging process of quitting. Some people also may lack the skills, resources, or capabilities to alter their behaviour.

Second, the social cognitive model places a strong emphasis on *observational learning* and *role models* in modifying the behaviour. If, for example, all of the people around a smoker decide to quit, offer their advice on how to do it effectively, and condemn smoking, it can motivate the individual to try quitting, to learn how to do it, and to re-evaluate his or her beliefs about the dangers of smoking. Alternatively, if all of those in an individual's social circle continue to smoke, it may make the effort to quit that much more challenging due to the social benefits of smoking.

It has been argued that a major benefit of this theory may also be its major drawback. Since the model covers the complex relationship among cognition, environment, and

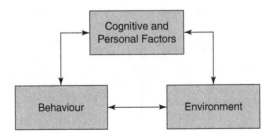

Figure 10.2 Social Cognitive Model

behaviour, operationalization becomes difficult (Stone, 1999). That is to say, how do we tell what is having a specific cause and effect on the health behaviour in question? It is unclear how we can study changes in behaviour when we need to take into account constantly changing social learning and interaction between various environmental factors and their influence on humans' cognition and behaviour.

Stages of Change Theory

Another model that looks at the process of behaviour change is the Stages of Change Theory. This model of health behaviour envisions the change as comprised of five sequential stages (Prochaska & DiClemente, 1983) (see Figure 10.3). The first stage, *precontemplation*, indicates that the person has not yet thought about changing or is not yet willing to make a change. During the second stage, *contemplation*, an individual begins to consider the possibility of making a change. The *preparation* stage signals small changes or readiness of the individual to try and change the behaviour and the *action* stage is where the change actually happens. The last stage, *maintenance*, refers to the need for continuous practice to preserve the new behaviour. As the arrows on the figure indicate, the goal is to achieve and maintain the change but at any stage there is a possibility of relapse. Thus critics claim that the process of change should be seen as cyclical with relapse being a recognized part of the behaviour change process (Zimmerman, Olsen, & Bosworth, 2000).

Each stage has its own goals and strategies that can be used to facilitate the desired behaviour (Zimmerman et al., 2000). Again referring back to the issue of smoking, at the precontemplation stage, the smoker would not indicate any desire to quit. At this point, health promotion efforts should be concentrated on education about the risks of smoking and the benefits of quitting to encourage the contemplation of quitting. When the smoker starts questioning the habit of smoking and considers the possibility of quitting, he or she

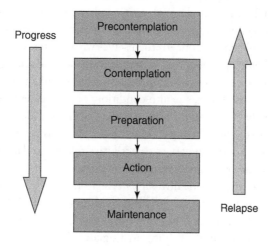

Figure 10.3 Stages of Change Model

has moved to contemplation. During the preparation stage, the individual begins to prepare for the quitting process by making small changes (such as not smoking in the car or in the house). At this point it is important that realistic goals be set to ensure a context of positive reinforcement for these goals. When the change—quitting smoking entirely—happens during the action stage, again, a context providing positive reinforcement is necessary (Zimmerman et al., 2000). Finally, during the maintenance stage, the individual must continue to be supported so as not to relapse. If relapse does happen here or at any other stage in the process, working back onto the stage of change is critical for ultimate success.

This model, although influential in program and policy development, because of its cyclical conceptualization, has also received its share of criticism. First, it provides little insight into how people make a change in the first place, what causes a person to successfully move from one stage to another, and why some individuals succeed while others do not (Munro, Lewin, Swart, & Volmink, 2007). Second, research demonstrates that actual applications of this model do not improve the chances of changing the behaviour (Horowitz, 2003). Other criticisms are oriented toward the assumptions made by this model that people are going through distinct stages and that the change in their behaviour is (much like the other models) based on a rational, well-calculated plan or series of actions. More importantly, all of these models focus on the illness and health behaviours at the individual level. While some of them (such as the social-cognitive model) do incorporate the importance of society on the decision-making of the individual, overall, the tendency is to analyze the change as happening to the individual.

HEALTH BELIEFS AND HEALTH PRACTICES

In previous chapters it was pointed out that health is unequally distributed across different segments of the population. In this section, we look at how health practices and beliefs shape the everyday lives of people from different social positions. We do so to better understand how social contact and social position shape the ways in which people perceive health and illness and pursue health care. Although there are exceptions (see Chapter 12), most people do not concern themselves with matters of illness and disease to the same extent as health professionals (Bury, 2005). Most people generally take good health and the absence of illness for granted and do not reflect on their health until threatened by symptoms of illness, a health condition, or an accident. Some people lead a healthy lifestyle, usually exhibited through everyday activities, such as healthy eating or exercising regularly. Therefore, the topic of health behaviour is better understood when it is contextualized in the routine practices or activities related to daily living rather than when it is presented as an open, general topic of inquiry.

Moreover, the attention to health varies based on the various social positions of people. For example, Michael Calnan and his colleagues (Calnan, 1987, 1994; Calnan & Williams, 1991) take this approach in examining health beliefs and health practices of working- and middle-class families living in England. Looking at diet, exercise, and health, Calnan argues that there are some important differences between working-class and middle-class respondents in the way health practices are conceptualized and incorporated into everyday life. For instance, whereas smoking was identified as a health-threatening behaviour among both groups of respondents, the connection made between smoking and ill health was made differently by individuals (Calnan & Williams, 1991). Middle-class respondents perceived smoking as a potential future harm to their health while working-class respondents conceptualized the link between smoking and health as actual, suggesting that smoking should be abandoned once ill health manifests itself. This difference in perception of smoking demonstrates how health rhetoric (e.g., smoking is bad for you) does not necessarily lead to action (e.g., quitting smoking) and can be interpreted differently by various groups.

Seeking to understand these differences in perceptions, Calnan looked at the social context in which health practices occur. For instance, in analyzing smoking, he demonstrated that the *meaning* of smoking was different for men and women (Calnan & Williams, 1991). Women saw smoking as a possibility to "get away" and relax, as a break from monotonous and stressful tasks that they performed in everyday life. Men defined smoking as a social and habitual activity. Therefore, Calnan and Williams (1991) suggest that "smoking has a differential meaning, place, and function according to gender" (p. 518).

Social class also predicted discernible differences in health beliefs and practices related to diet and exercise. Physical fitness, often cited as an essential component of a healthy lifestyle, was defined in "vocational" terms by working-class respondents and applied to their ability to perform everyday tasks and activities without physical limitation. Middle-class respondents, on the other hand, saw exercise as a means to maintain health and achieve well-being, as a recreational activity separate from their work. The markers of class and gender were also identified in the dietary practices of the households. In both situations, women bore primary responsibility for providing healthy diets to their families and struggled with lack of time and managing the eating preferences of their family members; however, working-class women were also burdened by the cost of healthy food (Calnan & Williams, 1991).

These findings indicate that the beliefs people hold about health and illness are not necessarily translated into everyday lives due, in part, to the structural barriers that people face while trying to implement a healthier lifestyle. Although health promotion often focuses on explaining the benefits of exercising or eating healthily, structural constraints (such as lack of time, a hazardous or stressful work environment, and lack of financial means) can prevent people from pursing healthy lifestyles. Moreover, people are often aware of these constraints. In a study conducted by Herzlich (2004) among middle-class individuals in France, the respondents made the link between health and "way of life." Urban living, which brings stress and anxiety to everyday life along with pollution and physical hazards, was perceived as causing illness and contributing to deterioration in health. Therefore, while individual lifestyles might have contributed to illness, the "way of life" in contemporary society was viewed as creating a paradox in which society demands health from individuals but at the same time it brings disease and distraction to health. A classic study started in Alameda County, California, in 1965 linked the following lifestyle behaviours to poor health and higher mortality twenty years later (Alameda County Study, n.d.):

- excessive alcohol consumption,
- smoking,
- obesity,
- hours of sleep (fewer or more than seven to eight hours per night),
- physical inactivity,
- eating between meals, and
- not eating breakfast.

Although dangers in the physical and social environment often permeate people's accounts of health and illness, when it comes to their everyday life, the definitions given to health can vary among individuals. Blaxter (1990) identified three ways in which people define health. The first is negative, defining health as the absence of disease. The second is functional, evaluating health based on the ability to perform everyday tasks. The third definition is a positive one, seeing health as overall well-being (Blaxter, 1990, p. 14). Interestingly, Blaxter also noted that having an illness or a chronic health condition is not necessarily defined by people as being "not healthy." Some individuals, despite their chronic health problems, see themselves as healthy based on a relative metric compared to people in similar positions. For example, this tendency was noted among older people who often tend to self-assess themselves as being healthy despite numerous health problems that come with old age (Cockerham, 2001).

Understanding the differences among the various definitions of health individuals make may explain this phenomenon. If health is defined negatively, such as an absence of disease, then by definition, the presence of disease means a person is "ill." Some people with chronic health conditions, however, have adapted to their illness by reorganizing their daily lives and redefining themselves and their bodies (see Chapter 11). Adapting to illness and continuing to perform their daily activities, these individuals may define their health functionally, assessing their ability to independently engage in daily activities. The frame of reference that people use in defining their health status is also important—we usually compare ourselves to our age groups and the general health status of people similar to us. That is why, as Cockerham (2001) notes, older people, who often see reaching old age itself as an indicator of health, can perceive themselves as healthy—the ability to be independent and to take care of themselves becomes a marker of health for them.

According to Cockerham (2001), we need to differentiate between illness behaviour and health behaviour (p. 90). **Health behaviour** is comprised of activities that seek to prevent illness and promote well-being; **illness behaviour** is oriented toward identifying the illness and seeking relief. So far we have described health behaviours and health beliefs and practices. We have also touched upon the theoretical models that describe how and why people decide to seek medical help. In the next section of this chapter we move on to describe illness behaviour and interaction with the health care system.

SOCIOLOGICAL APPROACHES TO THE STUDY OF ILLNESS AND HEALTH BEHAVIOUR

Unlike the conceptual models already discussed, broader sociological understandings of health and illness behaviour focus more on the social factors contributing to the illness experience and less on individual, psychological factors. For example, David Mechanic (1992), who studied people's decisions to seek medical help, emphasizes that many behaviours are actually constructed socially and culturally. Often our behaviours are not based on a conscious process of decision making but are a product of social culture. Therefore, instead of focusing on why individuals choose to smoke, Mechanic's approach is more aligned with understanding how and why some groups of people smoke while other groups do not. He encourages us to ask, what are the structural and the cultural differences between these populations? If we focus on societal influences and their impact on our understanding of health and illness, we can move beyond the **blaming the victim** approach that emphasizes personal failure in some individuals who do not adopt a healthy lifestyle.

This approach is also useful in analyzing the decision to seek medical help. According to Mechanic (1992), this process consists of two steps that can be experienced one after another or simultaneously. During the first step, the individual monitors the discomfort in her or his body, seeks to understand its nature, its severity, and its symptoms. During the second step, the individual seeks an explanation for the somatic experience and tries to understand its seriousness and its potential dangers. Should the assessment indicate that the discomfort signals a "serious" condition, the individual may decide to seek medical help (Mechanic, 1992). Moreover, the "seriousness" of the condition is not an objective, scientifically established fact. Rather, it is based on the personal familiarity of an individual with the experienced symptoms and his or her ability to explain them and includes four dimensions for assessment of the "seriousness" (see Figure 10.4).

Although Mechanic's approach does not deny the importance of individual characteristics, which may include sensitivity to bodily changes, levels of stress, or previous medical history, he still places the utmost importance on the role of social and cultural forces in shaping health and illness behaviour. For instance, the absence of medical insurance

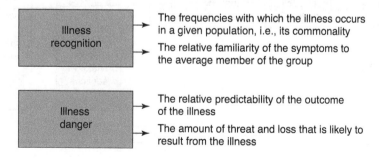

Figure 10.4 Mechanic's Four Dimensions for Assessing Illness

Source: Mechanic, D. (1961). The concept of illness behavior. *Journal of Chronic Disease, 15,* 189–194

(which is a more important factor in the United States context) may play a crucial role in making the decision to see a doctor. Similarly, if being sick disrupts the usual routine and places a serious burden on a person's family, the decision to seek medical help can be abandoned or at least postponed (Mechanic, 1992). Most notably, the illness recognition and illness danger components in this model are heavily influenced by cultural and social beliefs and the exposure to similar symptoms through a person's social network.

The Socio-Behavioural Model of Health Services proposed by Andersen (& Newman, 1973; Andersen, 1995) is another attempt to understand health-seeking behaviour and is particularly useful for identifying predictors of use to assess whether services are equitably distributed based on need or something else. The model identifies three sets of predictors, including predisposing, enabling, and need factors. Predisposing factors include, but are not limited to, demographic variables such as gender, marital status, race, age, and education. Enabling factors refer to both social and structural resources (e.g., social support from friends and family, and income) that facilitate or impede access to formal care. Need factors are the symptoms or experience of illness (including severity) that prompt an individual to seek help. The measurement of need can be based on evaluated (diagnostic) criteria or perceived criteria (see Figure 10.5).

The inclusion of predisposing and enabling factors in Andersen's model permits examination of a broad range of individual and social determinants of service use that may vary across various social-structural factors such as gender and family structure. For example, given their elevated risk for psychiatric morbidity, single mothers and fathers should be more likely to receive professional services for their mental health care needs (Wade, Veldhuizen, & Cairney, 2011). However they may not seek care because of a lack of enabling factors, such as lower income or social support. By examining the relative and combined contribution of these factors, we can assess which factors account for the greatest share of the variation in health care use.

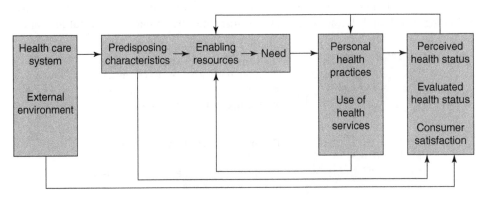

Figure 10.5 Andersen's Socio-Behavioural Model

Source: Andersen, R. M. (1995). Revisiting the behavioral model and access to medical care: does it matter? *Journal of Health and Social Behavior, 36*(1), 1–10, p. 8.

INTERACTING WITH THE FORMAL HEALTH CARE SYSTEM

Today, when we seek help to alleviate our pain and sickness, the decision to seek medical assistance is the most common practice. It was not so long ago that individuals seeking help would think to choose from a variety of health care providers that included not only physicians, but also homeopaths, naturopaths, traditional healers, and many more. Today, most Canadians access the physician-led health care system. (We discuss the resurgence of complementary and alternative medicine later in this chapter.)

While people have health beliefs, assess their health, and define the point at which they will consult a physician, doctors in our society have the power to "label" the individual as sick. With this label legitimized by the physician, the person enters the sick role, discussed in detail in Chapter 11. In seeking medical help, individuals acknowledge that they want to feel better, and it is the role of the physician to assess and treat them (Parsons, 1951). In this role, physicians gain access to a patient's body, access that in other everyday social encounters would be seen as inappropriate or too exposing. In the context of provider–patient interaction, the social contract between physician and patient permits the physician to engage in such an encounter with the patient. The model proposed by Parsons presumed a necessary level of trust between patient and physician. It is also based on the premise that knowledge about the disease and its treatment is in the hands of physician, leaving the patient to follow the physician's advice and comply with treatment.

Challenges to this traditional view of the medical encounter have been proposed from a number of theoretical angles. Some sociologists, such as Freidson (1970b), Zola (1994), and others criticize the physician-dominant position on which the interaction between the physician and patient is based. The power to define a discomfort as a "disease" instead of malingering is located in the hands of the health care provider. The patient can have little or no role in presenting his or her point of view on the issue. In addition, despite Canadians' universal access to health care, it has been often demonstrated that people of different social statuses receive different quality of care. Differences in socio-economic status also influence the ability to receive a medical diagnosis and to gain a referral to a medical specialist (Dunlop, Coyte, & McIsaac, 2000; McKinlay, 1996).

Criticism of the unbalanced distribution of power in the patient-provider encounter is not limited to medical sociologists. Increasingly, health care providers and health policy makers have started to acknowledge that patients should have more say in their own care. The move toward consumerism in health care has characterized the health care systems of many developed nations. This is most explicitly conceptualized by Haug and Lavin (1983), who describe how patients have become more like consumers who have the knowledge and the power to influence the medical encounter, to ask questions about their treatment, and assume the right to participate in their care. In many countries, including Canada, treatments suggested by physicians are ideally reached through discussion and **informed consent**. Patients now have a right to access their medical records and all the information in their medical chart through their province's freedom of information legislation. Moreover, with increasingly easy access to knowledge about medical issues from a variety of sources, most significantly the internet, some individuals come to their medical appointment armed with information (sometimes of variable quality) wanting to actively participate in decisions regarding their diagnosis and care. While the previous era of medical encounters was defined as the period of medical dominance (Freidson, 1970b), today many sociologists suggest that the profession of medicine is undergoing a process of **deprofessionalization** (Haug, 1988) which signifies the physician's loss of autonomy over the medical encounter and medical decision making.

As we argue in other chapters (Chapters 3 and 12), we are far from reaching the point where medicine has lost its autonomy or its dominance. Moreover, the availability of medical information on the internet does not necessarily mean that all Canadian patients have become active consumers participating in their own care. Availability of care and factors such as age, socio-economic class, gender, and ethnicity all play a role in shaping interactions in formal health care settings. In previous chapters we discussed the idea that access to health services is unequally distributed across several characteristics such as geography and demographics. When access to care is limited, it makes it practically impossible to "shop around" for a better health care provider. Access to medical information as well as the ability to negotiate the medical encounter and navigate through the health care system makes it easier for middle- and upper-class Canadians to become consumers in the health care system, leaving lower-status individuals at a disadvantage (Chappell & Penning, 2009, pp. 124–125). The lack of access to medical care and the lack of knowledge about navigating the health care system may also partially explain why the health of Canadian immigrants deteriorates over time once they settle in Canada (Pederson & Raphael, 2006).

Moreover, access itself does not mean that people receive equal treatment in communication with their health care providers. Gender, for example, has an enormous impact on the dynamic of the medical encounter (Lorber & Moore, 2002). Male physicians tend to spend less time with their patients and dominate the conversation more often than female doctors (Lorber & Moore, 2002). Female physicians prescribe more pap smears and mammography tests than male doctors (Lorber & Moore, 2002). The length and quality of conversation between doctors and patients are also marked by gender differences. For example, West (1984) found that female doctors interrupt male patients less frequently than they do their female patients.

Gender and ethnic inequality, which both play a role in medical encounters, should not be seen as affecting only physicians. Other health care providers are not immune to personal biases. In her ethnographic study analyzing interactions between midwives and South Asian women in the United Kingdom, Bowler (1994) found that racial discrimination influenced the interaction between midwives (who were all white and predominantly of British descent) and their South Asian clients and shaped the practices of care rendered to these women. Examining the impact of these stereotypes, she found that midwives saw their South Asian patients as problematic due to:

1. Difficulty in communication posed by language barriers and differences in cultural norms;

2. The women's lack of compliance with care and perceived abuse of health services;

3. Their tendency to complain about pain and headaches during and after labour; and

4. The women's perceived lack of "normal maternal instinct," which was explained as the women's unwillingness to breastfeed the baby right after delivery or through preferences for male infants.

These perceptions negatively influenced communication between women and midwives and further marginalized South Asian women (Bowler, 1994).

While social factors such as age, gender, and socio-economic factors undeniably set a context in which the interaction occurs, the medical encounter itself can shape the communication between health care provider and the patient. Examining the context of provider–patient communication, Heritage and Maynard (2006) demonstrated that physicians and patients actively construct their social encounter based on the differences in the types of questions asked by physicians and verbal and non-verbal communication. As well, the opportunities given to patients to present their medical problems not only impact patients' satisfaction, but also affect compliance with medical treatment and health outcomes overall.

At the same time, patients also influence the medical encounter and decision making of health care providers. In pediatric medical visits, for example, when physicians were under the impression that parents wanted antibiotics for their children, the doctors prescribed them more often and also diagnosed the illness as requiring a treatment with antibiotics more often (Heritage & Maynard, 2006).

Finally, it should be noted that patients sharing decision making in medical encounters is neither always possible nor desirable by the patients (Bury & Gabe, 2004; Charles, Gafni, & Walen, 1997). Although informed consent and active participation in the treatment process can be favourable in some situations, such as chronic illnesses or an ongoing medical problem, in the case of sudden heart attack or other acute problems that significantly incapacitate a person and require urgent medical attention, informed consent and participation in decision making during the medical encounter are moot. Moreover, patients' ability and willingness to ask questions and to actively participate in medical encounters varies by age and social class (Lupton, 2003). As Lupton (2003) shows, older people and patients from lower socio-economic backgrounds tend to be less "active" in their care. Analyzing interviews with African American teen mothers, Brubaker (2007) found that in some situations, young mothers were relieved when the decision making was in the "hands" of the physicians—following medical advice rather than making their own decision. This both allowed them to transfer the responsibility for their care to physicians and to demonstrate their compliance with the advice on pregnancy and childbirth, which is consistent with the image of a "good" mother.

Nevertheless, most researchers agree that we are no longer living in the era of overarching dominance of the medical profession (Coburn, Torrance, & Kaufert, 1983; Conrad, 2005; Light, 2000). Some attribute this shift to the increasing involvement of the state in the provision and regulation of health care services (Coburn et al., 1983), others to the triumph of capitalism, which succeeded in undermining the power of the medical profession (Navarro, 1988), and still others to the introduction of the market model into the health care system (Calnan & Rowe, 2007). The expansion of the role and scope of other health professionals, both within and outside of mainstream medicine, also had an impact. While all of these developments may have played a role in a social shift toward a medical model of care that is more balanced in its distribution of power, it should also be noted that the larger socio-historical context could have set in motion the erosion of medical authority. Similar distrust in authority is quite common in contemporary post-modern society and extends far beyond medicine. People are less likely to trust social institutions, such as politics and the legal system. Nevertheless, for many medical sociologists, the existence of trust between a patient and medical care provider seems to be a crucial component for successful health outcomes and any undermining of this trust would not necessarily benefit the patients (Calnan & Rowe, 2007; Heritage & Maynard, 2006; Lupton, 2000).

So far, we have demonstrated that the interactions between health care professionals and their patients in formal medical encounters are shaped by such social factors as gender, age, ethnicity, and culture. We also showed that the power imbalance in the medical encounter is influenced by the wider socio-cultural context and can shift between a patient and a physician. In the next section, we move on to the complementary and alternative medicine that is rapidly growing in popularity among Canadians.

COMPLEMENTARY AND ALTERNATIVE MEDICINE

Definitions

Complementary and alternative medicine (CAM) is typically defined "residually" as those therapeutic approaches that fall outside of orthodox Western biomedicine (see Chapter 4 for a discussion of naturopathy) (Achilles, 2001; Hirschkorn & Bourgeault, 2007). Conversely, CAM is also defined positively as a group of practices/practitioners embodying the characteristics of holism, vitalism, and individualized care (Kelner & Wellman, 2000). Not surprisingly, attempts at categorizing practices/practitioners as CAM are contested and vary according to political context, point of view, and study design (Achilles, 2001; Kelner & Wellman, 2000). Preliminary results from an internationally facilitated consensus process (Hirschkorn, Andersen, Bourgeault, 2009) identified the following as core practitioner-based or self-care CAM therapies/modalities:

- acupuncture
- traditional Chinese medicine
- homeopathy
- herbal supplements
- nutrition therapy

In Canada, chiropractic medicine was also included as a core therapy, and various other therapies/modalities were identified for other countries.

Who Uses Complementary and Alternative Medicine and Why?

In recent decades, there has been a large increase in the consumption of CAM in the Western world (Goldstein, 2000), including Canada (Kelner & Wellman, 2000). According to the 2003 Canadian Community Health Survey (CCHS), approximately 20% of Canadians 12 years old or older used some form of alternative medicine (Park, 2005). There is also some indication that the use of CAM is increasing, since in 1994–1995 only 15% of Canadians over 18 years old were reported to have used CAM (Park, 2005). Even more far-reaching than CAM, over 76% of Canadians have purchased natural health products such as vitamins, minerals, homeopathics, and herbal products. Sixty-nine percent of Canadian adults report having used one or more natural health products at least once in the past week prior to being surveyed (Health Canada, 2011) (see Researcher Profile 10.1).

The growing popularity of CAM can be explained by a number of factors. First, as we indicated in the previous section, the slow erosion of medical authority can partially account for why people look for alternative methods of treatment. Dissatisfaction with medical care, increasing public distrust in physicians, and the increased availability of information and greater awareness may have opened the doors to alternative forms of healing. Second, CAM is becoming more and more accessible. Globalization and the mixing of various culture-based health care providers has increased access to different forms of healing practice. Yoga, Chinese medicine, Reiki, and many other forms of healing are now more readily accessible to Canadians. Moreover, the formal health care systems in many Western countries has become more tolerant toward CAM (Kelner et al., 2006) and private insurance policies provided to employees in some workplaces have added CAM practitioners to their list of covered services. Adding further legitimacy, many CAM practitioners such as naturopaths, acupuncturists, and traditional Chinese medicine practitioners are now regulated by provincial regulatory bodies in Canada.

Arguably one of the most important additional factors contributing to the growth in the use of CAM is the increase in a variety of chronic health problems for which conventional medicine does not provide a cure. Among those reporting the use of CAM, 37% listed suffered from fibromyalgia, 36% had back problems, and 28% listed migraines and chronic fatigue syndrome as their health problems (Park, 2005). The use of CAM is also prevalent among patients with cancer and other terminal diseases (Bourgeault, 1996).

The use of CAM is unevenly distributed among the population. Studies done in the United States demonstrate that members of visible minority groups and those from lower socio-economic backgrounds are less likely to use CAM than are white, affluent individuals

Heather Boon

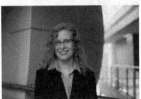

Courtesy of Heather Boon

Heather Boon, BScPhm, PhD, is a Professor and the Interim Dean at the Leslie Dan Faculty of Pharmacy, University of Toronto. She originally trained as a pharmacist and then completed a PhD in the field of Medical Sociology. Having helped to establish the Interdisciplinary Network on Complementary and Alternative Medicine (IN-CAM) in Canada, she now also holds the position of President of the International Society of Complementary Medicine Research (ISCMR). She previously served as the Chair of Health Canada's Expert Advisory Committee for Natural Health Products from 2006 to 2009. Her primary research interests are the safety and efficacy of natural health products as well as complementary/alternative medicine regulation and policy issues. She is the author of a textbook on natural health products and over 100 academic publications on CAM.

(McFarland, Bigelow, Zani, Newsom, & Kaplan, 2002). Geographic region is also a factor. In Canada, people in the Western provinces are more likely to use CAM more frequently and receive insurance benefits for their use (McFarland et al., 2002). As Park (2005) notes, however, these differences can be explained by the unequal distribution of health insurance coverage of CAM across Canadian provinces. For example, Manitoba pays for 12 visits to a chiropractor while Newfoundland and Labrador do not pay for any chiropractic services (Park, 2005).

Since CAM is not automatically covered under provincial health care plans (Medicare) or supplementary insurance, it is probably not surprising that income and education have an influence on the use of CAM. In 2003, 26% of Canadians from the highest-income households accessed CAM while only 13% from the lowest-income group did (Park, 2005). Higher levels of education are associated with higher income and with employment that has additional health insurance. However, it could also be explained within a *fundamental causes framework* (see Chapter 7) that different levels of education have a role in the awareness and access to CAM. People with higher education levels may know more about different forms of CAM, they have more resources to research alternative therapies, could be more open to alternative forms of treatment, and have more diverse social networks in which they can learn about CAM. The use of CAM is also unequally distributed by age and gender. Younger and older people are less likely to use CAM than people between 25 and 64 (Park, 2005) and women are more likely than men to consult CAM practitioners. It is evident, therefore, that differences in health care utilization are spread beyond the formal medical structure and persist in the use of CAM.

GLOBALIZATION AND MEDICAL TOURISM

Travelling to another country in search of a better treatment has always been practised to some extent. The phenomenon of **medical tourism**, however, is seen by many as a new development in self-care (Horowitz, Rosensweig, & Jones, 2007). Medical tourism is best understood as "a manifestation of an increasingly privatized global medical market arising in the wake of globalization and the diffusion of neoliberal economic policies that expanded space for private health care market growth in much of the world" (Hopkins, Labonté, Runnels, & Packer 2010, p. 193). Globalization and improvement in technology have made medical tourism more accessible. In the United States alone, close to 750 000 individuals a year are expected to seek medical care abroad (Horowitz et al., 2007). Although Canada has been a destination for Americans seeking treatment and pharmaceuticals at lower cost—and Canadians have sought access in the United States to treatments not available or treatments with long waiting lists in Canada, most of the growth in the medical tourism industry has been from the northern to the southern hemisphere. As Table 10.1 indicates, in each world region there is a number of countries that attract medical tourists, offering more sophisticated and/or less expensive care.

Where Are People Travelling and Why?

It is probably safe to assume that the majority of individuals would prefer to receive health care within their own home country. After all, travelling to another place to undergo a medical treatment can add uncertainty and concerns about recovering "on the road." Nevertheless, a growing number of individuals do travel abroad to receive medical treatment. In what follows, we describe the motives that drive people to look for medical care offshore (Hopkins et al., 2010):

Table 10.1 Countries of Destination for Medical Tourists by World Region

Africa	America	Asia	Europe	Middle East	Other
South Africa	Argentina	China	Belgium	Israel	Australia
Tunisia	Brazil	India	Czech Republic	Jordan	Barbados
	Canada	Malaysia	Germany		Cuba
	Colombia	Singapore	Hungary		Jamaica
	Costa Rica	South Korea	Italy		
	Ecuador	Philippines	Latvia		
	Mexico		Lithuania		
	United States		Poland		

Source: Horowitz, M. D., Rosensweig, J. A., & Jones, C. A. (2007). Medical tourism: Globalization of the healthcare marketplace: Medical tourism destinations. *Medscape General Medicine, 9*(4), 33.

- *Better quality of care*
  Traditionally, more industrialized countries also have more advanced medical care systems and medical technology. Although this path is only available to more affluent individuals who can afford not only the cost of medical treatment but also the cost of travel, some people travel abroad to receive a better quality of care.

- *Economic reasons*
  While the travel to more "developed" countries marked medical tourism of the past, today many individuals from richer countries travel to the global South to seek medical treatment at a reduced cost. Some scholars suggest that receiving medical treatment in India costs about 10% of the price that individuals would have paid for the same treatment in the United States (Horowitz et al., 2007).

- *Waiting times*
  Another argument in favour of using health services abroad could be the long waiting times for medical care that are a current reality of some health care systems. In Canada, as well as in the United Kingdom, waiting periods to see a specialist and undergo surgery could extend to months. Bypassing the system by travelling abroad allows individuals to receive health services without waiting.

- *Availability of procedures*
  Finally, many people travel abroad to undergo a medical treatment that is not available in their home country. Procedures such as sex reassignment, advanced fertility treatments, or new and untested medical techniques may not be offered or may be prohibited in some health care systems.

In addition to a variety of individual reasons that make medical tourism more accessible, it is also useful to understand the social context of the expansion of medical tourism. The availability of technology made access to international medical care more available. Today, surfing the internet in the comfort of their own homes, individuals can find what they see as the most suitable treatment, receive information on the quality of offered treatments, arrange for the date and time of the procedure, and book flight and travel accommodations (Horowitz et al., 2007). Moreover, recognizing the benefits of cost savings on medical expenses, some private health insurance companies are offering to cover the expenses of medical procedures performed abroad (Horowitz et al., 2007). Finally, an additional structural factor that should be considered is the unequal distribution of advances in medical treatment on a global scale.

Those who support the growth of medical tourism argue that it will have positive economic and development effects on the countries offering services. Others, however, raise concerns about patient safety, the ethics of specific types of care only offered abroad (e.g., **transplant tourism**), and the growth of private markets that medical tourism fosters in developing countries at the expense of adequately staffed and resourced public health care systems for the local population (Hopkins et al., 2010). There are also concerns about the effect on the local health care system when medical tourists return home and experience complications arising from out-of-country treatments. What all seem to agree upon is that medical tourism will not abate in the near future (Hopkins et al., 2010).

SUMMARY

This chapter highlighted how health and illness behaviours are shaped by social and cultural factors. We started with the description of health belief and health practices models that seek to understand the behaviours of individuals. These models, focusing on the individual, for the most part do not fully take into consideration the social and structural factors that influence behaviour. More sociological contributions to the field demonstrate the degree to which our "choices" and "practices" are constrained or shaped by our social milieu. Just as in other spheres of social life, age, class, gender, ethnicity, and other factors such as sexual orientation or disability influence access and use of formal and alternative health services. Disadvantaged groups usually do not have equitable access to the most advanced and most sophisticated types of health care, even when public funding to these services is provided and especially when it is not.

Key Terms

Blaming the victim—when applied to health beliefs and practices, emphasizes the personal failure of individuals to stay healthy

Consumerism—within the discussion of health care, the empowerment of the patient/consumer to guide and choose among different options of treatment and medical care

Deprofessionalization—the loss of autonomy of medicine over the medical encounter and medical decision making

Health behaviour—activities that individuals pursue to prevent illness and promote well-being

Illness behaviour—actions taken by individuals in identifying the illness and seeking relief

Informed consent—consent for treatment reached by the patient and the health care provider after the patient has been given an adequate explanation about the condition and the options for treating it

Medical tourism—a manifestation of an increasingly privatized global medical market arising in the wake of globalization and the diffusion of neoliberal economic policies that expanded space for private health care market growth in much of the world

Transplant tourism—commercialization of organ donor and transplants involving the marketing, selling, and purchasing of organs for transplants and the provision of medical treatments that use these organs

Critical Thinking Questions

1. Using obesity as a topic, compare and contrast the various models of health behaviour and health care seeking.

2. How does the practice of informed consent shape the power relations between health care providers and patients?

3. What are the advantages and disadvantages of introducing the politics of consumerism into health care services delivery?

4. What are the possible impacts of the development of medical tourism on the health care services and organization?

Further Readings and Resources

Calnan, M. (1987). *Health & illness: Lay perspective*. London and New York: Tavistock Publications.

Herzlich, C. (2004). The individual, the way of life and the genesis of illness. In M. Bury & J. Gabe (Eds.). *The sociology of health and illness: A reader* (pp. 27–35). London and New York: Routledge.

Lorber, J., & Moore, L. J. (2002). *Gender and the social construction of illness*. Walnut Creek, CA: Altamira.

Chapter 11
Health and Illness Experiences

Chapter Outline

Learning Objectives

After studying this chapter, you should be able to:

1. Examine how people experience illness;

2. Describe various ways of conceptualizing the illness experience;

3. Analyze the roles of social class, gender, and ethnicity in shaping the experiences of illness;

4. Demonstrate that rather than being an objective condition, the meaning of illness varies culturally and historically and is always shaped by society.

Every day we perform thousands of activities using our bodies. We usually do not reflect on the physiological processes that are required for walking, driving, eating, or engaging in other basic activities. In most cases, we use our body mechanically, unconsciously, without thinking through the physics, biology, mechanics, and chemistry behind the process. For many of us, the body is "just there" until it signals that something is wrong with it through manifestation of some unusual behaviour. After breaking an arm, for example, the person might suddenly realize to what degree his or her ability to be physically active becomes restricted and how many routine tasks the arm was performing before this unfortunate incident.

We have a complex relationship with our bodies. We *are* bodies in the sense that we cannot function in this world without a body. We also *have* bodies that we can use, decorate, make work hard, or diet. We *experience* our bodies and we experience the world through our bodies (Turner, 1996). Moreover, the way we see our bodies and the way we teach them to move, to talk, or to respond to the world around us is shaped by our society (Merleau-Ponty, 1962). Therefore, experiencing illness is always a social phenomenon because the way we see our bodies and interpret the signs given by them is mediated through meanings constructed in social interactions. It is also a social phenomenon because illness can limit the ability of individuals to fulfill their roles in society. Finally, different illnesses have different cultural meanings. While a person who recently had a heart attack, an individual with a broken limb, someone who had been diagnosed with cancer, or a patient with AIDS are all experiencing the physical dimensions of an illness (e.g., sudden, temporary, chronic, or potentially life threatening), they are also affected by the moral and cultural meanings attached to each of these conditions and this shapes the experience of illness for each one of them in unique ways.

In this chapter, we examine how people experience illness and discuss how illness changes the identity and the social roles of the individuals. We start by introducing sociological theorizing on the illness experience, which argues that health and illness are both socially constructed concepts. As such, they receive a specific meaning and shape the somatic (bodily) experiences of the individual's suffering from illness. Taking a chronology of the illness development, we reflect on the role of the body in signalling the existence of illness. In doing so, we differentiate among (1) routine illness (e.g., the common cold or a simple infection), (2) acute and serious illness, and (3) chronic illness because all of them have different meanings and different consequences for the lives of the ill individuals and the people around them. In the next part of this chapter, we discuss various sociological conceptualizations of the experiences of individuals suffering from illness within and outside the health care system. Starting from the classical conceptualization of Parson's sick role, we move on to current models that incorporate the "insider view" of illness. In the final part of this chapter we map out the socio-cultural variations in the experiences of illness. We demonstrate the impact of macro, structural relations on personal experiences of illness, looking at the role of social class, gender, and ethnicity in shaping the experiences of health and illness.

THE SOCIOLOGICAL VIEW OF HEALTH AND ILLNESS

When we talk about society, social relations, or social structures, we simultaneously refer to the individuals who comprise society. Individuals occupy statuses in which they carry out tasks and perform various roles and activities. These roles are guided by specific societal expectations about what are considered appropriate behaviours. Illness can disrupt the normal roles of individuals. If someone is sick, he or she may not be able to perform the usual tasks or activities. Moreover, the type of illness can have different effects on a person's capacity to perform the roles. The difference between a mild cold and a heart attack exists not only in the symptoms and physiology of these two conditions but also in the way they are experienced by individuals and accommodated by society. While a mild cold usually lasts four to seven days and then goes away, a heart attack can significantly change someone's life through changes in perception of self, social roles, social and economic status, and interactions with others. A sociological analysis of the illness experience lies in this intersection of the relationship between the body, the self, and society. In what follows, we present a number of conceptualizations of the illness experience, starting from the structural functionalist view of illness followed by interpretive approaches grounded in individuals' everyday lives.

The Sick Role

One of the most influential concepts in medical sociology, the **sick role**, was introduced by Talcott Parsons (1902–1979), an American sociologist, whose writings significantly contributed to the development of the structural functionalist study of society (Parsons, 1951). Parsons sought to understand the relationship between illness and social structures. He saw illness as both a biological and a social experience that changes the social roles normally performed by individuals. Parsons believed that individuals who are sick are unable to function properly, both physiologically and socially. The illness therefore requires the individual to deviate from usual activities, which changes the person's status to one of deviance. This new status is seen as undesirable and thus the individual wants to get well as soon as possible so as to return to his or her normal activities. The concept of the sick role normalized the deviance of the individual who is not well and defined the unique rights and obligations of that role (see Figure 11.1).

Based on this model, the individual is not required to perform or is otherwise exempt from usual social roles when he or she is sick. The more severe the disease, the longer or

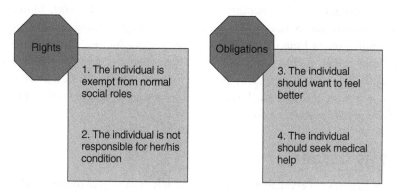

Figure 11.1 Talcott Parsons' Sick Role

Source: Adapted from Parsons, T. (1951). *The social system.* New York: The Free Press.

more extensive is the exemption from normal social roles. Moreover, the sick individual is seen as not responsible for having an illness and therefore the deviance is unintentional. The sick person, however, is obligated to seek out and comply with competent (i.e., medical) help in order to get well as soon as possible. The doctor's role, in turn, is to validate the sick role and assist the patient by administering treatment.

The four components of the sick role are interdependent. For instance, the exemption from normal social roles is based on the assumption that the person should not be blamed for contracting the disease and should have a desire to get well and reach out for medical help. Being sick but refusing to seek medical help can create a situation in which the individual is held responsible for sickness. Similarly, the exemption from normal social roles and responsibilities is predicated on seeking medical help. For example, being sick in and of itself does not give a student permission to miss an exam but a note from a medical doctor legitimizes the absence. Most importantly, the model developed by Parsons argues that disease does not only modify the body of an individual but also changes his or her social roles and social expectations.

Parsons' model was very influential in medical sociology, reflected in large part by the degree of attention and criticism it received (Bury, 1997). For instance, analyzing the experiences of illness among Italian Catholics, Protestants, and Jewish men residing in Rhode Island, Twaddle (1969) suggested that it is wrong to see a sick role as one, universal frame. Instead, his findings revealed that there are different ways in which individuals understand the concepts of being well or being sick, as well as different cultural and behavioural norms that render different conceptualizations that can all be defined as "sick roles." Criticism was also raised against Parsons' suggestion that sick individuals are not held responsible for their condition. Individuals are often blamed for contracting a disease (Varul, 2010). For example, people who contract STDs or chronic smokers who have lung cancer are typically not exempted from the responsibility of getting sick.

More relevant to this chapter's topic, however, is the criticism levelled against Parsons' model by scholars studying chronic illness (Bury, 2000; Crossley, 1998; Radley, 1994; Segall, 1976, 1997). Parsons' (1951) model assumes that illness is a temporary state that creates a disruption in the performance of everyday tasks. However, in many cases, illnesses and disabilities are not curable. People suffering from chronic illness and disability are not fully exempt from their social roles and responsibilities. The care and support they seek from formal and informal sources is to help them manage their sickness to allow them to fulfill these roles and responsibilities to the best of their abilities. In what follows, we present a number of sociological models that have sought to explain the unique manner in which people experience chronic illness.

Illness as Career

As much as Parson's conceptualization of the sick role contributed to the development of medical sociology (Williams, 2005), it can say very little about the experience of illness, or express an "insider view" on illness. The sick role does not explain what impact this exemption has on the individual's everyday life experiences. It also does not assist in understanding changes in social relations of the individuals.

Different diseases have different cultural and social meanings. Having epilepsy and having a cold can hardly be seen as similar experiences. Individuals with epilepsy have to organize their lives with a constant awareness of the possibility of an epileptic seizure. Their sense of self becomes constructed around the needs to monitor their bodies, conceal their experiences from others, and deal with the stigma attached to epilepsy (Conrad & Schneider, 1980). Having a cold may require a temporary change in roles and responsibilities but, in the absence of further complications such as pneumonia, it will not have a long-lasting effect.

Focusing on management of identity and the experiences of illness, many sociologists chose to study the experiences of chronic illness. The studies on chronic illness conceptualized **illness as a career** and as a process that requires adaption, reconstruction of self, and reorganization of daily life (Conrad, 1987; Young, 2004). This adaptation requires a restructuring of daily roles and responsibilities, changes in perception of self, and coping with stigma attached to illness (see Box 11.1 on the management of medical regimens). The onset of chronic illness challenges the taken-for-granted cycle of life and necessitates questioning of the meaning of the experienced symptoms, the need to reconstruct order in life, and the need to regain control over life (Charmaz, 2000).

Studying young people with rheumatoid arthritis (RA), Bury (1997) introduced the concept of **biographical disruption** into the study of illness experience. He showed that illness disrupts the socially expected chronological order of events and necessitates reorganization of social roles and responsibilities. As individuals, we are expected to take a

---

Box 11.1

The Management of Medical Regimens

In his 1985 article, "The meaning of medications: Another look at compliance," Peter Conrad (1985) re-examined the extent to which a person's behaviour complies with medical advice. He contrasted those suffering from chronic disease as more passively compliant with other patients who take a more active approach in which they manage their own regimens. In the case of epilepsy, Conrad spoke of *self-regulation* as opposed to *compliance;* how they undertook what he referred to as *medication practice* by which they attempted to assert control through such tactics as:

Testing—whereby they would intermittently take themselves off medication;

Control dependence—because their drugs were seen as a threat to self-reliance;

Destigmatization—by taking their drugs in private; and by

Practical practice—that is, adjusting the dosage by sometimes taking more or less medication depending on its effect.

Conrad argued that the *meaning of medications* should be emphasized in this management process.

certain trajectory in our lives (e.g., building a career, starting a family, and so on). Chronic illness disrupts this trajectory. People can feel that an illness threatens their sense of self, they can experience loss of control over their bodies and lives, and their relationship with others can be altered (Bury, 1982). The social situation and the availability of various resources among those suffering from chronic illness will facilitate the context in which the illness is reconsidered in everyday life.

As Charmaz (2000) notes, the diagnosis of an illness in and of itself does not necessarily define the *meaning* of the illness to the individual or those around the individual. Dealing with the body in everyday life becomes a process through which individuals learn what it means to have their illness. When the body refuses to complete previously taken-for-granted, routine activities, the illness manifests itself and becomes hard to ignore. The response varies from feeling alienated from your own body to adapting to the change. Regardless of the initial response, however, individuals have to learn to *live* with the illness, employing various strategies that will help them to adapt to it. Exploring how chronic and intrusive illness changes the lives of individuals, Charmaz (1995) identified three stages of adaptation. In the first stage, when illness is experienced, the body is often perceived as alien and out of control, which in turn disrupts the relationship between the body and self and creates a "loss of self." After recognition of illness, individuals start reassessing their lives and engage in what Charmaz terms "identity trade-offs." They revalue their goals and their lives in light of the change that the illness has brought into their lives. Finally, the person "surrenders" to his or her sick body. Paradoxically, "by freeing the self from the quest for control, it becomes possible to experience the moment and allow the boundaries of self to flow and expand" (Charmaz, 1995, p. 674).

Adaptation to the disease through the **reconstitution of self** (Bury, 2004; Charmaz, 1995; Conrad, 1987) is one of the major themes in the literature on chronic illness. When illness changes the body, it inevitably affects the self. Working mostly within the symbolic interactionist perspective, sociologists studying chronic illness demonstrate how the sense of self is changing during the course of illness and that time has a crucial influence on the way illness and self are experienced. As Charmaz (1995) showed, the discovery of illness creates shock and disorganization in life but as time progresses, individuals can adapt to illness. Corbin and Strauss (1991) referred to such processes of adjustment as "comeback." Similarly, interviewing individuals who had had rheumatoid arthritis for some time, Williams (1984) identified that talking about their illness, respondents build stories linking their disease to past stressful events in **narrative reconstruction**. Linking past (stressful events) to the present (living with illness) allowed these individuals to achieve some coherence in their lives and to "rupture" the link between the body and self.

The works of Arthur Frank (Frank, 1993, 2001) demonstrate how self can be reconstructed through an **illness narrative** (see Researcher Profile 11.1). Analyzing personal stories of people who had experienced illness, Frank (1993) shows that illness can contribute to the emergence of new perspectives on self. He identifies three processes through which the new self may emerge. First, there is a rediscovery of previous self. This refers to the

Arthur Frank

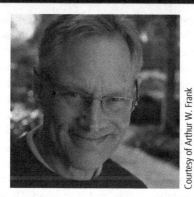

Courtesy of Arthur W. Frank

Dr Frank is a professor emeritus at the University of Calgary and has been a visiting professor at the University of Otago New Zealand, the University of Sydney, Keio and Ritsumeikan Universities in Japan, the University of Central Lancashire, and the University of Toronto. The author of numerous journal articles and book chapters, he has also published *At the Will of the Body: Reflections on Illness* (2002), which introduced the concept of "the remission society" to refer to the fact that people are never perceived of as cured of an illness even if they have overcome it; *The Wounded Storyteller: Body, Illness, and Ethics* (2013): which outlines a framework of the restitution, chaos, and quest narratives of illness that has become part of the vocabulary of medical sociology and humanities in medicine; and *The Renewal of Generosity: Illness, Medicine and How to Live* (2004), which expands the scope from illness experience to include stories of physicians and nurses and presents "generosity" as an antidote to demoralization in both the receiving and giving of medical care. Dr. Frank lectures internationally on illness experience, narrative, bioethics, and health care. He is an elected fellow of the Royal Society of Canada and also the winner of the Society's medal for bioethics, awarded for *Renewal of Generosity*.

process during which illness crystallizes the most important aspects of a person's previous self that are central to the new self. Second, there is a process of finding a new self. During this time, the experience of illness gives birth to a new self. The final process occurs when the person self-consciously becomes what he or she had always been. One of the new selves that may be discovered in the process of coming to terms with chronic illness is that of the expert patient.

Illness as Stigma

Chronic illness is a life-altering experience. It affects the body and self of individuals and their relationships with people around them. However the meaning of illness cannot be reduced to the physiological limitations the condition creates in the body. Foucault (1984), for example, argues that the experience of illness reflects the dominant system of thought within a culture. In all cultures, illness is associated with stigma and fear, with some diseases being more feared and stigmatized than others.

The concept of stigma, introduced into sociology by Goffman (1963), refers to the attribute that discredits the individual and transforms a "whole and usual person to a

Karen Yoshida

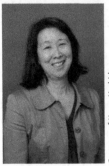

Courtesy of Karen Yoshida

Karen Yoshida is an Associate Professor in the Department of Physical Therapy, Graduate Department of Rehabilitation Science, and the Dalla Lana School of Public health, at the University of Toronto. In 2008, Dr Yoshida was a fellow in Columbia University's, Summer Institute on Oral History, topic: Narrating the Body: Oral History, Narrative and Embodied Performance.

As a disability studies scholar, her research over the past 20-plus years has emphasized the lived experience of disability and community research partnerships. In conducting her research and teaching, Karen uses an equitable partnership model based on disability rights principles with the diverse communities with which she engages. Her research interests focus on embodiment related to women living with disabilities, wellness issues, access to health services, disability activist life histories, and arts-based research and dissemination. She was a contributor to "Out From Under: Disability, History and Things to Remember," the first Canadian Disability History Exhibit, which has been exhibited at the Abilities Arts Festival in Toronto, 2007, the Royal Ontario Museum in Toronto in 2008, the 2010 Paralympics Games in Vancouver, and most recently in London, Ontario. The exhibit will become a permanent exhibit in the Human Rights Museum in Winnipeg that opened in September 2014.

tainted, discounted one" (Goffman, 1963, p. 3). Indeed, stigma can be seen as representing the gap between a person's virtual and actual social identify. Goffman describes two levels of stigma—the **discreditable stigma**, whose stigmatizing attributes are not immediately evident, and the **discredited stigma**, when the individual believes that his or her stigmatized attributes are visible or known to others (see Box 11.2 for another perspective on the dimensions of stigma). Goffman further describes three categories of an individual's relation to stigma: the stigmatized are those who bear the stigma, the "normals" are those who do not, and there are those among the normals who are "wise" to the stigmatized person's condition.

Being heavily influenced by symbolic interactionist theory, Goffman understood stigma not as an objective, permanent characteristic but as a label that is attached to the person in the course of social interaction that inevitably affects his or her sense of self. Different illnesses bear different stigma and many medical sociologists demonstrate how stigma and the illness experience shape the everyday lives of individuals. Accordingly, the meanings of diseases are socially and culturally constructed. For example, mental illness is heavily stigmatized in our society. A person who had been diagnosed with mental illness may prefer to hide the condition from others. Hiding a mental condition would not necessarily mean that

Box 11.2

Six Dimensions of Stigma

Jones et al. (1984) tease apart six dimensions of stigma that expand upon the two types outlined initially by Erving Goffman, the discreditable discredited. These six dimensions are:

1. *Concealable*, that is, the extent to which others can see the stigma.
2. *Course* of the stigma, indicating whether it becomes more prominent over time.

3. *Disruptiveness*, which refers to the degree to which the stigma get in the way of social interactions.
4. *Aesthetics*, or other's reactions to the stigma.
5. *Origin* of the stigma and whether others think the stigma is present at birth, accidental, or deliberate.
6. *Peril*, or the apparent danger of the stigma to others.

the person would be unaffected by the judgment about his or her condition. Indeed, the decision to hide mental illness stems out of the perception that having mental illness is shameful. Coping with illness in light of experiencing illness that is heavily stigmatized in our society may worsen the condition of the individual and limit his or her ability to reach out for social support and/or medical care.

When individuals have a medical condition that is stigmatized, they employ various strategies that help them manage their interactions with others and normalize their experiences. One of the major strategies used by individuals is controlling the extent to which they share the information about their illness with others. For example, examining the experiences of 80 individuals who have epilepsy, Schneider and Conrad (1980) borrowed the concept of being in the closet (the one that is usually used in reference to homosexuals who have not revealed their sexual orientation to others) to describe the strategy used to manage information about epilepsy. Coming out of the closet about their condition was not an easy task for many of the respondents. Epilepsy discredits a person's identity and many individuals were afraid that revealing their condition to others (friends, employers, neighbours) would negatively affect their relationships. The decision of whether or not to tell someone was carefully calculated. In many situations, the possibility of rejection was used as a test of the strength of the relationship (Schneider & Conrad, 1980). Regardless of the chosen strategy, however, the authors suggested that epilepsy was experienced in social isolation and the reactions of others were often more painful than having the disease itself.

Having HIV/AIDS can also require individuals to employ various strategies that help them deal with the stigma of the infection. Because of its association with homosexuality and drug use, HIV/AIDS is seen as a "morally despicable" disease. Thus, people who have HIV/AIDS have to deal with stigma while also coping with a potentially life-threatening condition. Not surprisingly, for many individuals who have HIV/AIDS, the process of managing the stigma attached to this disease becomes a part of learning to live with illness (Siegel, Lune, & Meyer, 1998). In a study looking into the experiences of gay and

Table 11.1 Stigma Management Strategies along the Reactive-Proactive Continuum

Reactive	Intermediate	Proactive
Concealment	Gradual Disclosure	Preemptive Disclosure
Selective Disclosure	Selective Affiliation	Public Education
Personal Attributional Style	Discrediting One's Discreditors	Social Activism
	Challenging Moral Attributions	

Source: Siegel, K., Lune, H., & Meyer, I. H. (1998). Stigma management among gay/bisexual men with HIV/AIDS. *Qualitative Sociology, 21*(1), 3–24, Springer Science + Business Media (formerly Kluwer).

bisexual men living in New York city, Siegel, Lune, and Meyer (1998) demonstrated the management of stigma is a complex process that requires careful consideration of various strategies (see Table 11.1).

The authors created a classification of stigma management strategies that builds a continuum from being "reactive" through "intermediate" (a more neutral stance) to being "proactive." Reactive strategies were usually employed to conceal the illness, avoiding the enactment of stigma. Protecting themselves from being stigmatized, these men hid their status from others, preferring to disclose their condition to a very small circle of people (e.g., other men with HIV/AIDS). Some also presented themselves as being different from other men with HIV/AIDS by, for example, claiming their innocence or absence of knowledge about the disease. All these strategies helped the individuals to prevent the enactment of stigma in their daily lives. This avoidance could have damaging effects on their self-identity. Concealing the illness could also add stress to an already compromised immune system. Such a strategy also ironically serves to reinforce the stigmatization of HIV in society.

Intermediate strategies used by HIV-positive men were based on disclosing their status but since the disclosure was usually managed gradually and with a select group of people, it had little effect on changing social attitudes toward individuals living with HIV. Proactive strategies, on the other hand, were publicly aimed at changing the way society sees HIV/AIDS, targeting changes in social attitudes toward individuals living with HIV/AIDS (Siegel et al., 1998).

Raising social awareness and becoming publicly active can allow people who are living with illness to build social networks, to find support, and potentially to reconstruct both their perception of self and the social meaning of the disease. Cancer is another illness for which, as some researchers noted (Bloom & Kessler, 1994; Klawiter, 2004), media and public awareness have contributed to changing the experience of the illness (see Box 11.3 regarding the ways in which complementary and alternative medicine [CAM] enables a reconceptualization of the experience of breast cancer). Cancer is often regarded as one of the most stigmatized diseases (Sontag, 1978), whereby the stigma associated with it can be

Box 11.3

Holistic Sickening: The Ways in Which Complementary and Alternative Practitioners Help Redefine Breast Cancer

Sered and Agigan (2008) introduced the concept of *holistic sickening* to refer to the way complementary and alternative medicine (CAM—see Chapter 10) practitioners who treat breast cancer redefine their patients' breast cancer in ways that expand and transform their illness. In contrast to mainsteam medical practitioners, CAM practitioners tend to espouse broad and complex causal frameworks that help give meaning to women's cancer. Sered and Agigan conclude that CAM practitioners "articulate holistic philosophies that describe healing as open-ended with correspondingly expansive definitions of what it means to be healed, [but at the same time] rarely articulating clear ways of conceptualising or measuring the efficacy of their own treatments" (p. 616). Their use of expansive and detailed etiological frameworks alongside vague and unelaborated efficacy frameworks is what made up the holistic sickening phenomenon.

seen as more damaging than the disease itself. The uncertainty of the causes of the disease, the general absence of a cure and resulting fatal nature, and the widespread concern about cancer in our society make this disease terrifying. Examining the cultural and moral aura that constructs the meaning of cancer, Sontag (1978) refers to the illness as a *metaphor*. Perceived as a disease of repression and suppressed emotions, the meaning attached to cancer becomes harmful and isolates individuals from their community, further stigmatizing them (Sontag, 1978). It is possible, however, that recent developments in the area of social activism and public awareness have changed the stigmatizing nature of cancer at least to some degree. While experiences of living with cancer can significantly affect a person's identity and social relations, public awareness has made cancer not only a personal problem, but also a serious social problem.

Illness as Secondary Gain

So far, we have shown that chronic illness changes the lives of individuals and has a profound impact on their self. Usually illness is perceived as an experience that has negative consequences on the life of the individuals. Occasionally, however, illness can be perceived as secondary gain and create social and interpersonal benefits for individuals (see Box 11.4). For instance, a sick person can receive compassion and support from others. Whereas before the person was not noticed, the illness can bring desired social attention and care. Illness can also provide a temporary "escape" from social responsibilities. Missing a day of work or a test at school can be a convenience derived from the unpleasant experience of being sick. Conceptualizing **illness as a secondary gain** brings us back to the Parsons' sick role model—being sick does often exempt us from our social roles and

Contested Illnesses: Occupational Overuse Syndrome (OOS) and Multiple Chemical Sensitivity (MCS)

The recognition of illness as secondary gain permeates the process whereby illnesses become socially and medically legitimized. Two interesting examples are Occupational Overuse Syndrome (OOS, otherwise known as repetitive strain injury) (Jaye & Fitzgerald, 2010) and Multiple Chemical Sensitivity (MCS) (Phillips, 2010). Each of these illnesses has been contested, and those who suffer from their affliction also experience the doubt as to the legitimacy of their claims. As Jaye and Fitzgerald (2010) argue in the case of OOS in New Zealand:

[B]attles were fought over diagnoses, over occupational health and safety in the workplace, and over entitlements to therapy and income compensation. However, participants were also battling to maintain their identities as hard workers, while resisting and challenging normalising technologies of self and morally charged negative identities offered them by employers, state-funded accident and injury insurance agencies, and the medical profession. (p. 1010)

responsibilities, which we potentially can even enjoy, but we also have an obligation to desire to feel better and to seek medical help, which defines the deviation from our social roles as only temporary and undesirable.

SOCIO-CULTURAL VARIATIONS IN THE EXPERIENCES OF HEALTH AND ILLNESS

While diseases are often perceived as universal (having similar symptoms and similar etiology), the meaning and experiences of illness are heavily influenced by society and cultural norms. In what follows, we examine the role of gender, ethnicity, and social class in constructing both health and illness experiences.

Gender

The gender ideologies that are embedded in our culture pertain to every aspect of social life. The socially constructed categories of femininity and masculinity are not only associated with particular character traits (e.g., women are perceived to be more nurturing and men are perceived to be more aggressive), clothing styles, and body type, but we can also see that certain diseases in our culture have become associated with a particular gender. Until recently, for instance, heart disease was perceived as a man's disease. The diagnosis of heart disease conjured the image of a white, middle class businessman with a stressful and demanding job. The perception of heart disease as a men's health problem affected the way in which women with heart disease were diagnosed and treated in a number of ways. First, since many doctors believed that women were less likely to suffer from heart disease, women presenting with symptoms consistent with heart problems were often dismissed, misdiagnosed, and not referred for follow-up testing (McKinlay, 1996). Second, the social construction of heart disease as a male problem not only masked heart disease among female patients from doctors, but it also became a part of the lay image of heart disease (Emslie, Hunt, & Watt, 2001). It is not surprising, therefore, that women tended to dismiss their symptoms and may not have sought immediate help when they experienced symptoms that could have been indicative of heart disease. Today, cardiovascular disease is recognized as one of the major causes of death and disability among both men and women in Canada. Moreover, it has been found that the symptoms of heart disease in women may be different from the ones that it manifests in men. While previous research on cardiovascular diseases was done predominantly on men, women are increasingly becoming a target of health research and health education campaigns. It is possible that this awareness can change the experiences of women with cardiovascular disease and improve women's experiences in the health care system (Adams et al., 2008).

Gender also plays a critical role in how individuals understand the meaning of the disease. Prostate cancer diagnosis and treatment can threaten a man's sense of masculinity (Chapple & Ziebland, 2002). Researchers in the School of Nursing at the University of British Columbia (UBC) (Halpin, Phillips, & Oliffe, 2009) examined over 800 prostate cancer articles published in *The Globe and Mail* and the *National Post* from January 2001 through December 2006. They identified three primary categories within these news articles: those reflecting illness perspectives, those reflecting medical perspectives, and those reflecting supplementary perspectives. Overall, they found that the descriptive content of most articles tended to reproduce hegemonic masculine ideals, such as competition and stoicism. Many articles also privileged the curative aspects of biomedicine and the medicalized nature of male bodies, which created what they referred to as the *treatment imperative*. The authors noted that "[a]ny discussion on the negative effects of treatment or explicit references to marginalised forms of masculinity was conspicuously absent" thus reinforcing "detrimental ideologies and perspectives of men's health" (p. 155).

Similarly for women, the diagnosis of breast cancer often forces them to face the challenge of potential body disfigurement. Clarke (2004) describes how the discovery of BRCA1 and BRCA2 has resulted in the members of certain families realizing there is an increased likelihood of breast cancer occurring. Being vulnerable to breast cancer has become equated with being "feminine" whereas being masculine is to be vulnerable to testicular cancer when young and prostate cancer when older. She argues:

> [T]he association of disease not just with personhood but also with the specifics of stereotyped masculinity and femininity may construct a more intimate, more personal link between disease and identity. This close attachment of gender and disease may shore up and exacerbate a fear reaction. It may also serve to diminish the awareness of other, more prevalent, causes of death for men and women. (p. 541)

When men are diagnosed with breast cancer, for example, they also have to deal with a stigma of having what society largely regards as a women's disease.

To summarize, because gender is at the centre of the social organization of societal roles, the responsibilities of individuals are always gendered, as are their identities and their sense of self. Therefore, analyzing the experiences of illness, it is important to consider the role of gender in shaping the experiences of the individuals who are living with illness. Some diseases may be perceived as affecting individuals of a specific gender. This, in turn, can affect both the orientation of health personnel and the personal experiences of people living with illness. In some cases, such as breast or testicular cancer, due to cultural constructs of femininity and masculinity the disease can affect the very sense of a person's gender. Finally, the daily experiences of individuals are shaped by culturally inscribed gender norms and therefore the experiences of the very same illness can be very different for men and women. Even pregnancy, a condition experienced only by women, is experienced differently by different women as they interact with others (see Box 11.5).

Box 11.5

The Social Embodiment of Pregnancy

Although pregnancy is a physiological transition, it also marks a significant change in women's social lives. Neiterman (2010) interviewed 42 women in order to understand how they experience their bodies during pregnancy and what impact their experiences have on their communications with others. The study showed that the meaning that pregnant women and people around them attach to pregnancy is constantly being re-negotiated through social interaction. The journey to motherhood is associated with changes women experience inside their bodies and it also facilitates a change in the social relationships of expectant mothers with their families, friends, co-workers, and even complete strangers. Women had to reorganize their lives to adjust to these changes, for example, feelings of nausea or being extremely tired. Sometimes, they would ask their family members to take on additional tasks to help them out. On other occasions, they would plan their days in a way that would allow them to continue their daily routines despite physical interruptions. The study also showed that moving from one social circle to another, expectant mothers and people around them are constantly re-defining the meaning of pregnancy and the same body in different situations can be perceived as "pregnant" or "not pregnant," labelled as "good" or "bad." Teen mothers, for example, were often stigmatized by strangers but received support and love from their family members and friends. Moreover, sometimes the pregnant body was not identified as pregnant by women themselves or by people around them. Especially in the cases of unplanned pregnancy, different physiological transformations were not interpreted as pregnancy by some women, who would, for example, mistake pregnancy nausea with an onset of the stomach flu. Other women told about their experiences of being identified as pregnant by complete strangers but not by closest friends who did not expect the women to have another child. It is apparent that despite the physiological transformation that women undergo during pregnancy, the pregnant body is not pregnant until it is socially defined as such through social interactions with others.

Ethnicity/Culture

Not only are illness experiences gendered, they are also heavily influenced by cultural beliefs and norms. In his famous work, *People in Pain*, Zborowski (1969) demonstrated that the reactions to pain are culturally learned. Analyzing white Anglo-Saxon American, Italian, and Jewish men's responses to pain, Zborowski showed that culture plays a role in how pain is experienced and expressed by individuals. The Italian and the Jewish patients tended to respond emotionally to their pain, but once the pain was gone, the Italians were able to return to their previous activities while Jewish patients often continued to worry about the underlying causes of their pain. White, Anglo-Saxon Americans tended to be stoic in their demeanour and were seen as more detached from their bodily experiences of pain.

Cultural variations in the experiences of menopause among Japanese and North American women have been examined by Lock (1993). Although the symptoms of menopause have been considered to be a universal experience, the meaning attached to menopause is culturally constructed. In our Canadian culture, menopause, a transition women undergo during their midlife, has been constructed as an illness requiring medical attention and treatment (see more about this in Chapter 12). In Japan, menopausal women are less likely to report hot flashes, a constant symptom of menopausal women in North America (Lock, 1993). Moreover, there is evidence that among some cultures, such as Mayan women living in Guatemala and some areas of Mexico or Cree women living in Canada, menopause is viewed as a positive event. Once these women move into menopausal age, they are regarded as "wise women" or "healers" who can contribute to the spiritual growth of their communities (Mills, 2013). The cultural significance of this transition makes the experience of menopause very different for women across different cultures (Mills, 2013).

Ethnicity can also be seen as a mediating factor in the experience of illness. Higginbottom (2006) studied the meaning and consequences of hypertension among middle-aged African Caribbean people living in England. The study participants had immigrated to England during the 1950s and 1960s as children or young adults. Not surprisingly, participants' understandings of their hypertension differed greatly from the common medical conceptualization of the condition. What was unique in their narrative accounts of illness, however, is the importance attributed to their ethnicity, their experience of migration and cultural adaptation, and their experience of racism and discrimination. The history of oppression and slavery, experienced by African Caribbean people for centuries, had left a long-lasting effect that was still manifested among many of the people of their generation (Higginbottom, 2006). Taken together, these factors can cause a major disruption in participants' life trajectories, within which the subsequent diagnoses and management of hypertension chronic illness needs to be contextualized.

Cultural differences in the experiences of health and illness point to the importance of the social norms, meanings, and practices in how a person experiences the disease. It shows that the ways we feel our bodies and understand them are always socially constructed. This becomes especially apparent when we compare our dominant experiences and perceptions of illness and the body with the ones adopted by other

Box 11.6

In Search of a Healing Place: Aboriginal Women in Vancouver's Downtown Eastside

Sociologist Cecilia Benoit and Aboriginal health consultants Dena Carroll and Munaza Chaudry (Benoit, Carroll, & Chaudry, 2003) examined whether Urban Aboriginal Health Centres that have emerged to address the unmet health concerns of Aboriginal people living in various metropolitan areas address the health care concerns of Aboriginal women. Their specific case study involved Aboriginal women who were clients of the Vancouver Native Health Society, its sister organization, Sheway, and residents of Vancouver's Downtown Eastside. Many of the Aboriginal women who took part in this study described themselves as being unable to direct major change in their lives but they nevertheless displayed incredible inner strength battling against poverty, disease, racism, sexism, and abandonment. The researchers found, however, that despite the efforts of various stakeholders to

more clearly articulate the health and social concerns of one of the country's most marginalized urban populations, existing services did not seem to be getting at the root causes of the problems experienced by these urban Aboriginal women. Instead, efforts to address the problems tended to adopt medical-oriented strategies that focused on symptoms as opposed to the root causes. As Benoit, Carroll and Chaudry (2003) noted,

> [m]any Aboriginal women expressed a strong desire for a Healing Place, based on a model of care where their health concerns are addressed in an integrated manner, where they are respected and given the opportunity to shape and influence decision-making about services that impact their own healing." (p. 821)

They continued to search for services that are both gender-sensitive and culturally appropriate.

cultures. For instance, we can see a different view of health and illness among Aboriginal communities (see Box 11.6). Although Aboriginal peoples in Canada have distinct conceptions of health and illness, there are also some key commonalities across them. Specifically, Aboriginal views about health and illness tend to be more holistic and include not only physical well-being but also the emotional, intellectual, and spiritual elements. Moreover, an individual's health cannot be understood in isolation from the collective well-being of a person's community (Commission on the Social Determinants of Health, 2007).

Social Class Differences

While the impact of class differences on health outcomes has been discussed in detail in Chapters 6 and 7, personal experiences of living with illness and disability can also be affected by social position. Illness, and especially chronic illness and disability, can be made more difficult when a person has fewer resources but their onset can also reduce future availability of material resources. Social class position can also have an impact on the availability of social support networks to individuals. For example, self-help movements and social activism that assist persons living with various chronic illnesses and disabilities are generally the domain of the middle class (Brown et al., 2004). The lack of social support among those in lower social positions can create a sense of isolation and deterioration of material conditions that can further stigmatize individuals living with illness, making it more difficult to function and cope with the disease.

Intersectionality

It should be noted that the division among gender, ethnicity, and class statuses on the experiences of illness is simply for analytical reasons. In real life, these characteristics intersect with each other creating unique social contexts within which individuals experience illness (see Chapters 6 and 7). The **intersectionality** among gender, culture, and social class is not merely the additive sum of each status (Cairney, Veldhuizen, & Wade, 2010). For example, in their study of the interaction of class and gender in constructions of gendered identity, Seale and Charteris-Black (2008) found that the class location of men and women have an impact on the way each "perform gender" in the face of the experience of illness. Men from a higher socio-economic class consider themselves (and perhaps others) to have a considerable degree of personal agency in the sphere of health and illness, more so than men from a low socio-economic class. Although illness was not experienced as a threat to conventional femininity by women from either class, reliance on existing networks of female friends and relatives for emotional and practical support was significantly greater for women from a lower socio-economic class. Thus, focusing on one specific aspect of socio-cultural relations brings a potential danger of not capturing the whole illness experience of individuals. To address this, the majority of scholars interested in the experience of illness delve into people's narratives to analyze how the concepts of self and identity are constructed through the intersection of multiple personal characteristics and social interactions.

SUMMARY

In this chapter, we moved beyond the physical aspects of health and illness to examine how people experience disease through the intersecting relationships among the body, the self, and society. We started by focusing on the human body, distinguishing between the lived experience of both having a body and being a body, between having a physiological disease and living with the illness. To help understand the social aspects of illness, we presented Parsons' sick role and highlighted its usefulness but also its limitations in understanding the social aspects of chronic illness. In the second part of this chapter, we focused on the contributions from symbolic interactionism to the study of the experiences of illness, discussing illness as a career. We demonstrated that while there are different conceptualizations of the illness experience based on different theoretical perspectives, the overall focus was centred on the relationship among body, self, and society. Illness can change the body and self but since both body and self are socially constructed and the meaning attached to illness is mediated through social and cultural norms, the relationships between the body and self are never unidirectional. Rather, the relationship between body and self is dynamic, changing each other and, potentially, generating an agency that can bring about change to society. Although societal change is possible, the experience of illness continues to deal with the issues of stigma and social isolation that become social characteristics of many chronic diseases and disabilities.

The experience of illness is a critical area of sociological investigation that some argue still requires a great deal of work. In a review and proposal for a *sociology of disease*, Timmermans and Haas (2008) argue that:

> "Social scientists have been reluctant to tackle disease in its physiological and biological manifestations. The result is an impoverishment of sociological analysis on at least three levels: social scientists have rarely made diseases central to their inquiries; they have been reluctant to include clinical endpoints in their analysis; and they have largely bracketed the normative purpose of health interventions. Consequently, social scientists tend to ignore what often matters most to patients and health care providers, and the social processes social scientists describe remain clinically unanchored. A sociology of disease explores the dialectic between social life and disease; aiming to examine whether and how social life matters for morbidity and mortality and vice versa." (p. 659)

Key Terms

Biographical disruption—disruptions of socially expected chronological order of life trajectory and events caused by illness

Discreditable stigma—a stigma when the stigmatizing attributes are not immediately evident

Discredited stigma—the individual believes that the stigmatized attributes are visible or known to others

Intersectionality—the simultaneous occupancy of multiple social positions that combine beyond the additive sum of each individual position to influence health status and experience of illness

Illness as a secondary gain—an illness that can create social and interpersonal benefits for individuals

Illness as a career—conceptualization of illness as a process that requires adaption, reconstruction of self, and reorganization of daily life

Illness narrative—the emergence of a new perspective of self, based on one's illness

Narrative reconstruction—when talking about a person's illness, respondents build stories linking their disease to past stressful events

Reconstitution of self—transformation of self as a process of adaptation to illness

Sick role—a conceptualization of illness that highlights the relationship between illness and social structure of society

Critical Thinking Questions

1. What are the strengths and weaknesses of the concept of the sick role in understanding the social dimensions of experiencing various types of illness?

2. What are the relationships between the physiological and social transformations associated with experiencing illness?

3. Analyze how the experience of diabetes can differ among people of different classes, ages, genders, and ethnicities. Does a focus on intersecting statuses help to better understand people's experience?

4. Compare and contrast reasons why both mental illness and cancer are stigmatized in our society?

Further Readings and Resources

Charmaz, K. C. (1991). *Good Days, Bad Days: The Self in Chronic Illness and Time*. New Brunswick, NJ: Rutgers University Press.

McElroy, A., & Jezewski, M. A. (2000). Cultural variation in the experience of health and illness. In *The Handbook of Social Studies in Health and Medicine* (191–209). *London: Sage*.

Timmermans, S., & Haas, S. (2008). Towards a sociology of disease. *Sociology of Health and Illness, 30*(5), 659–676.

Turner, B. (1992). *Regulating Bodies: Essays in Medical Sociology*. London: Routledge.

Chapter 12

The Medicalization and Pharmaceuticalization of Society

Chapter Outline

Learning Objectives

After studying this chapter, you should be able to:

1. Describe the concept of medicalization and identify the ongoing process of the medicalization of society;

2. Understand the history of medicalization and its transformation from a physician-driven to market-driven phenomenon;

3. Appreciate the development of healthism as a form of social control and a new measure of morality;

4. Discuss the role of the pharmaceutical and medical-device industries in contributing to the medicalization of society.

Every day[1] we are bombarded with reminders of how important it is to stay healthy. Radio and television ads fill the airwaves, newspapers and flyers fill our mailboxes, and

---

[1]An earlier version of this chapter was published in Frankel, B. G., Speechley, M., & Wade T. J. (1996). *The Sociology of Health and Health Care: A Canadian Perspective*. Toronto: Copp Clark

email and social media ads fill our inboxes and Twitter and Facebook accounts. Fitness clubs advertise that only through regular exercise at the gym we can truly feel "healthy" and achieve "wellness," and they eagerly sell us memberships. Advertisements for yoga counter the message from fitness clubs, arguing that only through meditation can you address your physical, mental, and spiritual discipline to reach "peace" and "wellness." Now it isn't enough to practise yoga, you have to do "hot" yoga. Even reality television has taken on the charge with shows such as *The Biggest Loser*.

On our quest to get healthy or stay healthy, we are provided with a variety of treatments offered by contemporary medicine. When our bodies manifest what we believe to be signs of illness, we have been conditioned to seek medical help. While the idea of seeking medical help when something is "wrong" with the body feels most natural, until relatively recently, this was not a common course of action for individuals (Turner, 1995). Today, we seek medical help not only for what ails us; today we seek help for improvements in health and performance. How and why we have come to this point where more and more aspects of our lives are being defined in medical terms is the topic of this chapter.

This chapter will focus on various aspects of the medicalization of society. **Medicalization** is the redefining of an aspect of our life or a behaviour or condition under the domain of medicine and away from other historical frames. Pregnancy, birth, and aging, for example, are now thought of as conditions that require medical attention instead of being perceived as natural life events and human processes. We begin the chapter by identifying some of the historical and social conditions that empowered medicine to position itself as a safeguard of individual health, and discuss how medicalization can be conceived as a form of social control, replacing the role of other societal institutions. Issues arising from the process of medicalization, including iatrogenesis, will be described as well as the changes in our understanding of the role of medicine in our lives. Finally, this chapter will discuss the industry surrounding the rising use of prescription drugs and medical equipment/technology and the evolution of prescriptive practices from diseases to newly defined conditions.

SOCIAL CONSTRUCTION OF MEDICAL KNOWLEDGE

Examining various diseases through a medical lens is not a universal social phenomenon. Of course, people have always had diseases and sicknesses, but the understanding of the *etiology* of disease, as well as the way of treating diseases, has varied greatly historically and culturally. Drawing on the works of Emile Durkheim (1921/1995), Turner (2004) suggests that in premodern societies, health and illness were often associated with the distinction between the **sacred**, objects or ideas that have been assigned a religious or a transcendent meaning, and the **profane**, those objects and ideas that lack sacred meaning (p. 86). The sick or disfigured body was seen as a polluted body resulting from a breach of social and cultural conventions. Exposure to dangers, restricted objects, or practices breaching these conventions were taboos that resulted in sickness. As such, sickness was generally perceived as a moral problem, a punishment for breaking some social or religious norm. Consequently, the treatment for sickness did not have to be directed at the body of the individual but instead focused on punishment for the breach of a taboo, usually requiring purification and religious rituals. Moreover, sickness was not necessarily seen as an individual condition. On many occasions, the "treatment" of sickness might require the participation of the whole community in a cleansing ritual. It is not surprising, therefore, that the prerogative of treating the sickness was located within religious institutions. Even today, some diseases evoke a sense of punishment for breaking social and religious norms (e.g., lung cancer and smoking; AIDS and risky, immoral sexual activity). While treatments generally no longer occur in religious institutions, the social stigma of some diseases persists.

Development of the Medical Model

In his famous book *The Birth of the Clinic*, Foucault (1975) described the transformation in our understanding of the meaning and nature of sickness. With the emergence of medical science, disease was redefined as a physiological pathology located within the human body. As medical knowledge advanced, the body itself ceased to be seen as one, single entity. It became fragmented into organs and parts, and the physician's task was to locate the diseased organ within the body. This biomedical, reductionist perspective functioned by isolating the disease from the whole body, separating the sick component and treating it apart from other parts. The ability to diagnose the disease and isolate the diseased organ belonged only to one with specialized training and qualifications trained to be able to "see" the problem—the physician. As discussed in Chapter 5, the **medical gaze** described by Foucault (1975) captured the process of the depersonalization of disease and the role of medical experts in gaining power over individuals through the possession of medical knowledge about human conditions. As a result, the personal troubles of the individual were not considered; no connection was made between physical illness and overall well-being. This detachment is further illustrated by the advent of the standardized system of classification of conditions and diagnoses that has become a central focus of medical knowledge, diagnoses, treatment, and, most importantly, billing. The most accepted classification system is the *International Classification of Diseases* (ICD) now in its tenth edition (WHO, 1992).

The history of medicine describes the emergence of the biomedical focus as a triumph of science, as a logical victory of scientific progress over other forms of knowledge. Sociologists highlight two issues that challenge this claim. First, all knowledge (including medical knowledge) can be seen as a socially and culturally constructed phenomenon (Berger & Luckmann, 1966). Therefore, rather than being an inevitable triumph of medical knowledge, the expansion of medicine can be attributed to a number of socio-historical conditions:

> The historical development of concepts of health and illness in Western societies is characterized by increasing secularization, the rise of scientific theories of health, the separation of mental and physical illness, the erosion of traditional therapies by scientific practices, and the differentiation of categories into specific micro notions. (Turner, 2004, p. 89)

Medicine has been very successful in expanding its domain of knowledge and jurisdiction into almost all the other life domains, including religion, criminal justice, aging, and other natural processes, daily activities and recreation, family form and functioning, and even sexuality and sexual desire. For example, many forms of deviance and crime have become redefined within a medical framework. It is legal to consume banned substances such as opioid-based narcotics and marijuana if you have received a supporting medical diagnosis and a prescription from a physician. Unruly and poorly focused behaviours in children, once deemed naughty and requiring discipline, have been redefined as a medical disorder requiring medication (either attention-deficit disorder (ADD) or attention-deficit hyperactivity disorder (ADHD)). In fact, as Friedson (1970a) argues, the medical profession has been successful in claiming jurisdiction over many phenomena irrespective of its ability to adequately address the source or symptoms of these phenomena.

Government and Regulation

Following logically from knowledge and jurisdiction, the second component of the triumphant expansion of medicine into everyday life relates to the question of regulative power. In addition to holding knowledge about disease and illness, medical professionals are also given the legislative authority to produce and protect this knowledge by institutionalizing it via the establishment of medical school curricula, board examinations and licensure, association membership and censure, and control of medical journals that legitimize particular things as medical conditions and illnesses while (potentially) dismissing others.

Physicians also have been given legislative power to control and regulate other health-related professions but enjoy self-regulation through their own associations. Although this is changing (see Chapter 4), physicians have had the almost exclusive right to diagnose illnesses and treat people. The very fact that the legitimacy of sickness can only be granted by physicians provides an example of medical dominance (Friedson, 1970b) or of "**diagnostic imperialism**" (Illich, 1976, p. 76). This power of physicians over people's lives is significant. For example, by providing genetic counselling or assisting women with fertility treatment, physicians often define who is to be born. By assigning a patient the "sick" label, physicians define who is afforded legitimate time away from school or work and who is not. Physicians even validate the status and actions of the deceased by pronouncing time and cause of death. Cause of death is especially important for several reasons; for example, the implications for receiving religious sacraments or validating insurance claims for suspected suicides, as well as the associated stigma.

MEDICALIZATION OF SOCIETY

According to Conrad, medicalization is "a process by which nonmedical problems become defined and treated as medical problems, usually in terms of illnesses or disorders" (Conrad, 2000, p. 324). There are at least three levels at which medicalization can

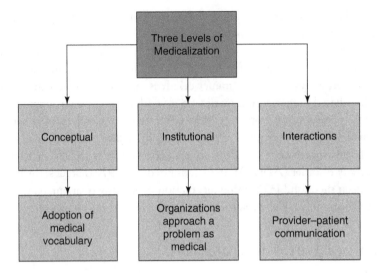

Figure 12.1 Levels of Medicalization

occur: (1) the *conceptual* level, when medical vocabulary has been adopted to define a problem as medical; (2) the *institutional* level when organizations approach a problem as medical; and (3) the level of *interactions*, when the problem is defined and/or treated as medical in the context of provider–patient communication (Conrad & Schneider, 1980) (see Figure 12.1).

Applying a social constructionist perspective to the study of medicalization, Conrad (2007) examines the process of medicalization as a transformation of human conditions into medical disorders. It is the relationship among various social actors that plays a role in defining any human condition as medical. Traditionally, medicalization has been seen as a form of social control that is introduced and enforced by medical professionals. However, the medical profession does not act in a social vacuum. Members' views and opinions, as well as their ability to legitimize a condition as medical, are always a result of social and cultural beliefs about the nature of a condition. For instance, Irving Zola claims that:

> [Medicalization] is not occurring through the political power physicians hold . . . but is largely an insidious and often undramatic phenomenon accomplished by "medicalizing" much of daily living by making medicine and the labels 'healthy' and 'ill' relevant to an ever increasing part of human existence. (Zola, 1994, p. 404)

The field of mental health is one area in which medicine has taken a dominant role in regulating human behaviour. Medical labels are increasingly applied to behaviours that were previously understood as resulting from other causes. For example, children with behavioural problems are now often labelled as suffering from ADHD and receive medical treatment to cure the problem. More recently, the diagnosis of ADHD has

expanded to include adults. Adults diagnose themselves with ADHD, actively participating in placing a label of a medical disease on their condition to justify underperfor-
mance (Conrad, 2007). Medical labels can legitimize undesirable behaviour, and,
therefore, lay people often actively participate in medicalizing certain conduct. If, for
instance, a child has been diagnosed with ADHD, we are told that the child's unruly
behaviour is a result of his or her medical condition and not a result of bad parenting
or unsuccessful teaching practices. Medicalization of alcoholism is another example of
medical definitions replacing other explanations for human behaviour. Previously,
excessive alcohol use was perceived as a person's lack of self-control. Now redefined as
alcohol abuse and alcohol dependence, it is a recognized diagnosis. Although hyperactive children and alcoholics are not new phenomena, medicalization of these behaviours transforms them into medical conditions, which then require treatment under
the medical model.

Although lay people can benefit from formally established diagnoses of their conditions, at the societal level we can see how medicalization is slowly taking over more and
more aspects of people's lives. To demonstrate how medicalization expands its influence, we
discuss in detail three different phenomena: (1) the medicalization of women's bodies,
(2) the demedicalization and the possibility of remedicalization of homosexuality, and
(3) healthism or healthization as a new terrain for medicalization.

Medicalization of Women's Bodies

Men's bodies, and especially aging men's bodies, are becoming increasingly medicalized
(Conrad, 2007), but women's bodies and their bodies' natural processes have been the
object of extensive medicalization from the beginning of medical expansion (Riessman,
1983). The female body was seen as not only "different" from the male body but also as
deviating from the "norm" for medical science (which the male body had become). (Only
within the past 10 to 15 years have publicly funded drug trials required the participation
of women as well as men, unless there is a rationale for sexual exclusion.) Every bodily
function that is exclusively female, such as menstruation, pregnancy, childbirth, and
menopause, has become a central object of medical investigation and control (Kohler-
Riessman, 1983/2003). Feminist scholars argue that the attention paid by medicine to
women's bodies, and specifically to women's reproductive health, cannot be understood
simply as a result of random scientific discoveries. As Turner (1996) notes, regulation of
human bodies requires institutionalization of social control over human reproduction.
The regulation of women's reproduction is tightly linked to the desire of our historically
patriarchal society to control and regulate women's sexuality (Kohler-Riessman,
1983/2003; O'Brien, 1989).

Many feminist scholars see the medicalization of women's bodies as a form of oppression based on the vulnerability of women. This is especially evident in the control that
medical professionals gained over the processes of pregnancy and childbirth. The rise of

biomedical discourse and the popularity of medical science, the struggle of physicians for political and professional dominance, and the willingness of some women themselves to medicalize pregnancy and childbirth in a relatively short period of time transformed this natural process into a medicalized condition, an "illness" requiring constant medical supervision (Davis-Floyd, 1990, 1992).

This shift has dramatically changed the experiences of women giving birth. For example, it changed the very "physics" of birth—redesigned from a sitting/squatting position, which was used historically by midwives and perceived as more convenient for the labouring woman, to having women lay in a supine position. The supine position was perceived as more modest and more convenient for a physician, who had to attend a woman's labour but at the same time make sure that his physical and visual contact with the woman's body was managed within professional boundaries (Featherstone, 2001). That is, the physician's focus was on the specific organs and not the woman as a whole, consistent with the reductionist trend in biomedicine. It also changed the process of birth, with the physician becoming an active agent while the birthing woman was left in the role of a passive recipient or a "patient" of medical treatment (Riessman, 1983). Finally, it changed the nature of birth, which ceased to be a part of a women's world managed for women by women in a community setting.

Today, despite the resurgence of midwifery and alternative methods of childbirth (e.g., home birth), most people continue to see childbearing as a medical condition that requires continual supervision. Moreover, understanding childbearing as a medical process, many women are themselves willingly adhering to medical regulation and control during pregnancy and birth. Although many scholars criticize the medicalization of childbirth (Davis-Floyd, 1992; Katz Rothman, 1993; Martin, 2001), others point out that medicalization of pregnancy (Brubaker, 2007) and medicalization more generally (Lock & Kaufert, 1998) have been helpful to women. Margaret Lock and Patricia Kaufert (1998) show how medicalization is viewed pragmatically by women depending on how it assists them in their daily lives (see Box 12.1 on Pragmatic Women).

Box 12.1

Pragmatic Women

In *Pragmatic Women and Body Politics,* Canadian anthropologists Margaret Lock and Patricia Kaufert (1998) present the complex case of women's relationship to medicalization and medical technology. Through thirteen essays examining women from a variety of countries and cultures, they present evidence that indicate that women can accept, resist, or be indifferent to the medicalization of their bodies in ways that make sense in their lives or according to their lived experiences. It is in this way that women react pragmatically to how medicalization and medical technology can assist them in their daily living.

Medicalization of women's bodies exemplifies how medical surveillance can become a form of social control. Medical attention paid to women's bodies comes at the price of losing personal autonomy (Katz Rothman, 1993). Menstruation, childbirth, menopause, and other routine physiological processes are defined in medical terms not only by medical practitioners but also by women themselves. Moreover, seeing female bodies mainly through their reproductive capacity becomes a reason to objectify, regulate, and control women's bodies more generally. The medicalization of childbearing as a physiological process that brings everything consumed by a mother to the womb where a child is developing has become the reason behind denying women employment in potentially hazardous environments, forcing them to undergo compulsory treatment in cases of alcohol or drug abuse during pregnancy, and defining them as "deviant mothers" if they do not conform to prenatal regulations and social expectations (Callahan & Knight, 1992; Maher, 1992; Toscano, 2005).

It would be wrong, however, to solely blame medicalization for placing restrictions on women's bodies and on their personal freedom. While it is hard to assess to what degree medicalization has furthered social control over women's bodies, it seems that the patriarchal ideology of our society has both inspired medical research on women's bodies and informed the interpretation given to any findings about female reproductive physiology (Katz Rothman, 1993; Kohler-Riessman, 1983/2003; O'Brien, 1989; Oakley, 1980). The conclusion that can be drawn from this example is that far from being value-neutral, medicalization works in the context of cultural and ideological beliefs about human nature and social relations that often lurk behind the medical terms and explanations that are applied to human conditions.

Demedicalization and Remedicalization of Homosexuality

The process of medicalization can also be reversed as some behaviours previously defined as medical conditions or disorders can be demedicalized (Conrad, 2007). One of the most commonly cited cases of **demedicalization** of a human condition is homosexuality. Historically, homosexuality has been variously defined as a normative sexual practice, as a sin, as a crime, and later on as a form of illness (Conrad, 2007). Conrad and Schneider (1980) and Turner (1995) track the process of defining homosexuality first as a sin under most religious doctrines and then as a psychiatric disorder in early versions of the principal guide for mental diagnoses (*Diagnostic Statistical Manual*, DSM-II, 1968). Due largely to social pressure and activism by the gay community, subsequent editions of the DSM (DSM-III, 1980 onward) delisted homosexuality as a psychiatric disorder and it is now generally thought to be a sexual preference, although certain political and religious movements challenge this claim.

The story of the demedicalizaton of homosexuality may not end here. Recent reports on the discovery of the "gay gene" have reopened the discussion on homosexuality as a physiologically based phenomenon (Conrad, 2007). While not discussed in terms of a psychiatric disorder, the potential existence of a gay gene is alleged to explain the predisposition for a homosexual orientation. Notwithstanding the fact that the scientific support behind this discovery is still being built and quite controversial, public attention surrounding the gay gene makes possible the remedicalization of homosexuality as a potentially treatable medical condition (Conrad, 2007).

The case of demedicalizing and potentially remedicalizing homosexuality demonstrates that labelling a condition as medical or removing it from the list of possible diagnoses can be the product of highly contested social, cultural, and political processes. It took years of lobbying by social activists to achieve the demedicalization of homosexuality. Today, while some members of the LGBTQ (lesbian, gay, bi-sexual, transgendered, and queer) community criticize research on the gay gene, others see it as a means to defend their sexual orientation in medical terms. Therefore, medicalization and demedicalization are fluid processes, defined and redefined in cultural or medical terms, and greatly dependent on several social influences, such as political activism, research, social stigma, power and disadvantage, and morality.

Healthism and the New Morality

So far we have generally discussed medicalization as a process, but it can also be thought of as an ideology (Becker & Nachtigall, 1992; Crawford, 1979; Hartley, 2003). As our understanding of what the "body" is and what "disease" is are transformed under the medical gaze (Foucault, 1975), so is our concept of "health." Some scholars see the growing emphasis on a healthy lifestyle as another process of medicalization (Crawford, 1979). We eat and do what we are told (often by medical experts) to avoid getting sick. Eating, drinking, exercising, breathing—more and more of our daily activities have come to the attention of medical experts. Some activities (e.g., drinking alcohol, smoking, eating fatty or processed foods, being overweight) are defined as "not healthy" or "risky"; other activities (e.g., walking, meditating, drinking green tea, eating vegetables) are seen as contributing to health. We share with doctors the most intimate details of our daily lives: what we eat, where we live, how (and with whom) we sleep. They, in turn, take on the responsibility to give advice on all these issues (and we often expect they will). By allowing a medical gaze into our daily lives, we give physicians the right to become experts in almost all domains that previously biomedicine could not (or did not want to) reach. It is possible that physicians, or some other health professional, will soon test most of our activities on some manufactured health/illness scale leaving us little space to wonder about the potential harms and benefits of our daily routines. Therefore, some scholars argue that **healthism** and prevention can legitimate the perception that individuals are personally obligated to stay healthy (Crawford, 1979).

By letting medicalization creep into the domain of disease prevention, we allow medical ideology to classify our behaviours as "risky" and "not risky" (Lupton, 2001). In this sense, health behaviours become the basis for a new morality, our lens to judge others as good or bad. Everyday behaviours are redefined; the meanings of "food," "drink," "dance," "exercise," and other human activities become evaluated in health or medical terms (Zola, 1994). Not only do we let the medical gaze scan our inner bodies, but we also allow it to probe the context in which we live; how our bodies are moving, breathing, and interacting outside the medical world. This permits our lives to be further medicalized, redefining and attaching a medical label to everything we do and dichotomizing between healthy or "good" choices and unhealthy or "bad" choices.

This facilitates a move beyond discrimination based on physically ascribed traits (such as race, ethnicity, deformity, and gender) to include discrimination based on lifestyles and behaviours such as smoking, eating, and obesity. For example, when you walk past someone smoking a cigarette, the first thought often is not about the behaviour but an evaluation of the morality of the person smoking. We perceive this person as a "bad" person based solely on the smoking behaviour. The same can be said when we pass someone who is morbidly obese, or when we come upon a mother bottle-feeding her newborn baby. These behaviours are defined as medically risky and become synonymous with immorality, weakness, and an indication of the lower worth of the individual.

Wellness and health become the new virtues to which we aspire, a new puritan ethic that denies individuals any guilt-free pleasure and indulgence (Klein, 2010). Now, instead of enjoying a bowl of ice cream or bag of potato chips, we reach for the low-fat or fat-free ice cream, or the low-fat or fat-free baked, sodium-reduced potato chips. This new form of puritanism or righteousness has replaced the old Protestant ethic form of puritanism based on one's dedication to work and success (cf. Max Weber, *The Protestant Ethic and The Spirit of Capitalism* Weber, 1958). In fact, Metzel (2010, p. 2) has gone so far as to argue against health, maintaining that health is not being used in our common perception as something good but, instead, as something that is used "to make moral judgements, convey prejudice, sell products, or even exclude whole groups of persons from health care." Men's health, women's health, sexual health, healthy living—we are inundated with messages about health and how we just do not measure up. Health has been reconceptualized into an increasingly unobtainable goal to which we must strive. Men's health is about perfect hair, perfect teeth, perfect abdominal muscles, and virility all in the interest of attracting women; women's health is about extreme beauty, plastic surgery, sexually pleasing your partner, perfect complexion, perfect toes, and that elusive perfect bra. Health is now something mythical, a marketing tool to sell products to reach an unobtainable goal. In fact, if someone truly believes he or she is healthy and without any problems, we could label that person as deluded, suffering perhaps from "healthy-person syndrome."

The role of medicalization in seeing and understanding human physiology remains central despite a growing dissatisfaction with medical care and the consumerist approach to health, and of the critical assessment of the role of health care providers in health maintenance. However, while some people may not trust physicians, rarely do people challenge the importance and accuracy of medical knowledge. To what degree medicine as a science has conquered our world is evident through reviewing research on the placebo effect. The **placebo effect** is an improvement in symptoms by taking a fake medicine or simulated treatment (see Box 12.2)

To summarize, medicalization is the process of defining various phenomena under the medical domain. While the research on medicalization touches upon many fields in which human conditions have been redefined within a biomedical framework, the common claim of most researchers is that medicine is increasingly taking over people's lives, especially people in more vulnerable social positions. In the following sections, we examine two more aspects of medicalization—the description of medicalization in the context of iatrogenesis (Illich, 1976), and a relatively new and very powerful driving force behind medicalization—the pharmaceutical and medical equipment industry.

Box 12.2

The Placebo Effect

The placebo effect is a fake medicine or simulated treatment administered to participants or patients in the control group of an experimental randomized control trial (RCT) study to compare their responses to those of participants in the intervention group who received the bona fide medicine or treatment (see Chapter 2). Differences between these two groups provide evidence as to the efficacy of treatment. The administration of a placebo quite often appears to have a curing effect (Markle & McCrea, 2008). For instance, examining the effectiveness of the medication fluoxetine (Prozac) administered for depression in the United States, the double-blind study design included groups that were given only the medication, the medication with therapy, a placebo pill in place of the medication, or a placebo pill with therapy. The results demonstrated that fluoxetine in combination with therapy was effective in 71% of cases, fluoxetine alone helped in 60% of cases, and the placebo alone helped in 35% of cases (Markle & McCrea, 2008). While it is true that the medication was more helpful than the placebo, it is interesting that the placebo alone was helpful in 35% of cases.

Another example of the placebo effect is *sham surgery*, in which an incision is made during the procedure in a control group but the actual surgery is not performed on the organ. The patients in the control group are led to believe that they did have the full surgery. A recent study examined the effect of sham surgery on patients with osteoporosis who were to undergo knee surgery, finding that patients who had the real surgery did no better than patients who underwent the sham surgery (Moseley et al., 2002).

There are a number of explanations that might account for the placebo effect (Markle & McCrea, 2008). Here, we want to emphasize the way in which this effect can be explained by medicalization. It could be argued that the power of medicine does not lie exclusively in its ability to cure but instead in the patients' *belief* in the ability of medicine to cure. The confidence that medical treatment will help is what allows people to feel better after they have been administered a placebo. While the placebo effect may challenge the necessity of providing some medical treatments and inventing new medicine to treat human conditions (Markle & McCrea, 2008), it also demonstrates how deeply our belief in the power of contemporary medicine is embedded in our society.

IATROGENESIS

Iatrogenesis is a term that has been used extensively in the contemporary study of medicine to refer to physician-induced illness. First popularized by Ivan Illich (1976) and derived from the Greek roots *iatros* (physician) and *genesis* (origins), iatrogenesis has been used to refer to a number of dimensions of the phenomenon. It must be emphasized that the discussion that follows applies as much to institutions that provide care as it does to individual physicians. Thus, where we say "physician-induced," we can easily substitute other health professionals or "hospital." Illich describes three types of iatrogenic illness: clinical, social, and structural.

Clinical Iatrogenesis

Clinical iatrogenesis refers explicitly to illness created by the direct involvement in treatment. Through a wrongful (although not necessarily purposefully wrong) prescription of drugs or treatment by the physician, the contracting of bacterial infections while in the hospital (see Box 5.5 in Chapter 5), or other problems, the patient ends up worse off than before his or her interaction with the system. Navarro (1976) argues that clinical iatrogenesis is a result of the "engineering" approach that many doctors and health care workers take toward medicine, treating health care as a mechanical process. Rachlis and Kushner (1989, p. 9) support Navarro, suggesting that the action-based orientation of modern medicine creates a situation where iatrogenic illness is commonplace. Many of the illnesses people experience are a direct or indirect result of either too much care or inappropriate care. For example, Dhalla et al. (2009) reports a marked increase in the number of deaths due to opioid analgesic overdose following the introduction of long-acting oxycodone into the Ontario drug formulary in 2000. Importantly, most of these deaths were deemed unintentional overdoses that could have been prevented.

Although physicians and hospitals are ultimately responsible for illnesses of this type, one cannot blame them entirely. The health care system functions within a broader social context. Contemporary social beliefs about the current health care system create the impetus for physicians to adopt the approach of always taking some action to respond to our ailments. Physicians may be eager to do anything that may appear, at least on the surface, to be directed toward alleviating the problem. The physician is under pressure from the patient to take action even in the absence of good evidence that a treatment will really help. Ultimately, the physician ends up wasting time and money with treatments that are ineffective, or worse, that may create an illness that was not there previously.

For example, modern medicine has yet to develop a cure for the common cold; however, during cold season the first thing many people do is see their doctor or go to urgent care. The doctor, under pressure to help the patient, may prescribe an antibiotic. This prescription will not help cure the cold and the money spent is wasted. Moreover, the frequent and inappropriate prescribing of antibiotics for viral instead of bacterial infections has rendered many of these drugs ineffective against conditions for which they were once the only effective treatment (see Chapter 5).

Clinical iatrogenesis resulting from wrongful prescribing of drugs is, in part at least, a result of the very limited amount of education that doctors receive on pharmaceuticals (Regush, 1987). Canadian physicians depend on two main sources of information for their knowledge of prescription drugs, medical school and drug companies, and both are problematic (Regush, 1987). Future doctors receive only a course or two about pharmaceuticals over their four-year program. The information that they receive from drug companies may be biased and misleading (Angell 2004; Rachlis & Kushner 1989). Drug companies are not in the business of philanthropy; they are in the business of making money to satisfy their shareholders. They are very successful at this: many of the major pharmaceutical companies are consistently ranked among the most profitable manufacturing companies in Canada and globally (Lexchin, 2001). This point will be revisited in greater detail later in this chapter.

Social Iatrogenesis

Social iatrogenesis refers to the social perception of the health care system and the control it has over our daily lives. Medicalization has been defined as the process of bringing more and more everyday behaviour under the control of medicine (see Zola, 1972). What is defined as illness becomes illness, and falls under the jurisdiction of the health care system. Riessman (1983) argues that the biomedical basis of the current medical system is neither necessary nor sufficient to justify the classification of many social experiences in terms of illness. Illich discusses six "symptoms" of social iatrogenesis, which we describe below:

1. *The Dependence of Society on "Care."* Illich argues that more damage is caused to our health not by illness, but by our belief that we cannot cope or live without the care that the modern health care system provides. As soon as we become ill, our first thought is to seek medical advice. As consumers, we are encouraged to depend on such advice and to willingly comply with any treatment offered.

2. *The Dependence of Society on Drugs.* The second symptom is our persistent desire to find the "magic bullet" that will eliminate even the smallest complaint. If we have a headache, we take a pill rather than seek other means of relief. In response to the (perceived) demand from their patients, physicians are quick to prescribe drugs, and we have become conditioned and eager to take drugs without much thought.

3. *Medicalization of the Human Lifespan.* Another result of the medicalization of our daily lives is the medicalization of our life stages. From the unborn to the old, each stage of our life course becomes an opportunity for the health care system to poke and prod, to test and retest. As Illich describes, "The doctor's grasp over life starts with the monthly pre-natal check-up when he decides if and how the fetus shall be born; it ends with his decision to abandon further resuscitation" (Illich, 1976, pp. 44–45). Besides invading every stage of our life cycle, medicine also invades every environment in which these life stages occur. We are instructed on how to

live, creating a dependence on the health care system to coach us in what should be "natural behaviour."

4. *Medicalization of Prevention and Early Diagnosis of "Illness."* Preventive medicine has become the newest form of conspicuous and often unnecessary consumption for the middle class. This fixation on health can be a most unhealthy thing. If, through the yearly physical, a problem is identified, it transforms people who previously felt healthy into anxious patients. Prevention and early diagnosis of a condition or disease place patients on a lifelong treatment regimen (usually, including drugs), reduce life satisfaction, and condition the individual to depend even more on the health care system. (The counter-argument is that it may well be possible to intervene early in the course of an illness, restore the patient to health, or at least limit any disability resulting from the condition. As well, early intervention costs the health care system considerably less money in the long run.)

5. *Medicalization of Expectation.* The fifth symptom concerns the promise of medical technology to improve or prolong life. Through new technologies and treatments, people are living longer lives. Sometimes, these lives are limited in many ways, but the measure of success is quantity instead of quality. Because we have seen much success in prolonging life, people begin to expect the same success in improving the quality of life. People do not come to hold this expectation haphazardly. They are encouraged by the system to maintain hope for the cure that is "just around the corner."

6. *Patient Majorities.* As we noted in Chapters 8 and 11, there is a long history of labelling deviance in society. Labelling serves to reduce the anxiety of society and to exert social control over the unknown and unexplainable. Illich notes that since the 1950s, most labelling has been done by the health care system. Some would argue that medical definitions of deviance may be less damaging to the individual than legal or religious definitions, but the fact that so much defining of behaviour falls to the health care system again underlines the power of medicine in modern society.

These symptoms of social iatrogenesis have removed matters of health from the individual. In the past, people were considered healthy until proven otherwise. Now this no longer seems to be the case. Health, located in the hands of the physician and other health care professionals, is an unobtainable goal toward which we continually strive, but that is always kept just slightly out of our reach.

Structural Iatrogenesis

Changes in the basic structural orientation of our culture are also a source of iatrogenesis. Traditional culture was based on acceptance of pain and suffering; modern "medical culture" is based on the elimination of pain and suffering. Traditional culture equips individuals to fight pain; medical culture equips individuals to remove pain. Traditional culture is premised on working to alleviate the source of pain; medical culture is premised on alleviating the symptom, sometimes ignoring the underlying cause. The patient is made to depend upon social institutions, including hospitals and health professionals, to deal with personal weaknesses or vulnerabilities. Individual responsibility is removed and placed in the hands of the medical industry, effectively absolving the social and political environment of all responsibility.

Waitzkin (1989) argues that, by reifying symptoms at an individual-level, the focus shifts to the personal troubles of the individual and away from the social issues that are often the underlying causes. By treating the symptoms, society renders the social factors and institutional sources that cause the personal troubles immune to criticism. Within our medical culture, we deaden pain through the use of treatments and prescriptions making the underlying causes acceptable instead of working to eliminate these underlying sources of the pain.

Women are frequent victims of illnesses related to structural iatrogenesis consistent with the medicalization in women's lives. They visit the physician more often than men and are more likely to receive prescriptions for relief of symptoms. Riessman (1983, p. 16) argues that prescribing for symptom relief ignores the social cause of illness. By removing the social cause from view, the political context of the issue is also stripped away, reducing any chance of social action. In this way, the deadening of women's pain takes political action away from them and reinforces the dominant patriarchal institutions. Recall the 1966 song by the Rolling Stones, "Mother's Little Helper" about women taking pills (barbiturates) to calm them down, allow them to escape their daily lives, and get through their busy days. Today, women are prescribed antidepressants to accomplish the same goal, again avoiding action to rectify the underlying source of the pain and stress.

MEDICALIZATION AND THE PHARMACEUTICAL INDUSTRY

Throughout this chapter, we present an alternative critical perspective that challenges the common view that medicine is based solely on scientific discoveries. Social and political forces have a very large role to play in the process of medicalization. In the concluding section of this chapter we introduce the economic domain as another powerful player in the arena of labelling human processes and behaviours as medical disorders—specifically the pharmaceutical industry (or *Big Pharma*). While physician and health care dominance have traditionally been criticized for medicalization, researchers are paying closer attention to the role of pharmaceutical and medical equipment companies in this process (Conrad, 2005; Hartley, 2003; Lexchin, 2001; Moynihan, Heath & Henry, 2002). (See Researcher Profile 12.1 on Joel Lexchin.)

Canada, and many other Western countries, has a drug and equipment regulatory system that is enforced by government officials. This role is taken by the Therapeutic Products Directorate (TPD), a branch of Health Canada (Lexchin, 2010). These agencies are mandated to evaluate new and existing medical products to ensure the safety of the population. As Lexchin notes, however, government regulations and oversight do not always ensure public safety. For the salient example of the painkiller Vioxx, a Cox-2 inhibitor, developed and marketed by Merck, see Box 12.3.

Joel Lexchin

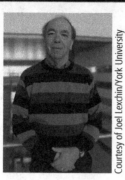

Courtesy of Joel Lexchin/York University

Joel Lexchin is an emergency physician, a Professor in the School of Health Policy and Management at York University, and an Associate Professor in the Department of Family and Community Medicine at the University of Toronto. His expertise focuses on issues surrounding pharmaceuticals, including physician prescribing, financing, and regulating pharmaceutical promotion and advertising; and conflict of interest and industry sponsorship in drug trials research. He has served as a consultant for pharmaceutical matters for a variety of governmental agencies at the provincial and federal levels as well as at the international level, including the World Health Organization and New Zealand and Australia. He argues that the Canadian government should establish more thorough policies and regulations in order to protect public safety and to control the escalation of health expenditures from drugs.

Driven by the profit from drug sales, the pharmaceutical industry is a very successful enterprise that generally exceeds the earnings for all other manufacturing industries in Canada (Lexchin, 2010). To make this profit, drug companies focus on marketing their products. In fact, the highest expenditure of these companies is not research or manufacturing, but marketing (Angell, 2004; Lexchin, 2010). New drugs that truly bring treatment innovation represent fewer than 10% of approved substances (Lexchin, 2010). Moreover, many new drugs are developed in universities and teaching hospitals and are partially subsidized by public funds through research grants. The bulk of new drugs that do come to market are "me-too" drugs that competing companies develop to closely replicate the initial discovery and market heavily to gain a share of sales. For example, as discussed in Box 12.3, Pfizer introduced their version of a Cox-2 inhibitor, Celebrex, to compete with Merck's Vioxx.

Marketing of new products is done in a number of ways targeting both physicians and consumers. Moynihan et al. (2002) identify various marketing strategies, including direct marketing to physicians, off-use marketing, medical education sponsorship, and direct-to-consumer marketing. To reach physicians, pharmaceutical companies advertise in medical journals and sponsor many continuing medical education events that Canadian physicians are required to attend regularly to keep their medical licence current and to learn new advances in medicine (Lexchin, 2010). It is worth noting that the Canadian Medical Association is a direct recipient of moneys paid by pharmaceutical companies through the funding for continuing medical education credits (CMEs) and through advertising in their medical journal, the *Canadian Medical Association Journal* (CMAJ).

Box 12.3

The Case of Vioxx

The drug *Vioxx* (rofecoxib, a Cox-2 inhibitor) developed by Merck, one of the largest pharmaceutical companies in the world, was originally approved for use in Canada and the United States in 1999 as a novel new pain medication. It was marketed as far superior to previous painkillers (NSAIDS, non-steroidal anti-inflammatory agents such as Naproxen) because of its lack of gastrointestinal side effects. It was later determined that Vioxx greatly increased the risk of heart attacks (Graham et al., 2005; Lévesque et al., 2006) prompting Health Canada to issue a warning in 2002. By 2004, Merck voluntarily pulled Vioxx from distribution following a number of successful and pending lawsuits in Canada and the United States. More importantly, evidence demonstrated that Merck knew about this increased risk and selectively withheld data about three cardiovascular deaths in their analysis published in a NEJM article (see Bombardier et al., 2000) about the gastrointestinal benefits of the new drug over other pain medication (Prakash & Valentine, 2006). Subsequent analysis of the original Merck sample, including the three missing cases (see Mukharjee et al., 2001), identified a significantly elevated risk of myocardial infarction (heart attacks) among those taking Vioxx versus both placebo and NSAIDs groups (Prakash & Valentine, 2006). However, in the face of this and other damning evidence, Merck continued to actively promote the drug until it finally pulled it from the market in 2004. The delay by Merck was completely understandable from a financial perspective. In 2003, it had over 20 million users worldwide (Eggertson, 2006) with annual global sales of $2.3 billion ("Vioxx, Celebrex," 2004). Interestingly however, Celebrex, the "me-too" Cox-2 Inhibitor drug created by Pfizer to capture part of this lucrative market, continued to be distributed even though it had the same side effects. After Vioxx was pulled, Celebrex prescriptions rose by over 100 000 in Canada ("Vioxx, Celebrex," 2004).

Pharmaceutical companies employ an army of salespersons referred to as "detail men" who visit and solicit business from physicians urging them to prescribe their products. They leave behind not only drug samples, but also promotional products and provide free lunches and goodies for staff. These detail men (and women) exert a strong influence on the prescribing habits of physicians, and, at times, create a false impression that a drug is safe and effective when this may not be the case (Angell, 2004). Although many doctors deny that they are influenced by the marketing of drugs, if it were not effective, it is doubtful that pharmaceutical companies would continue such an expensive and labour-intensive marketing strategy.

Off-label use, the prescribing of drugs for symptoms and illnesses for which the drug was not specifically tested, is another way pharmaceutical companies increase their sales. Although Health Canada prohibits companies from actively marketing drugs for off-label use, there is nothing stopping them from researching the use of these drugs for off-label use and presenting this evidence. In fact, since this research does not require the rigorous and expensive studies involved in the original work, it is another way for companies to increase market share at little cost. Moreover, there is nothing stopping physicians from prescribing medication for use other than the original purpose nor is there anything stopping the detail men from providing the drug. For example, Paxil, one of the SSRIs identified above, was newly developed to compete in the crowded market for treatment of depression. To increase its marketability, GlaxoSmithKline has directed its attention to the use of Paxil for anxiety and obsessive-compulsive disorder (OCD).

Direct-to-consumer marketing is another way in which pharmaceutical companies try to increase their market share. How often have you seen ads on television and in magazines that suggest you just "ask your doctor" if you are experiencing a specific problem with emotions or sexuality because the pharmaceutical company has a medication for that? Although this direct-to-consumer advertisement marketing strategy is not allowed in Canada, it is permitted in the United States, so we are still subject to its influence (Moynihan, Heath, & Henry, 2002). Using images that resonate with the majority of the public, this tactic promises the public a hope that a drug can cure personal troubles and improve the quality of life (Conrad, 2007). Headaches, sadness, pain, anxiousness, and almost every other human condition can be solved just by asking your doctor for a pill. Although sales still depend on physician prescribing, consumer demand is created by the suggestion that people contact their physicians, further pressuring the prescribing habits of physicians.

There are two consequences of this direct-to-consumer marketing tool. First, exposure to such advertisements makes drug consumption seem a mundane, universal tool for solving most of our problems (see social iatrogenesis). Second, pharmaceutical companies do not only promote their products as solutions to already existing medical conditions; they also play a part in "inventing" diagnoses by redefining natural and ordinary processes as diseases or conditions (Moynihan & Smith, 2002). One example for this trend is the invention of medications for sexual problems, perceived sexual inadequacy, and increased sexual desire. Sildenafil, commonly known as Viagra (Loe, 2004), was initially developed to treat coronary artery disease, but researchers noticed an interesting and unexpected side effect—increased blood flow to the genital areas (Loe, 2004). This "happy accident" (Loe, 2004, p. 43) was later labelled as a successful discovery of the drug Viagra that was helping to treat "erectile dysfunction" (ER), a diagnosis that was borrowed by Pfizer, the manufacturer of Viagra, from *DSM IV-R*, to market the new drug (Loe, 2004). As Loe (2004) suggests, Viagra brought about a change in sex life in America (and increasingly around the world). Expanding the marketing campaign from targeting the relatively small population of men who actually suffer from erectile dysfunction, to a larger population of men who seek to improve sexual performance, it challenges men's virility with claims of sexual fulfillment for yourself and your partner with ads that run during sports shows. The discussion of sexual performance, previously considered by many as private, if not taboo, has become the focus for marketing and advertising Viagra. It has also become a topic for discussion with your physician. As Loe (2004) notes, however, the invention of Viagra has its own dangers and problems. In addition to sexual satisfaction, Viagra also brought with it an increase in recreational use of the drug, unintended side effects, and a booming illegal market, all of which just increase manufacturing and sales.

Viagara wasn't necessarily the panacea it was advertised to be—a positive change in the sex life of all aging couples (especially for men's aging spouses). To address this gender imbalance or, more likely, in an attempt to create demand and market share among the missing 50% of the population (women), pharmaceutical companies have attempted to develop a similar magic pill for women. As Moynihan (2003) notes, in order to do this, they first needed to create a new syndrome called female sexual dysfunction or what others have labelled female sexual arousal disorder (FSAD, see *DSM IV-R and DSM-5*—see Box 12.4). An advertisement for "Vibrel" from Helm Pharmaceuticals stated:

Box 12.4

Female Sexual Arousal Disorder (FSAD)

DSM-IV-R definition of Female Sexual Arousal Disorder:

> The essential feature of Female Sexual Arousal Disorder is a persistent or recurrent inability to attain, or to maintain until completion of the sexual activity, an adequate lubrication-swelling response of sexual excitement (Criterion A). The arousal response consists of vasocongestion in the pelvis, vaginal lubrication and expansion, and swelling of the external genitalia. The disturbance must cause marked distress or interpersonal difficulty (Criterion B). The dysfunction is not better accounted for by another Axis I disorder (except another Sexual Dysfunction) and is not due exclusively to the direct physiological effects of a substance (including medications) or a general medical condition (Criterion C). (American Psychiatric Association, 2000, p. 543)

Compare the above clinical definition in *DSM-IV-R* with a study published in 1999 that analyzed the 1992 National Health and Social Life Survey (NHSLS), estimating female sexual dysfunction to be as being as high as 43% compared to only 31% for male sexual dysfunction (Laumann, Paik, & Rosen, 1999). The study prevalence rates were based on a positive response to any one of the seven following dichotomous (yes/no) questions (p. 538):

1. lacking desire for sex;
2. arousal difficulties (i.e., erection problems in men, lubrication difficulties in women);
3. inability achieving climax or ejaculation;
4. anxiety about sexual performance;
5. climaxing or ejaculating too rapidly;
6. physical pain during intercourse; and
7. not finding sex pleasurable.

How many of these items coincide with the DSM clinical definition above? The authors argue that, "taken together, these items cover the major problem areas addressed in the Diagnostic and Statistical Manual of Mental Disorders, Fourth Edition classification of sexual dysfunction" (p. 538). Although the authors do acknowledge that "[the] NHSLS data on critical symptoms do not connote a clinical definition of sexual dysfunction"(p. 540), Moynihan (2003) argues that this caveat has been conveniently ignored. Being able to claim such an inflated prevalence estimate allows physicians and pharmaceutical companies to create a perception of the great need for something to be done. It is notable that the authors of the 1999 study, Laumann and Rosen, did not disclose their financial relationships with various pharmaceutical companies, including Pfizer (the manufacturer of Viagra), in the original article. These were subsequently published in an erratum (which appears in [1999]. *JAMA, 281,* 1174).

An advertisement for "Vibrel" from Helm Pharmaceuticals *focused specifically on women who have, to this point, been neglected, that they too now have a solution—a proverbial pink pill—to improve their sex-life. (Helm Pharmaceuticals [advertisement], Dec, 2007)*

The whole idea is to increase the potential population to which a company can market its products. The population of "sick" people is relatively small compared to the population of "healthy" people. Moreover, healthy people are often more financially well off than sick people, having much more disposable income. As such, it only makes sense that pharmaceutical companies will try to expand their target population and market their products to those who can better afford them in order to increase profitability.

SUMMARY

In this chapter we describe the increasing medicalization of our lives. Our aim was to demonstrate that these processes both are informed by and influence social relations in society. Knowledge and its application, including medical knowledge, is not immune to the interplay and negotiation of social forces consisting of government agencies, political parties, social activists, corporate lobbying, and lay people's perceptions.

The continuing growth of medical dominance of our understanding of human processes and morality brought about a critique of medical imperialism. Being sick or being healthy is often defined in medical terms and less and less of our lives are immune to receiving a medical label. Moreover, some groups are more vulnerable than others to this redefining of natural processes as medical phenomena based on the differential distribution of power and control in society. Finally, some scholars suggest that professional dominance that has existed for decades is diminishing under the increased pressure of markets and capitalism where corporations take a leading role in defining disease and health.

Key Terms

Demedicalization—the reverse of medicalization, where medical problems are being defined as nonmedical problems

Diagnostic imperialism—the exclusive rights of physicians to diagnose and treat the disease

Healthism—increasing concern with health that is reflected in the tendency of defining the actions and practices in relation to potential benefits or risks to our health and in our moral evaluation of others

Iatrogenesis—physician, health professional, or health system–induced illness, an illness that would not have occurred if it were not for contact with the health care system in some capacity

Medicalization—the process by which problems previously defined as nonmedical become redefined and treated as medical conditions

Medical gaze—the inspection of disease by medical experts that is associated with the process of depersonalization of disease and increase in the power over individuals through the possession of medical knowledge about human conditions

Off-label use—the use of a drug to treat the conditions and diseases that it was not originally designed or tested to treat

Placebo effect—an improvement in symptoms by taking a fake medicine or simulated treatment

Profane—those objects and ideas that have no religious or transcendent meaning

Sacred—objects or ideas that have been assigned a religious or a transcendent meaning

Critical Thinking Questions

1. How can individuals' cultural beliefs shape their attitudes toward the medicalization of a particular social phenomenon?

2. Provide an example not previously mentioned that illustrates the process of medicalization and describe the how the process occurred.

3. What are the differences and similarities between healthism and medicalization of society?

4. Describe how structural iatrogenesis could be used to explain alcohol and tobacco use.

5. How is the consumption of pharmaceutical products shaped by gender, age, class, and ethnicity?

Further Readings and Resources

Angell, M. (2004). *The truth about drug companies.* New York: Random House.

Conrad, P. (2007). *The medicalization of society: On the transformation of human conditions into treatable disorders.* Baltimore: The John Hopkins University Press.

Goldacre, Ben. (2013). *Bad pharma: How drug companies mislead doctors and harm patients.* London: Fourth Estate.

Metzl, J. M. & Kirkland, A. (Eds.) (2010). *Against health: How health became the new morality.* New York: New York University Press.

Moynihan, R. (2003). The making of a disease: female sexual dysfunction. *BMJ 326* (4 January), 45–47.

Goldacre, Ben. (2012). *TED talks,* April 2012, on Bad Pharma
www.ted.com/talks/view/lang/en//id/1575

Chapter 13
Food and Agriculture

Chapter Outline

Learning Objectives

After studying this chapter, you should be able to:

1. Understand the importance of examining the social aspects of food as a factor for health among Canadians;

2. Describe the changes in the industrialized trends in agricultural and production patterns of the food supply;

3. Examine how changes in food production influence food consumption and some of the consequences;

4. Differentiate among recent movements and social responses to changes in agriculture and food production.

Why would a text on the social dimensions of health cover something as seemingly unrelated as food and agriculture?[1] There are numerous issues in agriculture and food that have a profound effect on our health. Changes in how our food is produced, processed, and consumed have a substantial effect on the health of the population, the environment, the workers, and the plants and animals being consumed. Moreover, many business and personal decisions that influence food production, processing, and consumption occur within the social, political, and economic environment.

Mass-produced food and foods processed outside the home for purchase are relatively new phenomena. In 1950, there were very few processed food products. Cheez Whiz, for example, wasn't introduced until 1953 (Hevesi, 2007). Grocery shelves contained few of the multitudes of prepared food products we see today and a large proportion of prepared foods for sale in grocery stores were prepared on site. Meat, for example, was typically cut in the store and most grocery stores had a staff of butchers. Most food was far more local than it is today. Tomatoes and strawberries, unless canned or preserved, were available only in season and were fragile, flavourful, and juicy. Watermelons had seeds. Local quality and availability of fresh produce changed with the seasons and regions. By default, most people were locavores, eating goods produced by local farmers.

Although retail frozen foods were introduced in 1930 by Clarence Birdseye, who, through his work with the Inuit in the Canadian Arctic, realized that quickly frozen fish retained its freshness (Pehanich, 2003), there were very few frozen products available for consumers. Even frozen dinners (previously referred to as TV dinners with the advent of television), today a common grocery staple, only began to appear in the 1950s and took several decades to infiltrate and replace home cooking. TV dinners took nearly a half hour to heat up since few people had microwave ovens until the 1970s. With a few exceptions related principally to ceremonies such as weddings and funerals, religious holidays, and to religious demands such as fasting and dietary restrictions, most people ate for sustenance. There were no advocates of slow food—virtually all food was "slow."

Today's grocery stores have far more, highly refined and processed products. They now have entire aisles dedicated to ready-to-eat frozen meals. Other aisles are dedicated to soft drinks, frozen confections such as ice cream, and refined high fat–based and high carbohydrate–based food such as crackers, cookies, and chips. The current shelf life of processed foods and produce (their ability to stay on the store shelf without spoiling) is far longer, which results in a much wider variety of goods and fresh produce no

---

[1]This chapter was co-authored with Paul Millar as primary author.

matter the season. Tomatoes and strawberries can be shipped from almost anywhere in the world and are always available. But they are far less juicy, less flavourful, and much tougher, even if they do last for weeks in the refrigerator. The products available in one store or region are now virtually identical to other stores and regions.

Products are marketed and located in grocery stores based on profitability. The most profitable foods are placed in the most accessible places and manufacturers pay for this privilege. Products at eye level and at the ends of aisles are those that are more profitable (Winson, 2004). Winson (2004) describes foods that are high in refined fats and carbohydrates and low in nutrients as "pseudo-foods." A survey of Canadian supermarkets found that 26 to 37% of shelf space was devoted to these foods; an average of 19 special displays for pseudo-foods were present in each store (Winson, 2004).

Schools in Canada in the 1950s did not generally have cafeterias or vending machines. Children brought lunches made at home. Today, many schools not only have vending machines, but have signed "pouring rights" contracts that give specific soft drink suppliers exclusive rights to market their products to the children at that school. In return, the school receives a payment from the soft drink supplier, a payment that makes the contract attractive to school administrators (Nestle, 2000). Generally, individual school boards set their own policies on food in the school: few schools in Canada supply free food. The situation in the United States is very different. There, most schools serve lunch as part of the services the school provides, including free and reduced-cost lunches for students whose family income is low enough to qualify. However, the menu is often more centred on cost considerations than providing good nutrition.

There are many societal factors that influence food production and consumption. We explore these to gain a sense of how much our food is governed by various social forces that may or may not be within our individual control.

FOOD AND FOOD CONSUMPTION

The world population continues to increase, with projections by the United Nations of 8 billion by the year 2025 (Population Division of the Department of Economic and Social Affairs of the United Nations Secretariat, 2010). Many analysts believe that it will be difficult to achieve an adequate diet for this population, even with advances in technology. This is compounded by the differential caloric distribution of foodstuff across countries. Developed countries currently derive 27% of their calories from animal products—which are agriculturally more expensive—versus only 13% in less developed countries. As less developed countries grow economically, so will the demand for more animal-based agriculture (Gilland, 2002). In other words, agricultural demand will increase even faster than the population due to the demand for animal-based food. Meeting these demands will be a challenge that will be difficult to achieve, even after accounting for efficiencies gained by using modern agricultural technologies.

While changes in the world population will greatly influence patterns of food production and consumption, these patterns will also change based on other, often competing, incentives between producers and consumers. Consumers, of course, usually want a product that costs less. However, they also want a product that is safe, nutritious, and tasty. Producers want to reduce production costs to improve their profitability. The cost-benefits achieved through improvements to the efficiencies of production sometimes negatively affect the characteristics of the products that consumers value. However, the message the consumer receives is "food—now at lower cost" instead of "food—now with reduced nutrients, bland taste, pesticide residue, and an increased chance of pathogens." Producers reduce costs by increasing yield (tonnage produced per acre), reducing labour costs, decreasing spoilage, and increasing the scale and efficiency of processing facilities. One of the ways to increase yield and reduce costs is through breeding plant varieties that meet the needs of producers. Consequently, breeds of tomatoes have been developed that can withstand mechanical harvesting (saving labour), sorting, and transportation (reducing spoilage), and be artificially ripened with ethylene gas (so they can be picked and shipped before they are ripe).

Lack of flavour is not an issue for processors since flavour is not so much derived from the fruits and vegetables being processed as by natural and artificial flavours that can be added. An unintended consequence of breeding plants for increased yield is to reduce nutrients through a process called *dilution*. That is, plants may produce more yield per acre under cultivation, but each plant has reduced nutrient value (Davis, 2009). The nutritive value of plants is also affected by depleted soils maintained through chemical fertilizers. Refining agricultural products also creates benefits for processors that are not necessarily in the interests of consumers. Perhaps the most familiar example is the refining of flour that, especially in the case of white flour, removes many of the original nutrients, for example, the bran in wheat. Sometimes these nutrients are removed because they are problematic for shelf life. For example, one of the more important nutrients contained in oil is omega-3 fatty acids, which are also the components that are the first to spoil, or turn the oil rancid. Further refining of the oil removes many of these components, resulting in a more uniform but blander tasting and less nutritious oil. Such oil lasts far longer on the grocery store shelf. Concerns about the use of these methods have led to the availability of "virgin" oils, especially olive oils that have not been highly processed. However, these products are priced higher because they are seen as having value added even though they are less processed.

Another way to add value to products is convenience, such as demonstrated by prepared frozen dinners. Again, this usually entails reduced nutritional value, high fat and sodium, and a taste that is bland or derived from artificial flavouring and chemical additives.

Regulation of Food and Agriculture in Canada and the United States

Inspection and regulation of food in Canada is the responsibility of the Canadian Food Inspection Agency (CFIA), part of the Department of Agriculture and Agri-Food (DAAF). Pesticides, drugs administered to animals, nutrition, and food-borne illness are the responsibility of Health Canada. Canada and the United States (each being the other's most important food trading partner) have made efforts to improve the consistency of their regulations to better enable agricultural imports and exports (Raj, 2011).

United States' regulation of food production involves several government agencies. The role of some departments is clear. For example, the Environmental Protection Agency (EPA) regulates pesticides used in agricultural production; the National Marine Fisheries Service of the U.S. Department of Commerce inspects seafood and certifies seafood-based animal feeds. However, the bulk of American food regulation is divided between the Food and Drug Administration (FDA) of the Department of Health and Human Services (DHHS) and the U.S. Department of Agriculture (USDA). The division of what is regulated by the USDA and the FDA is not always easy to determine. Overall, the USDA has a mandate for meat, poultry, and processed eggs while the FDA is responsible for regulating other food, drugs used on animals, and feed. For example, the USDA regulates spaghetti sauce with meat but the FDA regulates spaghetti sauce without meat.

Over time, differences in incentives between consumers and producers have changed the character of how we produce and consume food in ways that benefit producers and processors more than consumers. To explore this change, we take a closer look at both food production and food consumption.

CHANGES IN FOOD PRODUCTION
Technological Changes

Technologies and techniques have already dramatically transformed the way food is produced. Food in developed nations is now produced using technologically advanced methods on an industrial scale on increasingly larger farms. Foremost among these technologies is the development of new species of plants and animals through conventional breeding and genetic engineering. Conventional modifications entail selective breeding to develop the genetic characteristics desired. Cattle are bred to match changes in consumer tastes, for leanness or fat marbling. More commonly, however, breeding revolves around concerns of producers such as their ability to provide more meat, faster. In the case of beef cattle (cattle raised for meat, not dairy), both the average weight of the animal for slaughter and the time required to achieve that weight have changed radically. The average weight of cattle raised in Ontario has steadily risen from about 560 kg in the mid-1970s to about 820 kg (an almost 50% increase!) in the mid-2000s (Mussell, Oginsky, & Hedley, 2008). A similar trend is present for hogs. Cattle that in the 1800s took four years to raise on grass to reach slaughter weight (MacLachlan, 2001) now take fewer than 18 months (Pollan, 2006). These efficiencies are not just the result of breeding; hormones, antibiotics, and feed supplements are also involved. Antibiotics, often the same formulations humans use, are routinely given to healthy animals in their feed in order to prevent disease and increase growth rates (see Box 13.1 on bovine growth hormone). The antibiotics are given because the animals generally live in close confinement and in contact with their feces. Now, however, people are concerned that using antibiotics in this way may be helping pathogens to mutate into "superbugs" resistant to antibiotic treatment, such as certain strains of campylobacter

(Wegener, 1999; Smith et al., 1999). In fact, the FDA is now attempting to restrict routine antibiotic use in livestock to address this concern (Tavernise, 2013).

A more controversial aspect of technology is the creation of engineered **genetically modified organisms** (GMOs) involving the direct insertion of DNA from one species into another. The most common of these products are the Roundup Ready (RR) series of soybean and corn products from Monsanto (Monsanto, "Genuity Roundup Ready 2," n.d.) The RR series of seeds have been genetically modified to resist the Monsanto herbicide Roundup so that the control of weeds is much simpler, more effective, and—aside from spraying—virtually labour-free. Most of the corn and more than 90% of all soybeans grown in Canada and the United States now use RR seeds (Monsanto, "Soybean Facts,"

Box 13.1

Bovine Growth Hormone

One of the first genetically engineered products continues to be one of the most controversial. Monsanto genetically engineered a bacterium to synthesize bovine growth hormone (BGH), which has been sold in the United States since 1994 under the trade name Posilac® (Monsanto has since sold Posilac to the Eli Lilly Co.) (Monsanto, "Company History", n.d.). The synthetic product is called recombinant bovine growth hormone or rBGH (also called recombinant bovine somatotropin [rBST]). Injecting this hormone into dairy cows increases their milk production, but also negatively affects the health of the animal, increasing the likelihood of mastitis and other health problems, such as lameness and reproductive problems (Dohoo et al., 2003a; Dohoo et al., 2003b). Posilac was approved for use in the United States, but not in Canada, due, in part, to concerns about human health, such as possible hypersensitivity to milk from rBGH-treated cows (Royal College of Physicians and Surgeons of Canada, 1993). This denial was controversial, since it came after three Health Canada scientists (Shiv Chopra, Margaret Hayden, and Gerard Lambert) were fired after testifying against rBGH and complaining of pressure from Health Canada management to approve the hormone (Standing Senate Committee on Agriculture and Forestry,1999; Standing Committee on Health, 2005).

A recent legal case in Ohio, over whether labelling milk as "rBGH-free" was legal, ruled that there were three differences in milk produced using rBGH: elevated levels of insulin-like growth factor 1 (IGF-1); decreased nutritional content (higher fat and lower protein); and higher somatic cell counts (a consequence of pus from mastitis) (*International Dairy Foods Association v. Boggs*, 2010). This case illustrates another issue related to genetically modified organisms (GMOs): whether foods grown using this technology should be labelled so the consumer is aware. Companies marketing GMOs argue that labelling products derived from GMOs is not fair since the resulting product is not substantially different from the equivalent non-GMO product. In Canada, foods produced using genetic engineering are not labelled, so unless the product is certified organic, it may contain genetically engineered components. Although most developed nations have not approved the use of rBGH in dairy production, it continues to be used in the United States and many developing nations. Because of our reliance on prepared food, much of which comes from the United States, we end up consuming it even though Canada has not approved it.

n.d.; Monsanto, 2004). The greatly simplified weed management when growing RR soybeans does come with a price. These crops require more herbicide to be applied than conventional crops and have lower yields (Benbrook, 2001).

There are many concerns about the introduction of GMOs into nature and the food supply. Well-known scientist and broadcaster David Suzuki compares the use of genetic engineering within biotechnology to the discredited scientific discipline of eugenics, a discipline dedicated to improving human genes. Since we know so little about the effects of genetically modified organisms on nature and humans, their use is essentially an uncontrolled experiment on subjects who have not given their informed consent. Suzuki argues that GMOs may be more dangerous than nuclear waste since they are living organisms that can multiply instead of degrading over time (Suzuki, 2000).

The first genetically modified animal likely to be introduced into the food supply is a genetically modified Atlantic salmon that grows more than twice as fast as and much larger than conventional Atlantic salmon (Kopun, 2010). The fish has not yet received approval from the Food and Drug Administration (FDA) in the United States. This is only the first in a long line of potential food animals created through genetic engineering. Among the concerns with genetically engineering animals are the potential health effects on humans who consume them and the effects on other species if the newly created animal escapes into the wild. Genetically engineered salmon, for example, have the ability to breed with wild (non-GMO) salmon (Moreau, Conway & Fleming, 2011) with unknown consequences.

A newer technology targeting food safety is **irradiation**. Irradiation is the treatment of food with X-rays, gamma rays, or electron beams to kill pathogens (microbes and insects) that might be present in the food. It is a solution to the potential contamination of some foods, such as hamburger, that have been subject to outbreaks of food-borne illness such as E-coli bacteria (CFIA, "Food Irradiation," n.d.; CFIA, "Irradiation of Ground Beef," n.d.). Food in Canada that has been irradiated must be labelled with the logo shown in Figure 13.1. Industry sometime uses the term "cold pasteurization" to counter negative public perceptions of the use of radiation.

Canada is considering allowing the routine use of irradiation for foods such as mangos, poultry, shrimp, prawns, and ground beef (CFIA, "Food Irradiation", n.d.). Irradiation makes small changes in the food, including, for example, the production of small amounts of benzene (a carcinogen) and 2-alkylcyclobutanones. The amounts are much smaller, for example, than the amounts of benzene in non-irradiated eggs (CIFA, n.d.). One wonders, however, whether this information should make Canadians complacent about foods being irradiated instead of raising interest in why our eggs contain a toxic and carcinogenic chemical in the first place.

Industrialization of Animal-Based Food Production

The industrialization of the production of food animals is nothing new. Indeed the initial concentration of cattle slaughtering in the Chicago area in many ways presaged the challenges of current day meat production. Its assembly-line (or more accurately, its

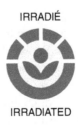

IRRADIÉ

IRRADIATED

Figure 13.1 Canadian Irradiation Logo

"The labelling requirements for irradiated food products are set out in section B.01.035 of the Food and Drug Regulations. Labeling provisions for prepackaged products, bulk retail units, shipping containers and the use of the internationally recognized radura symbol and label statement shall be followed. Information should be provided on the label which enables the tracking of individual lots of irradiated product sold to the consumer."

Source: Health Products and Food Branch. *Recommended Canadian Code of Practice for Food Irradiation*, Section 8. Health Canada and the Canadian Food Inspection Agency, Nov 19, 2002. Retrieved from www.hc-sc.gc.ca/fn-an/securit/irridation/code_of_practice-code_de_pratique01-eng.php#a5.2

disassembly-line) methods pre-dated Henry Ford's famous innovations in mass production of the automobile (Carlson, 2001). Prior to the centralized and industrialized slaughterhouses in Chicago in the late 1800s, most cattle were slaughtered in local butcher shops in each city or town. The problem of preserving the meat was avoided by slaughtering the animals as needed locally. The very large facilities developed in Chicago combined the technologies of railroad transportation and ice-based chilling (and later refrigeration) to rapidly bring pre-slaughtered meat at a much lower cost to consumers across the United States (Carlson, 2001). This led to the displacement of many local butcher shops, especially in larger cities. Despite the transportation cost, meat was cheaper due to the efficiencies of mass production. Slaughterhouses gained extra revenue from the sale of byproducts that were formerly wasted, such as bone, entrails, horns, and hooves (Carlson, 2001). However, this new mode of production had problems, most prominently in food safety, concentration of ownership (the "beef trusts"), and the treatment of workers. A popular novel of the time, *The Jungle*, illustrated these problems and led to a United States' presidential inquiry, the breaking up of the beef trusts, and the formation of the U.S. Food and Drug Administration (FDA) (Sinclair, 1906/2004).

Today Canada experiences many of the conditions in meat production that were present at the end of the nineteenth century. Ownership of meatpacking is concentrated into "shared monopolies" where the market is dominated by a few very large companies. Treatment of workers (discussed later in the chapter) remains a concern because of high rates of injury. Food safety, while no doubt an enormous improvement over the eighteenth century, remains near the forefront among concerns with meat production. The industrial production of meat is reaching levels unheard of in history. Canada's largest slaughterhouse, Lakeside Packers in Brooks, Alberta, for example, processes 1.4 million cattle per year or 28 000 per week (MacLachlan, 2001). The concentration of meatpacking into fewer, larger slaughterhouses is illustrated by changes in Alberta between 1987 and 1998. The weekly average slaughter rose from 22 900 to 56 550 cattle per week while the number of processing plants decreased from seven to three (MacLachlan, 2001).

Large slaughterhouses are not generally supplied directly from farms, but instead receive most of their stock from large feedlots (concentrated animal feeding operations—CAFOs). Most cattle are raised by farmers from birth and then sold to feedlots at anywhere from six to 16 months for "finishing" before slaughter. Feedlots fatten the calves with carefully controlled diets that are high in corn, soy, animal protein (some of the byproducts from slaughter houses), and other supplements such as vitamins and antibiotics calculated to enable the greatest growth in the shortest time. The use of feed that cattle do not naturally eat, such as corn, soy, and animal protein; the strain of being in close quarters with so many other cattle; and the ease with which contagious disease can spread are some of the reasons that antibiotics are used in a preventive fashion, as an ongoing component of their feed. Antibiotics also increase the growth rate of the cattle. Animal protein supplements have been controversial in the past, not just because cows are normally vegetarians, but also because of food safety, specifically as a cause of bovine spongiform encephalopathy (BSE) (see Box 13.2 on BSE).

Box 13.2

Bovine Spongiform Encephalopathy (BSE)

BSE, also known as mad cow disease, is a disease that gradually destroys the brains of cows and causes a related incurable and fatal disorder in humans called Creutzfeldt-Jakob disease (CJD). (CJD can also be caused genetically (fCJD) and can arise sporadically (sCJD). This discussion is related more specifically to variant Creutzfeldt-Jakob disease or vCJD, caused by prions, the most common form of the ailment.) Both are caused by *prions* (improperly folded proteins). These proteins are difficult to destroy and can transmitted by eating the tissue, especially neurological matter, of animals that already have prions. Prions survive autoclaving, normal sterilization processes, and pasteurization. Recently, it has been shown that CJD can be transmitted in humans via blood transfusions (Peden, Head, Ritchie, Bell, & Ironside, 2004).

BSE and CJD have received a lot of attention from the public, not because they are common,

but because their effects are devastating and incurable. Further, there is no test for either disease, except after death, though some are under development. When BSE was discovered in one cow in Alberta in 2003, most countries closed their borders to Canadian beef, essentially shutting down all exports of Canadian beef. To date, there have been 18 confirmed cases of BSE in Canadian cattle—at least one each year since 2003, with the exception of 2004. Testing is performed on a small proportion of cattle at higher risk—cattle with obvious symptoms and those over 30 months of age. Since BSE can take many years to develop, older cattle are most susceptible although Japanese testing has revealed BSE in male dairy cattle younger than two years of age (Food Safety Commission, 2004). Canada has implemented some safeguards to reduce the prevalence of BSE in Canadian cattle. These

(continued)

Box 13.2 (*Continued*)

include banning the feeding of the bodies of rumi-nants (cattle, sheep, goats, bison, elk, and others) to other ruminants and the removal of specified risk material (SRM) from meat destined for human consumption. SRM includes the distal ileum, brain, skull, and certain parts of the nervous system (CFIA, "BSE", n.d.). Cattle may still be fed ren-dered hogs or poultry, and cattle blood; these hogs and poultry may be fed rendered cattle.

There are some concerns about the adequacy of Canada's BSE prevention and surveillance strategies. For example, given the resilience of prions, the feeding of rendered cattle to swine, then feeding rendered swine to cattle may not eliminate the transmission of prions. Since the finding that human vCJD may be transmitted via blood, the feeding of cattle blood to cattle may also be risky. Canada's surveillance is not as stringent as Japan's, which tests 100% of cattle 24 months and older. Since Canada only tests a few percent of animals over 30 months, many cases may not be detected. In 2003, then Alberta Premier Ralph Klein advocated that cattle farm-ers should "shoot, shovel and shut-up" or, in other words, cover up any suspected cases of BSE (Cryderman, 2003).

Changes in Farm Size and Labour

The advances in technology paralleled the move from the traditional family farm to fewer and much larger industrial farms (see Table 13.1) (Stanton, 1993). This change has largely been seen in the area of livestock (Allen & Lueck, 2000). The cost of new technologies necessitates larger farms for efficiency. Farm machinery that reduces labour requires capital-ization to be spread over enough acres to be cost effective. As larger farms implement machinery, smaller farms find it more difficult to compete, since they cannot produce for the same cost. In addition to machinery, technologies such as GMO seeds (discussed previ-ously) allow a reduction in labour that enables both larger farms and lower costs.

The trend to larger and fewer farms is one result of the combination of politics around agriculture and technology. As farms get bigger and more corporate, not only does it dis-place a large percentage of the rural population and threaten the existence of many small farming communities, there is also a trend toward hiring cheaper, immigrant labour (Preibisch, 2007). In Canada, two major programs manage the importation of temporary labour, the Seasonal Agricultural Workers Program (SAWP) and the Temporary Foreign Worker Program (TFWP). These workers are paid at least the minimum wage in the juris-diction in which they are employed. However, they are not allowed to organize into unions, they are vulnerable to being deported at their employer's discretion, and they are not allowed to switch employers (Bauder, 2008).

The use of foreign labour for agriculture work—work that is often low status, dirty, and dangerous—is also a public health issue in that these workers are vulnerable to drug use, illness, and injury (General Accounting Office, 1992). *Fast Food Nation* (Schlosser, 2005), which documents the American situation, suggests that slaughterhouse workers—often illegal immigrants—frequently use drugs to mitigate the difficult working conditions and are pressured to under-report job-related injuries to minimize a company's worker

Table 13.1 Number of Farms by Number of Acres in Crops or Summer Fallow in Canada

Size of Farm (in Acres)	2001	2006	Change
0–759	177 556	160 524	−17 032
760–1999	29 694	25 063	−4 631
2000–3499	6 678	7 123	445
3500+	2 582	3 253	671
Total	216 510	195 963	−20 547

Source: Statistics Canada. (2006c). *Census of agriculture, farm data and farm operator data.* Ottawa: Author, catalogue no. 95-629-XWE.

compensation costs. Canadian workers at Canada's largest slaughterhouse, who claimed similar pressures to refrain from seeking medical attention, through a successful strike won the right to be represented by a union (Brethour, 2005). The strike was the subject of a documentary film by the Canadian National Film Board (Inkster & Thompson, 2007).

Changes to Agricultural Biodiversity

The degree of biodiversity in agricultural plants and animals has dramatically decreased over recent decades. Underlying this trend is the increased concentration in seed markets and the greater degree of control over animal reproduction, along with globalization of food markets. In the past, seeds were grown and saved by individual farmers and were specific to a region, with each variety chosen for its adaptation to local growing conditions. Likewise, animals such as cattle were chosen over generations for their ability to survive and thrive under local climates and ecologies. This ensured a great deal of variation in the world's agricultural biodiversity since each location had variants of each type fruit or vegetable. Genetic techniques, both traditional breeding and genetic engineering, have accelerated the pace of adapting agricultural species to human needs. These adaptations are not to local conditions, but because of producer concerns such as yield, ability to withstand shipping and handling, uniformity, and other attributes allowing improved efficiency in production. With these aims, genetic material is "improved" at a much faster rate than in the past, but it is also far less diverse.

Another trend that reduces the diversity of agricultural genetics is the consolidation of companies that provide seed and semen. For example, in order to ensure a global market for its products, Monsanto purchased a large number of seed distribution companies, the most prominent of which is Seminis, acquired in 2005 (Monsanto, 2005). Seminis, itself a consolidation of a number of seed companies, is the world's largest provider of seed, its slogan being, "If You've Eaten a Salad, You've Had a Seminis Product" (Seminis, n.d.). As companies become global in scope, fewer of them market and distribute seeds. Biotech conglomerates that produce new seed varieties own these companies. At the same time, the variety of seeds available to the world's farmers have decreased, as fewer and fewer species comprise the world's food supply. Another Monsanto 2005 acquisition was a genetic engineering company that produced so-called terminator seeds that can be planted only once, producing a plant with sterile seeds, (Monsanto, "Terminator seeds", n.d.). So far Monsanto has not incorporated this technology into any of its products (Monsanto, n.d.).

Animal breeding is also affected by the trend toward less biodiversity. For example, cattle in developed countries are increasingly bred through the central production of bull semen from relatively few bulls, producing standard animals with reliable characteristics. The bull semen is then used to artificially inseminate cows to produce calves and milk. To a greater and greater degree, scientific techniques and equipment are involved with animal reproduction to ensure that the resulting offspring have the traits sought by producers. As with vegetables, the diversity of the genetic pools from which our agricultural animals are drawn is decreasing and will continue to do so.

Capture Fishery and Aquaculture

The final change in food production that we discuss is the transition of the world's production of fish from the capture fishery to an increasing reliance on **aquaculture** (fish farming). This transition to farmed fish is partially due to the world reaching a plateau in the catch of fish in the wild. Since the early 1990s, the world's capture fishery has peaked at just over 90 million metric tonnes annually, representing the maturity of most of the world's fisheries (see Figure 13.2). This plateau stabilized despite improvements in fishing technology and the overall increase in the capacity of the world's fishing fleet. So, even with our improved ability to capture fish, the amount caught has remained more or less constant.

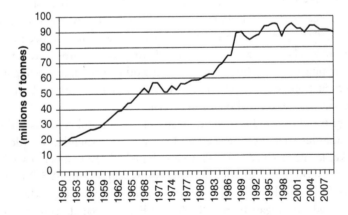

Figure 13.2 World Capture Fishery Production 1950–2009

Source: United Nations Food and Agriculture Organization (UNFAO), "Global Capture Production," n.d.

The danger of collapse of species-specific capture fisheries due to over-fishing is illustrated by the collapse of Canada's Atlantic cod fishery (see Figure 13.3). Despite an overall decrease in the world's take of Atlantic cod, Canada began to drastically increase its harvesting of cod beginning in the mid-1970s. This led to the collapse of the cod fishery that has yet to recover. The resulting fishing moratorium imposed by the federal government has had drastic consequences on the people of Newfoundland, many of whose livelihoods were intertwined with the cod fishery.

Aquaculture is the future of most of the world's seafood. It has recently reached 50% of the world's fish production and, given the maturity of the capture fishery, will only become larger. Aquaculture also has the advantage of providing a reliable, consistent product that is more suitable to mechanical production. That is, the resulting fish require less labour and expense to grow, harvest, and prepare for consumption. There are several issues around the use of aquaculture. For example, even though farmed fish are fed by the farmer, much of this feed is derived from the capture fishery, since many of the farmed fish such as salmon, shrimp, and trout are carnivores needing fish meal and fish oil as a part of their feed. Thus aquaculture can place additional stress on the capture fishery. Seaside farming of shrimp often involves the destruction of mangroves and coastal wetlands that serve as breeding grounds and safe havens for juvenile finfish. This is a concern in countries like Thailand that have installed shrimp ponds along much of their coastline, raising concerns about pressure on finfish. Also, while some aquaculture fish are raised from roe (eggs), others use captured seed fish from the wild, reducing the supply for the capture fishery. Finally, the highly concentrated effluent levels from aquaculture facilities can degrade local water quality (Naylor et al., 2000).

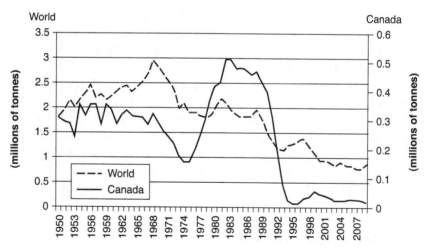

Figure 13.3 The Atlantic Cod Fishery

Source: United Nations Food and Agriculture Organization (UNFAO), "Global Capture Production," n.d.

Even the possible solutions to some of these problems may be problems in themselves. For example, a reduction in the amount of fish oil in feed can be achieved by replacing it with canola oil. However, the omega-3 fatty acid profile in people who eat salmon reflect the fatty acid profile in the fish. When fish oil is replaced by canola oil in the fish feed, the proportion of omega-3 fatty acids decreases in the fish and consequently also decreases in consumers (Seierstad et al., 2005). Farmed salmon also have higher levels of organochlorine contaminants than wild salmon (Hites et al., 2004). Normal economic forces may help provide solutions for reducing fish meal and fish oil in fish feed, since prices for these are rising and are likely to increase in the future (Tacon & Metian, 2008). However, the reduced demand on the capture fishery may come at the expense of human nutrition.

CHANGES IN FOOD CONSUMPTION

As a result of changes and innovations in food production, the cost of food compared to disposable income has steadily decreased. Moreover, the proportion spent on eating and drinking outside the home has nearly tripled since 1950, from 12% of total food expenditures to 35% in 2010 (United States Department of Agriculture [USDA], n.d.). In 1950, Americans spent 17% of their disposable income on food consumed in the home; that was reduced to about one-third (5.5%) by 2010; in the same period, food consumed outside the home rose only marginally in terms of proportion of disposal income—from 3.1 to 3.9% (USDA, n.d.). Even after accounting for the increase of food eaten outside the home, food as a proportion of disposable income has steadily decreased.

While this is a good news story, it also comes with several caveats. As prices for food have decreased, the overall contents of our diet have changed. These changes are not only in the macro-components of our food (fat, carbohydrate, and protein) but also in the quality of these macro-components as they become more highly refined and processed. Increasingly, families have to choose not between processed and non-processed food but between which manufactured foods they consume. The greater prevalence of food consumed outside the home and the food that is eaten at home being fully or partially prepared outside the home removes individual control over a person's diet. The choice of what to put into our bodies is made by producers and restaurants whose interest is not necessarily in nutrition, food safety, or even taste, but in products that will bring the greatest return to them and for their shareholders. For example, average sodium intake in Canada is about 3400 mg per day compared to the 2300 mg upper limit set by the Canadian Sodium Working Group (Conference Board of Canada, 2012). The bulk of our sodium (estimated at 77%) comes not from salt added at the table or during cooking, but in the processed foods we eat.

Technological Changes

Many of the technologies we have discussed have also transformed the way food is consumed. Most people do not even equate the meat they purchase at the grocery store with the animals that were slaughtered. Beef, chicken, pork, lamb are all just cuts of meat, disconnected (figuratively and literally) from the animal. Some meat is even further disconnected after additional processing has resulted in many new products debuting each year. The result is that some people find it odd, for example, to eat chicken that has bones or resembles the parts of the animal from which it came. Instead, we consume "nuggetized" chicken, formed into whatever shape the manufacturer wishes (usually for ease of eating without cutlery), flavoured with chemicals to make it taste virtually like anything the consumer might desire. The ingredients on these packages include terms like "mechanically de-boned chicken," which is essentially chicken meat slurry that can be pressed and moulded into various shapes, including dinosaurs, to make food "fun" for children. Although these changes have happened gradually, when they are viewed over a period of decades, they constitute a dramatic change, and, arguably, an uncontrolled experiment with the diets of millions of people.

Caloric Intake and Obesity

The increased processing of food has further consequences beyond a reduction in nutrients. The number of average calories consumed has increased by about 26% from 3100 per day in 1950–1959 to 3920 in 2000–2004 (Hiza & Bente, 2007). These calories, meanwhile, are increasingly energy-dense while at the same time nutrient poor (Grotto & Zied, 2010). Often, the more nutrient-poor and calorie-rich a food is, the more profitable it is for the manufacturer and the cheaper it is for the consumer.

A study of the relationship between obesity and poverty found that the highest rates of obesity occur in areas with the highest poverty. Both education level and income were correlated with the healthiness of diets and this relationship might be mediated by the low cost and high palatability of foods containing large proportions of fats, sodium, and refined carbohydrates (Drewnowski & Specter, 2004). Part of the story of the relationship between poverty and obesity is the lack of availability of nutritious foods in poorer neighbourhoods. This phenomenon has been termed *food deserts*, areas of "relative exclusion where people experience physical and economic barriers to accessing healthy food" (Reisig & Hobbis, 2000, p. 137). While there might be more food deserts in the United States, there is evidence they also exist in Canada (Apparicio, Cloutier & Shearmur, 2007; Larsen & Gilliland, 2008; Smoyer-Tomic, Spence, & Amrhein, 2006). For example, in Edmonton, researchers found that while most neighbourhoods had accessible groceries, some high-need neighbourhoods did not (Smoyer-Tomic et al., 2006). Food deserts result partly from the trend in food retailing that focuses on fewer but larger stores in suburban areas where the consumer base is more affluent.

Canada's overall nutrition situation, while likely similar to the United States, is more difficult to gauge. Unlike the United States and countries such as the United Kingdom, Australia, and New Zealand, Canada has no national nutrition-monitoring program. The national Nutrition Canada Survey in 1970–1972 was originally proposed as a longitudinal survey to track the dietary intake of Canadians using a 24-hour recall of food consumption, but the survey was never repeated (McAmmond, 2000). Subsequent surveys use other more simplified measures of diet and food consumption, such as eating habits (e.g., the 1981 Canada Fitness Survey) or food frequency (e.g., 1984–1985 Canada

Health Attitudes and Behaviours Survey), and fruit and vegetable consumption and food security (e.g., the 2004 Canadian Community Health Survey, Cycle 2.2 Nutrition). (See Chapter 2 for a discussion of Canadian health surveys.)

The principal concern about the increase in average caloric intake is the rising rate of obesity. Obesity is essentially a result of an energy imbalance where more energy is taken in than is needed for living. The body stores any excess as fat. Obesity, defined clinically for adults is a body mass index (BMI) of 30 kg/m² or more, and has been identified as a *pandemic* and one of the "top 10 risk factors for the burden of disease" (James, 2008). Obesity rates have been increasing rapidly in Canada with the overall percentage of obese Canadians rising from 13.8% in 1978–1979 to 23.1% in 2004 (Tjepkema, 2006). Rates in the United States are even higher. In 1999–2003, 29.7% of the population was obese, with the difference among Americans compared to Canadians being largely due to higher obesity rates among American women (Tjepkema, 2006).

Body mass index (BMI) is calculated by a person's weight measured in kilograms divided by his or her height measured in metres squared:

$$\text{Weight(kg)}/(\text{Height(m)})^2$$

While caloric intake is part of the equation for obesity, the other part is caloric expenditure and the balance between them. Some research suggests that it is the expenditure side, that is, the lack of physical activity, that is the problem (Blair, 2009; Temblay & Willms, 2003). Although lack of physical activity is connected to obesity, interventions that increase physical activity in children, for example, have not been effective in reducing BMI (Harris, Kuramoto, Schulzer, & Retallack, 2009) lending more support to the solution of reducing caloric intake. This may be due to the body's ability to change energy intake versus energy expenditure. Most calories are burned simply to keep a person alive; exercise only demands a small percentage above that. However, the average person consuming 3920 in 2000–2004 (Hiza & Bente, 2007) can reduce caloric intake by 50% (as much as 2000 calories per day). We are not discounting the health benefits of regular exercise, but this may explain why all major commercial diet interventions are based on diet alone.

Food-Borne Illness

Although food-borne illnesses have always been with us, the character and dynamics of these illnesses are changing with the way food is produced and consumed. As agriculture becomes more industrialized, a number of bacteriological illnesses that are deadlier and more difficult to treat have arisen (Nestle, 2003). These include listeria, campylobacter, and E. coli O157:H7. Some authors are concerned about these new threats to human health and their relation to changes in agricultural practices, such as the routine addition of antibiotics to animal feed (Gorbach, 2001).

The changing nature of how we consume food also affects the dynamics of food-borne illness. Since fewer meals are prepared in the home, the number of outbreaks (multiple people from a single source) of food-borne illness is increasing. That is, a contaminant introduced at a food-processing plant could reach thousands of people across a wide geographic area. A contaminant introduced in the home will likely affect only those in that home. For example, in 2008 a listeria outbreak in a Maple Leaf meat processing plant in Toronto resulted in 22 Canadians dead and 57 other confirmed cases across seven provinces of which the majority were elderly residents in Ontario (Chief Medical Officer of Health's Report on the Management of the 2008 Listeriosis Outbreak in Ontario, 2008). An editorial in the *Canadian Medical Association Journal* attributed the problem to a recent federal government decision to transfer inspection responsibilities from government inspectors to self-inspection by the meat-processing industry (Attaran et al., 2008). Although we run the risk of more severe outbreaks, the capacity to improve food safety in a systematic way could also increase. For example, the City of Toronto achieved a significant reduction in food-borne illness by implementing a stricter regime of restaurant regulation (Arthur, Gournis, McKeown, & Yaffe, 2009).

Keep in mind that the true rates of food-borne illness are usually underestimated. Some people who contract one of these pathogens may not exhibit symptoms serious enough for them to seek medical attention. If a person seeks medical attention, the doctor must order a stool sample to be analyzed by the laboratory and the patient must comply and provide the sample before a case can be recorded (Scallan et al., 2011). Consequently, medical authorities only detect a proportion of cases in the population.

Food-borne illness is a public health concern that has important economic consequences. A recent study estimated that "foods consumed in the United States that were contaminated with 31 known agents of foodborne disease caused 9.4 million illnesses, 55,961 hospitalizations, and 1,351 deaths each year"(Scallan et al., 2011, p. 7). Food-borne illness is estimated to cost nearly $7 billion annually in the United States and about $1.1 billion per year in Canada (Todd, 1989). Although most pathogens that cause food-borne illnesses originate in animals, fresh produce appears to be a growing source of outbreaks of food-borne illness, caused by contact with water that has been contaminated with animal feces (Sivapalasingam, Friedman, Cohen, & Tauxe, 2004). Bacteria have been identified, for example, in produce such as spinach imported from Mexico. Cases of the contamination of community drinking water are also more common, as in Walkerton, Ontario, where seven people died and more than 2300 people became seriously ill due to E. coli poisoning resulting from water contamination by farm animal feces (O'Connor, 2002). The cause was chlorination problems by the Walkerton Public Utilities Commission operators due to lack of training and poor government oversight and monitoring (O'Connor, 2002) (see Box 13.3 on the Walkerton Inquiry).

Pesticides

Pesticides, including insecticides, fumigants, fungicides, and herbicides, are an important enabling technology for modern agriculture. It is estimated that for every dollar spent on pesticides, three to five dollars are returned to the farmer in the form of increased yields (Andow & Davis, 1989). Although pesticides provide important benefits in conventional

Box 13.3

The Walkerton Inquiry

The Honourable Dennis O'Conner headed the Walkerton Inquiry to investigate the events leading up to the E. coli water contamination in May, 2000, and to examine issues with respect to the ongoing safety of Ontario drinking water (O'Conner, 2002). The outbreak in Walkerton, a small town in the Bruce Region, resulted in seven fatalities and almost half the population of the community (over 2300 of 4800) becoming ill. Needless to say, the scope of this tragedy had a profound effect on the community, the province, and the country.

The outbreak occurred after a few days of heavy rainfall resulting in runoff from a farmer's field into the Walkerton water source. The farmer was found to be innocent of any wrongdoing, having complied with all safe practices. However, the Inquiry identified chlorination problems by the Walkerton Public Utilities Commission operators as the principle cause of the E. coli outbreak as well as poor oversight and monitoring by the Walkerton Public Utilities Commissioners and the provincial government.

The operators of the water system had no malicious intent in placing the residents of Walkerton at risk. However, they were found to be guilty of improperly operating and maintaining the water system, failure to check chlorine levels, doctoring logs, and withholding information on water tests that were positive for bacteria from the Health Unit in the face of increasing incidence of intestinal illnesses. Moreover the operators' lack of training in and knowledge about the

potential severity of a bacterial outbreak was a significant factor. The Commissioners, having little expertise in the operations, were concerned principally with the financial aspects. After receiving reports from the Ministry of the Environment about water system operational problems and the presence of E. coli in numerous samples long prior to the events of May, 2000, the Commissioners took the operations manager at his word that changes would be made, neglecting their due diligence to follow up.

The provincial government and the Ministry of the Environment (MOE) were held partially responsible due to a variety of issues. First, in 1996, the government moved to private sources for municipality laboratory testing services. Although the Bruce-Grey–Owen Sound Health Unit received assurances from the Owen Sound MOE office that reporting of adverse tests would continue as in the past, this was not done. The Inquiry also identified other omissions and lack of action by the MOE in following up after inspections identified significant problems with the Walkerton water system. The last inspection had occurred in 1998 after which there was no follow-up to ensure compliance and changes to the operational procedures at Walkerton.

To conclude, there was a string of errors at all levels from the micro to the macro level, from local personnel to government policies and initiatives that contributed to this tragedy. This illustrates both how important and how vulnerable food and water safety is for the population.

food production, they also represent a major problem in global public health. These problems include deaths from direct acute pesticide poisonings as well as longer-term health problems such as cancer, birth defects, stillborn babies, Parkinson's disease, diabetes, and other illnesses that have been associated with pesticide exposure (Gunnell, Eddleston, Phillips, & Konradsen, 2007).

Direct effect of pesticides on human health   The World Health Organization reports a total of 355 000 deaths globally due to poisonings (all causes) each year (World Health Organization [WHO], 2003), of which 220 000 (62%) are due to pesticides (Hart & Pimental, 2002). It is estimated that there are from one million (Jeyaratnam, 1990) to 26 million (Richter, 2002) cases of unintentional poisonings due to pesticides worldwide annually, with the problem being most severe in developing countries.

Indirect environmental effects of pesticides on human health   Pesticide residues can be detected in our food and water supply, so avoiding exposure to pesticides is becoming increasingly difficult, if not impossible. There is strong evidence that pesticides used in agriculture migrate to streams and well water. A United States national survey of streams and groundwater found that 97% of streams in both urban and agricultural areas contained pesticide residue, as did a third (33%) of wells tapping major aquifers (Gilliom et al., 2006).

In a sample, representative of the United States, organochlorine pesticides such as DDE and hexachlorobenzene were detected in 100% (all) of the pregnant women tested. Most pregnant women had DDT in their blood or urine despite the fact that DDT has been banned for use in the United States and Canada for more than 40 years (Woodruff, Zota, & Schwartz, 2011). According to a review article published in *The Lancet*, there is increasingly strong epidemiological evidence of a link between pesticides and diabetes (Jones, Maguire, & Griffin, 2008). Pesticides have also been linked to Parkinson's disease (Tanner et al., 2011). Moreover, a range of widely used pesticides have been shown in the laboratory to be anti-androgenic and may play a role in degradation of male reproductive health (Orton, Rosivatz, Scholze, & Kortenkamp, 2011).

An American study of stillbirths (late fetal deaths) suggests exposure to pesticides through application in the vicinity of the maternal home between the third and eighth weeks of pregnancy increases the risk of stillbirth (Bell, Hertz-Picciotto, & Beaumont, 2001). A study of 1299 cases of four different birth defects (and 734 controls) in California found elevated risks of birth defects associated with living near an agricultural crop and with professionally applied pesticides in the home (Shaw, Wasserman, O'Malley, Nelson, & Jackson, 1999). A study of 4565 birth defects in 192 417 births in Norway found higher risks of birth defects among children through pesticide exposure of farmers, particularly orchard, greenhouse, and grain farmers (Kristensen, Irgens, Andersen, Bye, & Sundheim, 1997).

Pesticides and cancer   The U.S. Environmental Protection Agency (EPA) classifies 60% of herbicides, 90% of fungicides, and 30% of insecticides as oncogenic (tumour causing) (Committee on Scientific and Regulatory Issues Underlying Pesticide Use Patterns and Agricultural Innovation of the National Research Council, 1987). A study of 538 cases of neuroblastoma (the most common cancerous tumour among children) in Canada and the United States found an association between the use of residential pesticides and incidence in children older than one year (Daniels et al., 2001). In Australia, a study of 694 cases and the same number of controls found a three-fold increase in risk of non-Hodgkin's lymphoma in those with exposure to pesticides (Fritschi et al., 2005). Exposure to non-arsenic pesticides was associated with an increase in lymphoma among farmers in Spain (van Balen et al., 2006). Pesticides may also be associated with a number of other cancers, including prostate, lung, colorectal, and pancreatic cancer (Alavanja, Ward, & Reynolds, 2007).

In sum, the range of diseases linked to pesticide exposure may become more certain as more research is conducted, but it is clear that there are increased risks of several diseases as a result of exposure to pesticides. However, the hundreds of different chemical compounds that are used as pesticides complicate research on the effects of environmental exposure on humans. The possible complex interactions across the cocktail of substances become almost unimaginable. Much more research is required before the effects on humans of specific pesticides and links to specific disorders can be estimated accurately.

SOCIAL RESPONSES TO CHANGES IN AGRICULTURE PRODUCTION

Public concern over the changes in the food supply and production processes as well as the underlying economic, global, and political forces have given rise to several social movements. These movements are in response to issues that are more important to consumers than to producers and distributors of food, such as the taste and nutrition of the food at the point of consumption, the ecological footprint and sustainability of food production, public health concerns, concerns around the treatment of animals used as food, and issues around food security. Producers do attempt to jump on these trends if they think there is some way to profit from them.

Organic Foods

According to the International Federation of Organic Agriculture Movements [IFOAM], organic agriculture is defined as "a whole system approach based upon a set of processes resulting in a sustainable ecosystem, safe food, good nutrition, animal welfare and social justice." (IFOAM, 2006). Organic production entails more than simply refraining from using synthetic fertilizers and pesticides. The specific requirements to meet organic standards are controlled and regulated nationally, with each country developing a set of standards and regulations that define what constitutes "organic." In Canada, organic agriculture is regulated by the Organic Products Regulations, 2009—regulations under the Canada Agricultural Products Act (Canada Agricultural Products Act (R.S.C., 1985, c. 20 (4th Supp.)) that determine whether a product can bear the logo designating that the product is certified organic (see Figure 13.4).

The organic market has seen rapid and sustained growth in recent years, with the American market recently surpassing that of the European Union (Organic Monitor, 2010). From 2001 to 2006, there was a 60 percent increase from 2230 to 3555 farms that devote at least some of their production to certified organic crops. Despite the broad

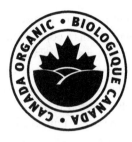

Figure 13.4 Canadian Organic Certification Logo

Source: Canada Organic Logo. Reproduced by permission of the Canadian Food Inspection Agency.

definition developed by the International Federation of Organic Agriculture Movements (IFOAM), the primary factor underlying consumers' preference for organically produced food is concern for their safety and health (Yiridoe, Bonti-Ankomah, & Martin, 2005). In other words, consumers buy organic food primarily because they believe it is more nutritious and contains fewer harmful substances. This self-interested motivation dominates other possible reasons, such as the environmental benefits of improved soils and reduced pollution.

Considering the emphasis that the people who buy organic products place on the health and safety provided by organic foods, we might ask if these benefits are real: have they been confirmed by scientific studies? While lamenting the lack of carefully controlled studies, one early review of the literature found that the nutrient content of organic products was not consistently superior to conventionally grown products (Bourn & Prescott, 2002). Subsequent studies, however, have shown benefits from organic production methods. For example, a study of three major datasets in the United States found that "organically grown foods consistently had about one third as many [pesticide] residues as conventionally grown foods" (Baker, Benbrook, Groth, & Benbrook, 2002). A study that compared organic versus conventional methods of tomato production on the same farm found that organic soils increase in nutrients over time and contained higher levels of carbon, nitrogen, phosphorus, calcium, and potassium than soil where conventional growing methods were used. Moreover, tomatoes grown organically had higher levels of phosphorus and calcium, while conventionally grown tomatoes were richer in nitrogen and sodium (Colla, Mitchell, Poudel, & Temple, 2002). A similar, ten-year study found that organically grown tomatoes had higher levels of some nutrients when compared with conventional tomatoes and that flavonoid levels increased over time in organic production (Mitchell et al., 2007). Other researchers found that organic kiwifruit grown on the same farm in California and harvested at same stage of maturity as conventionally grown kiwifruit had higher levels of minerals and antioxidants (Amodio, Colelli, Hasey, & Kader, 2007). With respect to organically produced meat, one study found that the concentration of omega-3 fatty acids was higher in range-fed beef than feedlot beef (Rule, Broughton, Shellito, & Maiorano, 2002). Although more research is needed, there seems to be a growing body of evidence to suggest that organic methods produce products with higher levels of some nutrients.

Some authors, including Nobel prize-winning scientist Norman E. Borlaug, argue that in order to feed a rapidly growing human population, new techniques of biotechnology such as genetically modified organisms are required and to insist otherwise is "anti-science" (Borlaug, 2000). Others contest this and argue that the entire world's agricultural demands could, in theory, be met by organic farming methods based partly on the fact that much of the world's food supply is currently produced at productivity levels far below that of modern organic agriculture (Badgley et al., 2007).

Locavorism

Locavorism is a recent social movement that is about eating foods that are grown nearby, and about changing the relationships between farmers and consumers. The movement was greatly affected by recent books such as *The 100-Mile Diet* (Smith & MacKinnon, 2007) and *Animal, Vegetable, Miracle* (Kingsolver, 2008). Locavorism is motivated in part by ecological reasons, such as reducing the amount of transportation involved in bringing food to the table. One estimate puts the average distance an item of produce has to travel at around 2414 km (1500 miles) before it gets to the consumer (Pirog & Benjamin, 2004). Another aspect of locavorism is rearranging agricultural relationships, making the connection between farmer and consumer more direct. One way to do this is to buy produce at a local farmer's market where farmers market their products directly (or nearly so) to the consumer. A more permanent relationship between farmers and consumers is the recent phenomena of community shared agriculture (CSA) in which farmers contract with consumers in advance for the farm output for the year. Under a typical CSA arrangement, a consumer will buy a share of the farm's output for a fixed monthly fee. Each week, the consumer gets a share of whatever is in season and harvested from the farm that week. With this arrangement, the farmer has a guaranteed income and transfers some of the crop risk to the consumer. The consumer gets fresh seasonal produce grown locally but also assumes some risk of potential crop loss due to weather and other factors. Often the consumer is able to go to the farm to see how the food is grown and even participate in the work.

Vegetarianism

Vegetarianism is a social movement that predates recent changes in food production but has witnessed a resurgence in recent years. Vegetarians range from vegans, who eat no animal products, to semi-vegetarians, who eat some meat or fish. Semi-vegetarians eat a predominantly vegetarian diet, supplemented by fish (in the case of a pescevegetarian or pesco vegetarian) or meat such as chicken (pollovegetarian). Lacto-vegetarians eat no meat, fish, or eggs, but do consume milk and milk products such as cheese or yogurt. Ovo-vegetarians, on the other hand, eat eggs but no milk products while lacto-ovo vegetarians eat both eggs and milk products. Vegans have the most restricted of vegetarian diets, eating nothing that is produced by animals. Hence they abstain not only from milk and eggs, but also animal products such as honey and any product containing an animal product as an ingredient such as marshmallows that contain gelatin. The rationales for vegetarian diets vary but centre on three main areas: the potential health benefits from not eating meat, the environmental impact of meat production, and ethical or religious concerns about eating meat.

Vegetarianism and health Consuming meat is associated with a range of potential health concerns, or, stated differently, vegetarianism is associated with potential beneficial health outcomes. For example, a study of more than 52 000 American women identified an elevated risk of breast cancer in women who consumed red meat (Ferrucci et al., 2009). Another study of more than 61 000 in the United Kingdom found lower rates of cancer among vegetarians and fish-eating semi-vegetarians. Rates were particularly reduced for stomach, ovarian, and bladder cancers, after adjusting for age, smoking, alcohol, body mass index, physical activity level, and, for women only, parity and oral contraceptive use (Key et al., 2009). A systematic review of the literature by the American Institute for Cancer Research found strong evidence of an elevated risk of colorectal cancer associated with the consumption of red meat, as well as a likely reduction of a variety of cancers associated with the consumption of fruits, non-starchy vegetables, and an assortment of vegetable-based nutrients (American Institute for Cancer Research, 2007). Vegetarian diets are also generally associated with lower weight and body mass index (BMI), and lower rates of obesity, heart disease, hypertension, and diabetes (Berkow & Barnard, 2006). A natural experiment in diet change at a population level occurred in Denmark during World War I as a result of an Allied blockade of shipping to that country. In a response to the food shortages caused by the blockade, the wartime Danish government ordered abrupt changes to the Danish diet, nearly eliminating pork and beef. As a result, deaths due to disease were significantly reduced (Table 13.2) (see Box 13.4) (Hindhede, 1920).

Vegetarianism and the environment Health benefits, however, are not the primary motivation for some vegetarians' dietary choices. Many vegetarians cite environmental reasons for not eating meat. Meat production consumes more resources such as energy, water, land, topsoil, pharmaceuticals, fertilizers, and insecticides; and produces

Table 13.2 Mortality Rate per 100 000 Males between 25 and 65 Years of Age, Denmark 1900–1918

	All Disease	Communicable Disease	Non-Communicable Disease
1900–1916	14.2	3.3	10.9
1917	12.3	3.3	9
1917–1918*	9.9	2.7	7.2

*1 Oct. 1917–1 Oct. 1918

Source: Hindhede M. (1920). The effect of food restriction during war on mortality in Copenhagen. *Journal of the American Medical Association, 74*(6), 381–382.

The Danish Natural Experiment

During World War I, Denmark was blockaded by the Allied Forces resulting in severe food shortages. As a response to this crisis, the Danish government made drastic changes to the way food was used and the diet of about 3 000 000 Danes. Instead of grain crops being fed to animals, the grains were diverted to human consumption, with the result that most Danes were forced onto a (mostly) lacto-ovo vegetarian diet. Beer production was reduced by half, and food crops used for hard liquour production (brandy) were eliminated. According to Hindhede (1920):

> Our principal foods were bran bread, barley porridge, potatoes, greens, milk, and some butter

... People of the cities and towns got little or no pork. Beef was so costly that only the rich could afford to buy it. . . . (p. 381)

Traditional whole grain rye flour was supplemented with wheat bran and barley meal, to make rye bran bread, making the diet especially rich in bran. This program was phased in between March and October 1917 and was associated with a dramatic reduction on death rates due to non-communicable disease. Rates of non-communicable disease dropped by 34% compared to the Danish average from 1900–1916 (see Table 13.2). Hindhede (1920) estimates that, ironically, the Allied blockade saved about 6300 Danish lives.

more waste, including methane, carbon dioxide, and water and air pollution, than do non-meat sources of human food. A meat-based diet entails a higher demand on natural resources than a plant-based diet. For example, each kilogram of beef produced requires an input of 13 kg of grain. Chicken requires only 2.3 kg grain for each kilo of meat, while one kilo of lamb requires 21 kg of grain in its production (Pimentel & Pimentel, 2003). Eating meat, simply based on the amount of grain required as an input in modern agriculture, requires far more resources than directly eating grains, especially when you account for the greater need for energy, water, topsoil, pesticides, and fertilizer. This equation, however, does not always apply in the case of traditional and alternative agriculture. For example, cattle grazed on non-arable land, such as the foothills of the Rocky Mountains in Alberta, do not consume grain, nor do they displace other crops. This type of land use extends agricultural productivity of an area by making non-productive land produce meat. However, most meat in North America is produced using the modern industrial process.

Meat production is not only inefficient in grain use, it also puts more demand on water resources. Potatoes require only 500 L of water per kilogram of potatoes, while wheat requires 900 L and soybeans 2000 L per kilo. Chicken requires 3500 L of water per kilo, while cattle demand 100 000 litres of water per kilo of beef (Pimentel et al., 1997). Meat production places a greater strain on limited water resources, with agricultural demand accounting for the majority of freshwater use in the United States (Pimentel et al., 1997).

In addition to the higher inputs when compared with what is required to grow vegetables, meat—and particularly meat produced in modern concentrated animal feeding operations (CAFOs)—also increases the environmental hazard for food-borne illnesses. Traditional and alternative agricultural practices can absorb the normal production of manure as fertilizer; however, because of the density of animals in CAFOs, the amount and concentration of manure are more difficult to manage in ways that are harmless to the environment. Runoff from these facilities has been blamed for water contamination. An example is a recent lawsuit that alleges that runoff from a large chicken farm in Maryland has violated water pollution laws, contributing to a massive "dead zone" in the Chesapeake Bay estuary (*Assateague Coastkeeper et al. v. Alan and Kristin Hudson Farm, 2011*).

Vegetarianism and religion and ethics   Perhaps the original reason for vegetarianism is rooted in the traditional spiritual beliefs of many of the world's religions. For example, Muslims and Jews do not eat pork and Hindus do not eat beef for religious reasons. Modern vegetarians in the Western world are more likely to cite reasons of ethics or animal welfare. More recently, the vegetarian cause has been bolstered by organizations like People for the Ethical Treatment of Animals (PETA), which stages high-profile events that raise awareness about the plight of animals, and by ethicists and philosophers such as Pete Singer (2002) and Jonathon Safran Foer (2009).

Slow Food

The slow food movement is centred on the dinner plate: food that arrives there should be good (tasty and nutritious), clean (free of contaminants and sensitive to the environment), and fair (to those who work to bring it to the table). It is a response to modern agriculture that values production volumes and efficiencies over taste. The founder of this movement, Carlo Petrini, recalls some of the events that led him to advocate for slow food in his book *Slow Food Nation* (Petrini, 2005). A change in the taste of a favourite food in a particular area of Italy led him to find that the local red peppers that formed the basis of the dish had been replaced by peppers grown in Holland and imported to Italy. The imported peppers were very uniform, inexpensive, and visually appealing, but tasteless. Because they cost more, local peppers were unable to compete. The local farm that produced them had been converted to growing—of all things—tulips. Another encounter was with the disappearance of a special cheese produced in a mountainous area of France. Local cattle, that were adapted to grazing on the difficult mountain terrain and produced milk that gave the local cheese its special flavour, had been replaced by Holsteins. The Holsteins produced twice as much milk but the milk tasted different, was not as nutritious, and the Holsteins could not survive the mountain environment without the construction of dairy barns. Proponents of slow food aim to preserve the diversity of food, not just for food security, but also because of the diversity it provides to the human palate.

SUMMARY

This chapter provides an overview to the production and consumption of food products and how they may influence our health. This is a novel chapter in a book that examines the social dimensions of health and health care use. However, since food is so central to our lives and has such an impact on our health, we thought it important to at least begin a discussion on it. We have focused on food generally but this does not infer that other environmental aspects are less important or unimportant. Our water and air, in combination with the foods we eat, are all vital for our overall health. Each one could easily fill books on the topics that would be far beyond our intent. Moreover, there are several other aspects of food and consumption that we could include and expand upon for which we just do not have the space. For example, the issue of global inequalities in food consumption and production is becoming increasingly important. Another example is that of food insecurity, a growing problem in Canada that is clearly demonstrated by the rise of community food banks. Touched upon briefly in the section on caloric intake and obesity, the ability of some families to eat nutritious and healthy food is becoming more and more difficult. There are a number of further resources for interested readers to explore in greater detail how our health is linked to our food, water, and air.

Key Terms

Aquaculture—fish and seafood farming

Body Mass Index (BMI)—a formula to calculate and classify people as obese or overweight based on weight divided by height squared [Weight (kg) / (Height (m)^2]

Genetically modified organisms (GMOs)—genetic engineering involving the direct insertion of DNA from one species into another to enhance a desired characteristic

Irradiation—the treatment of food with X-rays, gamma rays, or electron beams to kill pathogens such as microbes and insects that might be present in the food

Locavorism—a recent social movement that is about eating foods that are grown nearby, motivated in part by ecological reasons such as reducing the amount of transportation involved in bringing food to the table

Vegetarianism—ranges from vegans who eat no animal products to semi-vegetarians, who eat some meat or fish

Critical Thinking Questions

1. Has reading this chapter made you rethink your current food consumption habits? Why or why not?

2. What are the consequences of processed prepackaged dinners and fast food on the individual, the family, society, and overall population health?

3. What are some of the possible links between the technological changes in food production and consumption and current disease trends?

4. Identify what steps you would be able to take in your community to become a locavore and how this would influence your food choices.

Further Readings and Resources

Books

Conference Board of Canada, Centre for Food in Canada. (2012). *Improving health outcomes: The role of food in addressing chronic diseases*. Ottawa: Author.

Kingsolver, B. (2007). *Animal, vegetable, miracle: A year of food life*. New York: HarperCollins.

Moore-Lappé, F. (1971/1991). *Diet for a small planet*. Toronto: Random House.

Patel, R. (2007). *Stuffed and starved: Markets, power and the hidden battle for the world's food system*. Toronto: HarperCollins.

Pawlick, T. F. (2006). *The end of food: How the food industry is destroying our food supply and what you can do about it*. Vancouver: Greystone.

Petrini, Carlo (2005). *Slow food nation: why our food should be good, clean and fair*. New York: Rizzoli.

Pollan, M. (2006). *The omnivore's dilemma*. London, UK: Penguin.

Schlosser, E. (2001). *Fast food nation*. New York: HarperCollins.

Smith, A. & MacKinnon, J. B. (2007). *The 100-mile diet: A year of local eating*. Toronto: Vintage Canada.

Electronic Sources

Beck Institute for Cognitive Behavior Therapy. (2012, March 30). *Aaron T. Beck, M.D. interviewed by Judith S. Beck, Ph.D.* [Video file]. Retrieved from www.youtube.com/watch?v=7BZp7ZiAE3c

Canell, M., & Remerowski, T. [Directors]. (2005). Frankensteer. [Television series episode]. In *The passionate eye*. Toronto: Canadian Broadcasting Corporation. www.cbc.ca

The Council of Canadians—Acting for Social Justice. (2014). *Water* [website]. Available at www.canadians.org/water

Cowan, S. [Director]. (2002). *Empty oceans, empty nets*. [Video file]. Available at www.pbs.org/emptyoceans/

Cowan, S., & Schienberg, B. [Directors]. (2004). *Farming the seas*. PBS. [Video file]. Available at www.pbs.org/farmingtheseas/

Encounter Generation Conference. (2007, December). *Ann Cooper talks school lunches on TED* [video file]. Available at www.ted.com/talks/lang/eng/ann_cooper_talks_school_lunches.html

Environmental Working Group. (2014, April). *EWG's list of produce with the most pesticide residue* [website]. Available at www.ewg.org/foodnews/summary/

Geyrhalter, N. [Director & Cinematographer]. (2009). *Our daily bread* [Video file]. Mongrel Media. Available at http://vimeo.com/55321525

Inkster, D. [Director]. (2007). *24 days in Brooks* [Video file]. National Film Board, Canada. Available at www.nfb.ca/film/24_days_in_brooks

Kenner, R. [Director]. (2008) *Food inc.* [Video file]. Magnolia Pictures. Available at http://vimeo.com/25310835

Palfreman, J. [Writer, Producer, & Director], & Servan-Schreiber, C. [co-Director]. (2004). Diet wars. [Television series episode]. *Frontline*. Available at www.pbs.org/wgbh/pages/frontline/shows/diet/

Robin, M-M. [Director]. (2008). *The world according to Monsanto*. [Video file]. Mongrel Media. Available at http://vimeo.com/37811912

Spurlock, M. [Writer & Director]. (2004) *Supersize me* [DVD]. Alliance Films.

Suzuki, D. [Producer]. (2003). *Alternative agriculture: Food for life*. [Television series episode]. *The nature of things*. Toronto: Canadian Broadcasting Corporation. www.cbc.ca

Whiting, G. [Director]. (2003). *The weight of the world*. [DVD/online]. Toronto: CBC/NFB/Heart and Stroke Foundation of Canada, and Physical and Health Education Canada. nfb.ca.

References

Abbott, A. (1988). *The system of professions*. Chicago: University of Chicago Press.

Achilles, R. (2001). *Defining complementary and alternative health care. Perspectives on complementary and alternative health care*. Ottawa: Prepared for Health Canada, I.1–5.

Adams, A., Buckingham, C. D., Lindenmeyer, A., McKinlay, J. B., Link, C., Marceau, L., & Arber, S. (2008). The influence of patient and doctor gender on diagnosing coronary heart disease. *Sociology of Health & Illness, 30*(1), 1–18.

Adams, T., & Bourgeault, I. L. (2003). Feminism and female health professions. *Women's Health, 38*(4), 73–90.

Alameda Country Study. (n.d.). Preventing heart attack and stroke: a history of cardiovascular disease. Retrieved from www.epi.umn.edu/cvdepi/study.asp?id=40.

Alavanja, M. C., Ward, M. H., & Reynolds, P. (2007). Carcinogenicity of agricultural pesticides in adults and children. *Journal of Agromedicine, 12*(1), 39–56.

Alberta Health Services. (2011). *New specialty clinics boost role of nurse practitioners*. Retrieved from www.albertahealthservices.ca/5963.asp.

Alberta Health Services. (2013). *AHS apps for iPhone and Android*. Retrieved from www.albertahealthservices.ca/mobile.asp.

Allen, D. (1997). The nursing-medical boundary: A negotiated order? *Sociology of Health & Illness, 19*, 498–520.

Allen, D. (2001). Narrating nursing jurisdiction: "Atrocity stories" and "boundary work." *Symbolic Interaction, 24*, 75–103.

Allen, D. (2002). Time and space on the hospital ward: Shaping the scope of nursing practice. In Allen, D., & Hughes, D. *Nursing and the division of labour in health care* (pp. 23–51). Basingstoke: Palgrave.

Allen, D. W., & Lueck, D. (2000). Family farm inc. *Choices: The Magazine of Food, Farm and Resource Issues, 15*(1), 13–17.

Ali, J. S., McDermott, S., & Gravel, R. G. (2004). Recent research on immigrant health from statistics Canada's population surveys. *Canadian Journal of Public Health, 95*(3), I9.

Amato, P. R. (2001). Children of divorce in the 1990s: an update of the Amato and Keith (1991) meta-analysis. *Journal of Family Psychology, 15*(3), 355.

Amato, P. R., & Keith, B. (1991). Parental divorce and the well-being of children: A meta-analysis. *Psychological Bulletin, 110*(1), 26.

American Institute for Cancer Research. (2007). Foods and drinks. In *Food, Nutrition, Physical Activity and the Prevention of Cancer: a Global Perspective*. Washington DC: AICR, 66–197.

American Psychiatric Association. (1968). *Diagnostic and statistical manual of mental disorders* (2nd ed.). Washington, DC: Author.

American Psychiatric Association. (1980). *Diagnostic and statistical manual of mental disorders* (3rd ed.). Washington, DC: Author.

American Psychiatric Association. (2000). *Diagnostic and statistical manual of mental disorders* (4th ed. TR). Washington, DC: Author.

American Psychiatric Association. (2013). *Diagnostic and statistical manual of mental disorders* (5th ed.). Washington, DC: Author.

Amodio, M. L., Colelli, G., Hasey, J. K., & Kader, A. A. (2007). A comparative study of composition and postharvest performance of organically and conventionally grown kiwifruits. *Journal of the Science of Food and Agriculture, 87*(7), 1228–1236.

Andersen, R. M. (1995). Revisiting the behavioral model and access to medical care: Does it matter? *Journal of Health and Social Behavior, 36*, 1–10.

Andersen, R. M., & Newman, J. F. (1973). Societal and individual determinants of medical care utilization in the United States. *Milbank Memorial Fund Quarterly Journal, 51*, 95–124.

Andow, D. A., & Davis, D. P. (1989). Agricultural chemicals: Food and environment. In Pimental, D., & Hall, C. W. (Eds.), *Food and Natural Resources* (pp. 192–235). San Diego, CA: Academic Press.

Aneshensel, C. S., Rutter, C. M., & Lachenbruch, P. A. (1991). Social structure, stress, and mental health: Competing conceptual and analytic models. *American Sociological Review, 56*, 166–178.

Angell, M. (2004). *The truth about drug companies*. New York: Random House.

Angus, J., & Bourgeault, I. L. (1998/99). Medical dominance, gender and the state: The nurse practitioner initiative in Ontario. *Health and Canadian Society, 5*(1), 55–81.

Antonovsky, A. (1979). *Health, Stress and Coping*. San Francisco: Jossey-Bass Publishers.

Antonovsky, A. (1987). *Unraveling the mystery of health— How people manage stress and stay well*. San Francisco: Jossey-Bass Publishers.

Apparicio, P., Cloutier, M. S., & Shearmur, R. (2007). The case of Montréal's missing food deserts: Evaluation of accessibility to food supermarkets. *International Journal of Health Geographics, 6*(1), 4–16.

Armstrong, D. (2000). Social theorizing about health and illness. In Albrecht, G. L., Fitzpatrick, R., & Scrimshaw, S. (Eds.), *The handbook of social studies in health & medicine* (pp. 24–35). London: Sage.

Armstrong, P. (2002). *Exposing privatization: Women and health care reform in Canada*. Toronto: Garamond.

Armstrong, P., & Armstrong, H. (2002). *Wasting away: The undermining of Canadian health care* (2nd ed.). Toronto: Oxford University Press.

Aronson, J., Denton, M., & Zeytinoglu, I. (2004). Market-modeled home care in Ontario: Deteriorating working conditions and dwindling community capacity. *Canadian Public Policy, 30,* 111–125.

Arthur, A., Gournis, E., McKeown, D., & Yaffe, B. (2009). *Foodborne illness in Toronto.* Toronto: Toronto Public Health. Retrieved from www.toronto.ca/health/moh/pdf/staffreport_april15_2009_appx_a.pdf.

Assateague Coastkeeper et al. v. Alan and Kristin Hudson Farm. U.S. District Court for the District of Maryland. (2011).

Association of Ontario Midwives. *Midwifery Led Birth Centres: An innovative solution to improve care and cut costs.* Retrieved from www.ontariomidwives.ca/images/uploads/documents/Final - MPP pamphlet.pdf.

Attaran, A., MacDonald, N., Stanbrook, M. B., Sibbald, B., Flegel, K., Kale, R., & Hébert, P. C. (2008). Listeriosis is the least of it. *Canadian Medical Association Journal, 179*(8), 739–740.

Audas, R., Ross, A., & Vardy, D. (2005). The use of provisionally licensed international medical graduates in Canada. *Canadian Medical Association Journal, 173*(11), 1315–1316.

Avison, W. R. (2010). Incorporating children's lives into a life course perspective on stress and mental health. *Journal of Health and Social Behavior, 51*(4), 361–375.

Avison, W. R., & Gotlib, I. H. (Eds.). (1994). *Stress and mental health: Contemporary issues and prospects for the future.* New York: Plenum Press.

Aylward, D. (2011, March). How mobile phones can transform healthcare. *Harvard Business Review.* Retrieved from http://blogs.hbr.org/innovations-in-health-care/2011/03/david-aylward-the-mobile-phone.html.

Badgley, C., Moghtader, J., Quintero, E., Zakem, E., Chappell, M. J., Aviles-Vazquez, K., . . ., & Perfecto, I. (2007). Organic agriculture and the global Food Supply. *Renewable Agriculture and Food Systems, 22*(2), 86–108.

Badgley, R., & Wolfe, S. (1967). *Doctor's strike: Medical care and conflict in Saskatchewan.* New York: Atherton Press.

Baker, B. P., Benbrook, C. M., Groth III, E., & Benbrook, K. L. (2002). Pesticide residues in conventional, IPM-grown and organic foods: Insights from three U.S. data sets. *Food Additives and Contaminants, 19*(5), 427–446.

Barber, B. (1963). Some problems in the sociology of professions. *Daedalus, 92*(4), 669–688. Retrieved from www.jstor.org/stable/20026806.

Barnes, J. E., Noll, J. G., Putnam, F. W., & Trickett, P. K. (2009). Sexual and physical revictimization among victims of severe childhood sexual abuse. *Child Abuse & Neglect, 33*(7), 412–420.

Barrington, E. (1985). *Midwifery is catching.* Toronto: New Canada Publishers.

Bauder, H. (2008). Foreign farm workers in Ontario (Canada): Exclusionary discourse in the newsprint media. *Journal of Peasant Studies, 35*(1), 100–118.

Beck, U. (1992). *Risk society: Towards a new modernity* (Vol. 17). Thousand Oaks, CA: Sage.

Becker, G., & Nachtigall, R. D. (1992). Eager for medicalisation: The social production of infertility as a disease. *Sociology of Health & Illness, 14*(4), 456–471.

Becker, H. S. (1963). *Outsiders: Studies in the sociology of deviance.* New York: The Free Press.

Becker, H. S. (1970). *Sociological work: Methods and substance.* Chicago: Aldine.

Becker, H. S., Hughes, E. C., Geer, B., & Strauss, A. (1961). *The boys in white.* Chicago: University of Chicago Press.

Bell, E. M., Hertz-Picciotto, I., & Beaumont, J. J. (2001). A case-control study of pesticides and fetal death due to congenital anomalies. *Epidemiology, 12*(2), 148–156.

Benbrook, C. M. (2001). *Troubled times amid commercial success for Roundup ready soybeans: Glyphosate efficacy is slipping and unstable transgene expression erodes plant defenses and yields.* Sandpoint, ID: Northwest Science and Environmental Policy Center.

Bengtson, V. L., Burgess, E. O., & Parrott, T. M. (1997). Theory, explanation, and a third generation of theoretical development in social gerontology. *Journal of Gerontology, SS 52B*(2), S72–S88.

Benoit, C. (1991). *Midwives in passage.* St. John's, NL: Institute of Social and Economic Research.

Benoit, C., Carroll, D., & Chaudry, M. (2003). In search of a healing place: Aboriginal women in Vancouver's downtown eastside. *Social Science & Medicine, 56,* 821–833.

Berger, P. L., & Luckmann, T. (1966). *The Social Construction of Reality: A Treatise on the Sociology of Knowledge.* New York: Doubleday.

Berkow, S. E., & Barnard, N. (2006). Vegetarian diets and weight status. *Nutrition Reviews, 64*(4), 175–188.

Berta, W., Laporte, A., Zarnett, D., Valdmanis, V., & Anderson, G. (2006). A Pan-Canadian perspective on institutional long-term care. *Health Policy, 79,* 175–194.

Bezruchka, S. (2010). Staying alive: Critical perspectives on health, illness, and health care. In Bryant, T., Raphael, D., & Rioux, M. H. (Eds.), *Epidemiological approaches to population health* (pp. 13–40). Toronto: Canadian Scholars Press.

Biggs, L. (2004). Rethinking the history of midwifery in Canada. In Bourgeault, I. L., Benoit, C., & Davis-Floyd, R. (Eds.), *Reconceiving midwifery* (pp. 17–45). Toronto: McGill-Queens University Press.

Binney, E. A., Estes, C. L., & Ingman, S. R. (1990). Medicalization, public policy and older persons: Social services in jeopardy? *Social Science & Medicine, 30*(7), 761–771.

Black Report. (1980). *Inequalities in Health.* Report of a Research Working Group. London, UK: Department of Health and Social Security [DHSS].

Blair, S. N. (2009). Physical inactivity: The biggest public health problem of the 21st century. *British Journal of Sports Medicine, 43,* 1–3.

Bland, R. (2010). The history of psychiatric epidemiology in Canada: The development of community surveys. In Cairney, J., & Streiner, D. (Eds.), *Mental disorder in*

Canada: An epidemiologic perspective (pp. 29–47). Toronto: University of Toronto Press.

Bland, R. C., Orn, H., & Newman, S. C. (1988). Lifetime prevalence of psychiatric disorders in Edmonton. *Acta Psychiatrica Scandinavica, 77*(S338), 24–32.

Blane, D. (1985). An assessment of the Black Report's explanations of health inequalities. *Sociology of Health & Illness, 7*(3), 423–445.

Blaxter, M. (1990). *Health and lifestyles.* London: Routledge.

Blishen, B. R. (1991). *Doctors in Canada: The changing world of medical practice.* Toronto: Statistics Canada and University of Toronto Press.

Bloom, J., & Kessler, L. (1994). Emotional support following cancer: A test of the stigma and social activity hypothesis. *Journal of Health and Social Behavior, 35,* 118–133.

Bloom, S. W. (2002). *The word as scalpel: A history of medical sociology.* New York: Oxford University Press.

Blumer, H. (1969). *Symbolic Interactionism: Perspective and method.* Englewood Cliffs, N.J.: Prentice-Hall.

Bolger, N., DeLongis, A., Kessler, R., & Schilling, E. A. (1989). Effects of daily stress on negative mood. *Journal of Personality and Social Psychology, 57,* 808–818.

Bombardier, C., Laine, L., Reicin, A., Shapiro, D., Burgos-Vargas, R., Davis, B., . . ., & Schnitzer, T. J. (2000). Comparison of upper gastrointestinal toxicity of rofecoxib and naproxen in patients with rheumatoid arthritis. *New England Journal of Medicine, 343*(21), 1520–1528.

Boon, H. (1998). The holistic and scientific orientations of Canadian naturopathic practitioners. *Social Science & Medicine, 46,* 1213–1225.

Boon, H., Welsh, S., Kelner, M., & Wellman, B. (2003). Complementary/alternative practitioners and the professionalization process: A Canadian comparative case study. In Tovey, P., Easthope, G., & Adams, J. (Eds.), *Mainstreaming of complementary and alternative medicine in social context: An international perspective* (pp. 123–139). London: Routledge.

Boreham, P. (1983). Indetermination: Professional knowledge, organization and control. *The Sociological Review, 31,* 693–718.

Borlaug, N. E. (2000). Ending world hunger: The promise of biotechnology and the threat of antiscience zealotry. *Plant Physiology, 124*(2), 487–490.

Bourgeault, I. L. (1996). Physicians' attitudes toward patients' use of alternative cancer therapies. *Canadian Medical Association Journal, 155*(12), 1679–1685.

Bourgeault, I. L. (2006). The provision of care: Professions, politics and profit. In Raphael, D., Bryant, T., & Rioux, M. (Eds.), *Staying alive: Critical perspectives on health, illness, and health care.* (pp. 263–282). Toronto: Canadian Scholar's Press.

Bourgeault, I. L. (2014). Canada: Healthcare delivery system. In Cockerham, W. C., Dingwall, R., & Quah, S. R. (Eds.), *Wiley-Blackwell Encyclopedia on Health and Illness* (pp. 790–795). Hoboken, NJ: Wiley-Blackwell.

Bourgeault, I. L., Dingwall, R., de Vries, R. (2010). *The SAGE handbook of qualitative methods in health research.* Thousand Oaks, CA: Sage.

Bourgeault, I. L., & Mulvale, G. (2006). Collaborative health care teams in Canada and the U.S.: Confronting the structural embeddedness of medical dominance. *Health Sociology Review, 15*(5), 481–495.

Bourn, D., & Prescott, J. (2002). A comparison of the nutritional value, sensory qualities, and food safety of organically and conventionally produced foods. *Critical Reviews in Food Science and Nutrition, 42*(1), 1–34.

Bowler, I. (1994). They're not the same as us: Midwives' stereotypes of South Asian descent maternity patients. *Sociology of Health & Illness, 15*(2), 157–178.

Boyle, M. H., Offord, D. R., Hofmann, H. G., Catlin, G. P., Byles, J. A., Cadman, D. T., . . ., & Szatmari, P. (1987). Ontario Child Health Study: I. Methodology. *Archives of General Psychiatry, 44*(9), 826.

Brante, T. (1988). Sociological approaches to the professions. *Acta Sociologica, 31,* 119–142.

Brethour, P. (2005, October 17). Bitter strike divides Alberta town: Tempers have flared five days into dispute. *The Globe and Mail,* A1.

Breton, J. J., Bergeron, L., Valla, J. P., Berthiaume, C., Gaudet, N., Lambert, J., . . ., & Lepine, S. (1999). Quebec Child Mental Health Survey: Prevalence of DSM-III-R Mental Health Disorders. *Journal of Child Psychology and Psychiatry, 40*(3), 375–384.

Brown G. W., & Harris, T. O. (Eds.). (1989). *Life events and illness.* New York: Guilford Press.

Brown, P., Zavestoski, S., McCormick, S., Mayer, B., Morello-Frosch, R., & Altman, R. G. (2004). Embodied health movements: New approaches to social movements in health. *Sociology of Health & Illness, 26*(1), 50–80.

Browne, A. J., & Fiske, J. A. (2001). First Nations women's encounters with mainstream health care services. *Western Journal of Nursing Research, 23*(2), 126–47.

Brubaker, S. J. (2007). Denied, embracing, and resisting medicalization. *Gender & Society, 21*(4), 528–552.

Bruhn, J. G., Cordova, F. D., Williams, J. A., & Fuentes Jr, R. G. (1977). The wellness process. *Journal of Community Health, 2*(3), 209–221.

Brunner, E. (1997). Stress and the biology of inequality. *BMJ: British Medical Journal, 314*(7092), 1472.

Bryant, T., Raphael, D., Schrecker, T., & Labonte, R. (2011). Canada: A land of missed opportunity for addressing the social determinants of health. *Health Policy, 101*(1), 44–58.

Bury, M. (1982). Chronic illness as biographical disruption. *Sociology of Health & Illness, 4,* 167–182.

Bury, M. (1997). *Health and illness in a changing society.* London: Routledge.

Bury, M. (2000). On chronic illness and disability. In Bird, C. E., Conrad P., & Fremont, A. M. (Eds.), *Handbook of medical sociology* (5th ed.) (pp. 173–183). New Jersey, PA: Prentice Hall: Pearson Education.

Bury, M. (2005). *Health and illness.* Cambridge, UK: Polity Press.

Bury, M., & Gabe, J. (2004). Part 3. Professional and patient interaction. In Bury, M., & Gabe, J. (Eds.),

The sociology of health and illness: A reader (pp. 173–241). London: Routledge.

Cairney, J., & Streiner, D. (Eds.). (2010). *Mental disorder in Canada: An epidemiologic perspective*. Toronto: University of Toronto Press.

Cairney, J., Veldhuizen, S., & Wade, T. J. (2010). Intersecting social statuses and psychiatric disorder: New conceptual directions in the social epidemiology of mental disorder. In Cairney, J., & Streiner, D. (Eds.), *Mental disorder in Canada: An epidemiologic perspective* (pp. 48–70). Toronto: University of Toronto Press.

Callahan, J. C., & Knight, J. W. (1992). Prenatal harm as child abuse? In C. Feinman (Ed.), *The criminalization of a woman's body* (pp. 127–155). New York, London: The Haworth Press.

Calnan, M. (1987). *Health & illness: Lay perspective*. London and New York: Tavistock Publications.

Calnan, M. (1994). Lifestyle and its social meaning. *Advances in Medical Sociology*, 4, 69–87.

Calnan, M., & Rowe, R. (2007). Trust and health care. *Sociology Compass*, 1(1), 283–308.

Calnan, M., & Williams, S. (1991). Style of life and the salience of health: An exploratory study of health related practices in households from differing socio-economic circumstances. *Sociology of Health & Illness*, 13(4), 506–529.

Canada Agricultural Products Act (R.S.C., 1985, c. 20 (4th Supp.)). Retrieved from http://laws-lois.justice.gc.ca/eng/acts/C-0.4/.

Canadian Alliance of Community Health Centre Associations. (2009). *Community health centres: An integrated approach to strengthening communities, and Improving the health and wellbeing of vulnerable Canadians and their families*. Toronto: CACHCA.

Canadian Association of Community Health Centres. (2012). About community health centres. Retrieved from www.cachc.ca/?page_id=18.

Canadian Association of Retired Persons. (2001). *Report on home care*. Ottawa: Author.

Canadian Cancer Society. (2012a). *Canadian tobacco statistics* (updated October 9, 2012). Retrieved from www.cancer.ca/Canada-wide/Prevention/Smoking and tobacco/Canadian tobacco stats.aspx?sc_lang=en.

Canadian Cancer Society. (2012b). *Lung cancer statistics at a glance* (updated May 8, 2012). Retrieved from www.cancer.ca/canada-wide/about cancer/cancer statistics/stats at a glance/lung cancer.aspx

Canadian College of Naturopathic Medicine. (n.d.). Home page. www.ccnm.edu/about_ccnm/about_ccnm.

Canadian Community Health Survey. (2002). *Cycle 1.2, Derived variable (DV) specifications*. (Public Use Microdata File). Ottawa: Statistics Canada. Retrieved from www23.statcan.gc.ca/imdb/p2SV.pl?Function=getSurvey&SurvId=1630&InstaId=3359&SDDS=3226

Canadian Food Inspection Agency. (n.d.). *Bovine Spongiform Encephalopathy (BSE)*. Retrieved from www.inspection.gc.ca/animals/terrestrial-animals/diseases/reportable/bse/eng/1323991831668/1323991912972.

Canadian Food Inspection Agency. (n.d.). *Food Irradiation*. Retrieved from www.hc-sc.gc.ca/fn-an/securit/irridation/index-eng.php.

Canadian Food Inspection Agency. (n.d.). *Irradiation of ground beef: Summary of submission process*. Retrieved from www.hc-sc.gc.ca/fn-an/alt_formats/hpfb-dgpsa/pdf/securit/gbeef_submission-soumission_viande_hachee-eng.pdf.

Canadian Health Care Association. (2004). *Organization and governance of facility-based long term care within each province/territory*. Ottawa: Author.

Canadian Health Coalition. (2004). *Found: Federal funding. Missing: A plan to stem privatization*. Canadian Health Coalition's analysis of the First Ministers' Health Care Agreement: A 10-Year Plan to Strengthen Health Care. Ottawa: Author. Retrieved from http://healthcoalition.ca/wp-content/uploads/2010/12/health-reportcard.pdf.

Canadian Health Services Research Foundation. (2011). *Myth: The aging population is to blame for uncontrollable healthcare costs*. Retrieved from www.cfhi-fcass.ca/Libraries/Mythbusters/Myth_AgingPopulation_EN_FINAL_1.sflb.ashx.

Canadian Home Care Association. (2003). *Canadian home care human resources study, final report*. Mississauga, ON: Author. Retrieved from www.cdnhomecare.ca/media.php?mid=1030.

Canadian Index of Wellbeing. (2012). *How are Canadians really doing? The 2012 CIW report*. Waterloo, ON: Author and University of Waterloo.

Canadian Institute for Health Information. (2005a). Hospital trends in Canada. *Results of a project to create a historical series of statistical and financial data for Canadian hospitals over twenty-seven years*. Ottawa: Author.

Canadian Institute for Health Information. (2005b). *National health expenditure trends, 1975–2005*. Ottawa: Author.

Canadian Institute for Health Information. (2007a). *Canada's health care providers*. Ottawa: Author.

Canadian Institute for Health Information. (2007b). *Public-sector expenditures and utilization of home care services in Canada: Exploring the data*. Ottawa: Author.

Canadian Institute for Health Information. (2008). *National health expenditure trends, 1975–2008*. Ottawa: Author.

Canadian Institute for Health Information. (2010a). *Annual report*. Ottawa: Author. Retrieved from www.cihi.ca/cihi-ext-portal/internet/en/document/health+system+performance/indicators/performance/release_16dec10.

Canadian Institute for Health Information. (2010b). *Canada's health care providers, 2000–2009*. Ottawa: Author.

Canadian Institute for Health Information. (2010c). *National health expenditure database*. Ottawa: Author.

Canadian Institute for Health Information. (2010d). *National health expenditure trends, 1975–2010*. Ottawa: Author.

Canadian Institute for Health Information. (2011). *CMDB hospital beds staffed and In operation, fiscal year 2010–2011*. Ottawa: Author. Retrieved from www.cihi.ca/CIHI-ext-portal/internet/EN/Quick_Stats/quick+stats/quick_stats_main?xTopic=Spending&pageNumber=1

&resultCount=10&filterTypeBy=undefined&filterTopicBy=14&autorefresh=1.

Canadian Life and Health Insurance Association. (2012). *CLHIA Report on long-term care policy*. Toronto: Author.

Canadian Medical Protection Association. (n.d.). *Disclosure of information*. Ottawa: Author. Retrieved from www.cmpa-acpm.ca/cmpapd04/docs/resource_files/ml_guides/consent_guide/com_cg_informedconsent-e.cfm.

Canadian Institute for Health Sciences. (2009). *International medical graduates in Canada: 1972 to 2007*. Analysis in brief; Taking health information further. Ottawa, p. 18.

Canadian Museum of History. (2010). *Making medicare*. Ottawa: Author. www.historymuseum.ca/cmc/exhibitions/hist/medicare/medic-1c02e.shtml.

Capponi, P. (1985). How psychiatric patients view deinstitutionalization. Canadian Council on Social Development (Ed.), *Deinstitutionalization: Costs and Effects*, Ottawa, 7–10. Ottawa: Canadian Council on Social Development.

Carlson, L. W. (2001). *Cattle: An informal social history*. Chicago: Ivan R. Dee.

Carpiano, R., Lloyd, J., & Hertzman, C. (2009). Concentrated affluence, concentrated disadvantage, and children's readiness for school: A population-based, multi-level investigation. *Social Science & Medicine*, 69, 420–432.

Carrière, G. (2006). *Seniors' use of home care*. Health Reports, 17, No. 4. (Catalogue 82-003). Ottawa: Statistics Canada.

Carroll, D., & Benoit, C. (2004). Aboriginal midwifery in Canada: Ancient traditions and emerging forms. In Bourgeault, I., Benoit, C., & Davis-Floyd, R. (Eds.), *Reconceiving midwifery* (pp. 263–286). Montreal: McGill-Queen's University Press.

Cassel, J. (1974). Psychosocial processes and "stress": Theoretical formulation. *International Journal of Health Services*, 4(3), 471–482.

Cassel, J. (1976). The contribution of the social environment to host resistance. *American Journal of Epidemiology*, 104(2), 107–123.

Castagna, M., & Dei, G. S. (2000). An historical overview of the application of the race concept in social practice. In Calliste, A., & Dei, G. S. (Eds.), *Anti-racist Feminism: Critical Race and Gender Studies* (pp. 19–38). Halifax: Fernwood.

Chan, B. (2002). *From perceived surplus to perceived shortage: What happened to Canada's physician workforce in the 1990s?* Ottawa: Canadian Institute for Health Information.

Chan, P., & Kenny, S. R. (2001). National consistency and provincial diversity in delivery of long-term care in Canada. *Journal of Aging & Social Policy*, 13(2/3), 83–99.

Chaoulli v. Quebec (Attorney General) [2005] 1 S.C.R. 791, 2005 SCC 35.

Chapman, D. P., Perry, G. S., & Strine, T. W. (2005). PEER REVIEWED: The vital link between chronic disease and depressive disorders. *Preventing Chronic Disease* [electronic resource], 2(1).

Chapple, A., & Ziebland, S. (2002). Prostate cancer: Embodied experience and perceptions of masculinity. *Sociology of Health & Illness*, 24(6), 820–841.

Chappell, N., & Penning, M. J. (2009). *Understanding health, health care and health policy in Canada: Sociological perspectives*. Don Mills: Oxford University Press.

Charles, C., Gafni, A., & Whelan, T. (1997). Shared decision-making in the medical encounter: what does it mean? (or it takes at least two to tango). *Social Science & Medicine*, 44(5), 681–692.

Charmaz, K. (1991). *Good days, bad days: The self in chronic illness and time*. New Brunswick, NJ: Rutgers University Press.

Charmaz, K. C. (1995). The body, identity, and self: Adapting to impairment. *Sociological Quarterly* 36(4), 657–680.

Charmaz, K. C. (2000). Experiencing chronic illness. In Albrecht, G. L., Fitzpatrick, R., & Scrimshaw, S. (Eds.), *The handbook of social studies in health and medicine* (pp. 277–290). Thousand Oaks, CA: Sage.

Chief Medical Officer of Health. (2009). *Report on the management of the 2008 listeriosis outbreak in Ontario*. Toronto: Author. Retrieved from www.health.gov.on.ca/english/public/pub/disease/listeria/listeriosis_outbreak_rep.pdf.

Clark, D., & Seymour, J. (1999). *Reflections on palliative care (facing death series): Sociological and policy perspectives*. Buckingham, UK: Open University Press.

Clarke, J. N. (2004). A comparison of breast, testicular and prostate cancer in mass print media (1996–2001). *Social Science & Medicine*, 59(3), 541–551.

CNW. (2008, January 15). Canadian medical association launches major campaign for more doctors. Retrieved from www.newswire.ca/en/story/343895/canadian-medical-association-launches-major-campaign-for-more-doctors.

Cobb, S. (1976). Social support as a moderator of life stress. *Psychosomatic Medicine*, 38, 300–314.

Coburn, D. (1987). I see and am silent. In Coburn, D., D'Arcy, C., Torrance, G., & New, P. (Eds.), *Health care and Canadian society: Sociological perspectives* (pp. 441–462). Markham, ON: Fitzhenry and Whiteside.

Coburn, D. (1988). The development of nursing in Canada: Professionalization and proletarianization. *International Journal of Health Services*, 18, 437–456.

Coburn, D. (1999). Phases of capitalism, welfare states, medical dominance and health care in Ontario. *International Journal of Health Services*, 29 (4), 833–851.

Coburn, D. (2006). Medical dominance then and now: critical reflections. *Health Sociology Review*, 15(5), 432–443.

Coburn, D., & Biggs, C. L. (1986). Limits to medical dominance: The case of chiropractic. *Social Science & Medicine*, 22, 10, 1035–1046.

Coburn, D., D'Arcy, C., & Torrance, G. M. (1998). *Health and Canadian society*. Toronto: University of Toronto Press.

Coburn, D., Denny, K., & Mykhalovskiy, E. (2003). Population health in Canada: A brief critique. *American Journal of Public Health*, 93(3), 392–396.

Coburn, D., Rappolt, S., & Bourgeault, I. L. (1997). Decline versus retention of power through restratification: The case of medicine in Ontario. *Sociology of Health & Illness, 19*(1), 1–22.

Coburn, D., Torrance, G. M., & Kaufert, J. M. (1983). Medical dominance in Canada in historical perspective: The rise and fall of medicine? *International Journal of Health Services, 13*(3), 407–432.

Cockerham, W. (2001). *Medical sociology* (8th ed.). Upper Saddle River, NJ: Prentice Hall.

Cockerham, W., & Ritchey, F. (1997). *Dictionary of medical sociology.* Westport: Greenwood.

Colgrove, J. (2002). The McKeown thesis: A historical controversy and its enduring Influence. *American Journal of Public Health, 92*(5), 725–729.

Colla, G., Mitchell, J. P., Poudel, D. D., & Temple, S. R. (2002). Changes of tomato yield and fruit elemental composition in conventional, low input, and organic systems. *Journal of Sustainable Agriculture, 20*(2), 53–67.

Collier, C., & Haliburton, R. (2011). *Bioethics in Canada: A philosophical introduction.* Toronto: CSPI.

Collier, K. (2011). Cottage Hospitals and Health Care in Newfoundland. Newfoundland and Labrador Heritage Web Site. Retrieved from www.heritage.nf.ca/society/cottage_hospitals.html.

Collins, P. H. (1990). *Black feminist thought.* New York: Routledge.

Collins, P. H. (2000). *Black feminist thought: knowledge, consciousness and the politics of empowerment.* New York: Routledge.

Colombotos, J. (1988). Continuities in the sociology of medical education: An introduction. *Journal of Health and Social Behavior, 29*(4), 271–278.

Commission on the Social Determinants of Health. (2007). *A conceptual framework for action on the social determinants of health.* Department of Equity, Poverty and Social Determinants of Health, Evidence and Information for Policy Cluster. Geneva: World Health Organization.

Committee on Scientific and Regulatory Issues Underlying Pesticide Use Patterns and Agricultural Innovation of the National Research Council. (1987). *Regulating pesticides in food: The Delaney paradox.* Washington, DC: National Academy Press.

Conference Board of Canada, Centre for Food in Canada. (2012). *Improving health outcomes: The role of food in addressing chronic diseases.* Ottawa: Author.

Connel, R. W. (1987). *Gender and power: Society, the person and sexual politics.* Cambridge, MA: Polity.

Connidis, I. A. (2010). *Family ties & aging* (2nd ed.). Los Angeles: London: New Dehli: Singapore: Pine Forge Press.

Connor, J. T. H. (1994). Larger fish to catch here than midwives': Midwifery and the medical profession in nineteenth century Ontario. In Dodd, D., & Gorham, D. (Eds.), *Caring and curing: Historical perspectives on women and healing in Canada* (pp. 103–134). Ottawa: University of Ottawa Press.

Conrad, P. (1985). The meaning of medications: Another look at compliance. *Social Science & Medicine, 20*(1), 29–37.

Conrad, P. (1987). The experience of illness: Recent and new directions. *Research in the Sociology of Health Care, 6,* 1–31.

Conrad, P. (2000). Medicalization, genetics and human problems. In Bird, C. E., Conrad, P., & Fremont, A. M. (Eds.), *Handbook of medical sociology* (5th ed.) (pp. 322–333). Prentice Hall: Pearson Education.

Conrad, P. (2005). The shifting engines of medicalization. *Journal of Health and Social Behavior, 46*(1), 3–14.

Conrad, P. (2007). *The medicalization of society: On the transformation of human conditions into treatable disorders.* Baltimore: The John Hopkins University Press.

Conrad, P., & Schneider, J. W. (1980). *Deviance and medicalization: From badness to sickness.* Philadelphia, PA: Temple University Press.

Corbin, J., & Strauss, A. A. (1991). Nursing model for chronic illness management based upon the trajectory framework. *Scholarly Inquiry for Nursing Practice, 5,* 155–174.

Cranswick, K. (2005). *Caring for an aging society.* Ottawa: Statistics Canada Housing, Catalogue 89-582-XIE.

Crawford, R. (1979). Healthism and the medicalization of everyday life: An evaluation of self help, holistic health and the new health consciousness. *International Journal of Health Services, 10,* 365–388.

Crenshaw, K. (1995). Mapping the margins: Intersectionality, identity politics and violence against women of colour. In Crenshaw, K. (Ed.), *Critical Race Theory: The Key Writings that Informed the Movement* (pp. 357–383). New York: New Press.

Crompton, R. (1987). Gender, status and professionalism. *Sociology, 21,* 413–428.

Crossley, M. (1998). 'Sick role' or 'empowerment'? The ambiguities of life with an HIV positive diagnosis. *Sociology of Health & Illness, 20*(4), 507–531.

Cryderman, K. (2003, Sept. 17). Klein feels heat over mad cow quip. *Calgary Herald,* p. A1.

Dahlgren, G., & Whitehead, M. (1991). *Policies and strategies to promote social equity in health:* Background document to WHO–Strategy paper for Europe. *Equity in health.* Stockholm: Institute for Future Studies.

Daniels, J. L., Olshan, A. F., Teschke, K., Hertz-Picciotto, I., Savitz, D. A., Blatt, J., . . ., & Castleberry, R. P. (2001). Residential pesticide exposure and neuroblastoma. *Epidemiology, 12*(1), 20–27.

Davis, D. R. (2009). Declining fruit and vegetable nutrient composition: What is the evidence? *Horitcultural Science, 44*(1), 15–19.

Davis-Floyd, R. E. (1990). The role of obstetrical rituals in the resolution of cultural anomaly. *Social Science & Medicine, 31*(2), 175–189.

Davis-Floyd, R. E. (1992). The technocratic body and the organic body: Cultural models for women's birth choices. *The Anthropology of Science and Technology, 9,* 59–93.

Dei, G. J. S. (1996). Critical Perspectives in Antiracism: An Introduction. *Canadian Review of Sociology and Anthropology, 33*(3), 247–267.

Denton, M. (2009). The provision of health care for older people in Canada. In Bourgeault I. L., Atanackovic, J., LeBrun, J., Parpia, R., Rashid, A., & Winkup, J. *The role of immigrant care workers in an aging society: The Canadian context & experience* (pp. 14–30). Toronto: Ministry of Health and Long-Term Care, Ontario.

Denton, M., Walters, V., & Prus, S. (2004). Gender differences in health: A Canadian study of the psychosocial, structural and behavioural determinants of health. *Social Science & Medicine, 58*, 2585–2600.

Denton, M., Zeytinoglu, I. U., Davies, S., & Lian, J. (2002). Job stress and job dissatisfaction of home care workers in the context of health care restructuring. *International Journal of Health Services, 32*(2), 327–357.

Denton, M., Zeytinoglu, I., & Davies, S. (2003). Organizational change and the health and well-being of home care workers. Social and economic dimensions of an aging population research papers (Ed.). Research paper no. 110. Hamilton: McMaster University.

Denton, M., Zeytinoglu, I. U., Davies, S., & Hunter, D. (2006). The impact of implementing managed competition on home care workers' turnover decisions. *Healthcare Policy/Politiques de Sante, 1*(4), 106–123.

DesMeules, M., Turner, L., & Cho, R. (2003). *Morbidity experiences and disability among Canadian women: Women's health surveillance report.* Ottawa: Public Health Agency of Canada.

Dhalla, I. A., Mamdani, M. M., Sivilotti, M. L., Kopp, A., Qureshi, O., & Juurlink, D. N. (2009). Prescribing of opioid analgesics and related mortality before and after the introduction of long-acting oxycodone. *Canadian Medical Association Journal, 181*(12), 891–896.

Dohoo, I. R., Leslie, K., DesCôteaux, L., Fredeen, A., Dowling, P., Preston, A., & Shewfelt, W. (2003b). A meta-analysis review of the effects of recombinant bovine somatotropin: 1. Methodology and effects on production. *Canadian Journal of Veterinary Research, 67*(4), 241.

Dohoo, I. R., DesCôteaux, L., Leslie, K., Fredeen, A., Shewfelt, W., Preston, A., & Dowling, P. (2003a). A meta-analysis review of the effects of recombinant bovine somatotropin: 2. Effects on animal health, reproductive performance, and culling. *Canadian Journal of Veterinary Research, 67*(4), 252.

Dohrenwend, B. P. (1990). "The problem of validity in field studies of psychological disorders" revisited. *Psychological Bulletin, 109*, 5–24.

Dohrenwend, B. P., Levav, I., Shrout, P. E., Schwartz, S., Naveh, G., Link, B. G., . . ., & Stueve, A. (1992). Socioeconomic status and psychiatric disorders: The causation-selection issue. *Science, 255*, 946–952.

Drewnowski, A., & Specter, S. E. (2004). Poverty and obesity: The role of energy density and energy costs. *American Journal of Clinical Nutrition, 79*, 6–16.

Dunlop, S., Coyte, P. C., & McIsaac, W. (2000). Socioeconomic status and the utilization of physicians' services: Results from the Canadian national population health survey. *Social Science & Medicine, 51*(1), 123–133.

Durkheim, E. (1897/1951). *Suicide: A study in sociology* (J. A. Spaulding & G. Simpson, Trans.). New York: The Free Press of Glenco.

Durkheim, E. (1912/1995). *The elementary forms of religious life* (K. E. Fields, Trans.). New York: The Free Press.

Eaton, W. W. (2000). *The sociology of mental disorders* (3rd ed.). New York: Praeger.

Edginton, B. (1989). *Health, disease and medicine in Canada: A sociological perspective.* Toronto: Butterworths.

Eggertson, L. 2005. Vioxx award good news for Canadian lawsuits. *Canadian Medical Association Journal, 173*(7), 744.

Elder, G. H. (1998). The life course as developmental theory. *Child Development, 69*, 1–12.

Emslie, C., Hunt, K., & Watt, G. (2001). Invisible women? The importance of gender in lay beliefs about heart problems. *Sociology of Health & Illness, 23*(2), 203–233.

Engels, F. (1845/1987). *The conditions of the working class in England.* New York: Penguin Classics.

Epp, J. (1986). *Achieving health for all: A framework for health promotion.* Ottawa: Health and Welfare Canada.

Erikson, E. H. (1950). *Childhood and society.* New York: Northern.

Erikson, E. H. (1959). *Identity and the life cycle.* New York: International University Press.

Erikson, E. H. (1968). *Identity: Youth and crisis.* New York: WW Norton & Company.

Erikson, E. H., & Erikson, J. M. (1987). *The life cycle completed.* New York: WW Norton & Company.

Esland, G. (1980). Professions and professionalism. In Esland, G., & Salaman, G (Eds.), *The politics of work and occupations* (pp. 213– 50). Toronto: University of Toronto Press.

Estes, C., & Binney, E. (1989). The biomedicalization of aging: Dangers and dilemmas. *Gerontologist, 29*, 587–596.

Etzioni, A. (Ed.). (1969). *Semi-professions and their organizations.* London: Collier Macmillan.

Evans, R. G. (2010, June). Sustainability of health care. Myths and facts. *Just the Facts.* Ottawa: Health Coalition of Canada.

Evans, R. G., Barar, M. L., & Marmor, T. R. (Eds.). (1994). *Why are some people healthy and others not?: The determinants of health of populations.* New York, NY: Aldine De Gruyter.

Featherstone, L. (2001). The kindest cut? The caesarean section as turning point, Australia 1880–1900. In Porter, M., Short, P., & O'Reilly, A. (Eds.), *Motherhood: Power and oppression* (pp. 25–40). Toronto: Women's Press.

Federal, Provincial and Territorial Advisory Committee on Population Health. (1999). *Toward a healthy future: Second report on the health of Canadians.* Ottawa: Minister of Public Works and Government Services Canada. Retrieved from http://publications.gc.ca/collections/Collection/H39-468-1999E.pdf.

Feldman, E. A. (2000). Blood justice: Courts, conflict, and compensation in Japan, France, and the United States. *Law and Society Review, 34*(3), 651–701.

Felitti, M. D., Vincent, J., Anda, M. D., Robert, F., Nordenberg, M. D., Williamson, M. S., . . ., & James, S. (1998). Relationship of childhood abuse and household dysfunction to many of the leading causes of death in adults: The Adverse Childhood Experiences (ACE) Study. *American Journal of Preventive Medicine, 14*(4), 245–258.

Ferraro, K. F., & Farmer, M. M. (1996). Double jeopardy to health hypothesis for African Americans: Analysis and critique. *Journal of Health and Social Behavior, 37*, 27–43.

Ferrucci, L. M., Cross, A. J., Graubard, B. I., Brinton, L. A., McCarty, C. A., Ziegler, R. G., . . ., & Sinha, R. (2009). Intake of meat, meat mutagens, and iron and the risk of breast cancer in the Prostate, Lung, Colorectal, and Ovarian Cancer Screening Trial. *British Journal of Cancer, 101*(1), 178–184.

Fierlbeck, K. (2011). *Health Care in Canada: A Citizen's Guide to Policy and Politics.* Toronto: University of Toronto Press.

Fisher, J. (2009). Morality and ethics. In Fisher, J. (Ed.), *Biomedical ethics: A Canadian focus* (pp. 1–23). Don Mllls: Oxford University Press.

Foer, J. S. (2009). *Eating animals.* New York: Little, Brown and Company.

Food Safety Commission. (2004). *Measures against bovine spongiform encephalopathy (BSE) in Japan.* Government of Japan. Retrieved from www.fsc.go.jp/sonota/measure_bse_injapan.pdf

Forget, E. (2011). The town with no poverty: The health effects of a Canadian guaranteed annual income field experiment. *Canadian Public Policy, XXXVII*(3), 283–305.

Foucault, M. (1975). *The birth of the clinic: An archeology of medical perception.* New York: Random House.

Foucault, M. (1984). *The Foucault reader.* London: Random House LLC.

Fox, R. C. (1959). *Experiment perilous; physicians and patients facing the unknown.* Glencoe, Ill: The Free Press.

Fox, R. C. (1994). The medicalization and demedicalization of American society. In Conrad, P., & Kern, R. (Eds.), *The sociology of health and illness: Critical perspectives* (pp. 414–418). New York: St. Martin's Press.

Frank, A. W. (1993). The rhetoric of self-change: Illness experience as narrative. *The Sociological Quarterly, 34*(1), 39–52.

Frank, A. W. (2001). Can we research suffering? *Qualitative Health Research, 11*(3), 353–362.

Frank, A. W. (2002). *At the will of the body: Reflections on illness.* Boston: Houghton Mifflin Harcourt.

Frank, A. W. (2013). *The wounded storyteller: Body, illness, and ethics.* Chicago: University of Chicago Press.

Frank, A. W. (2004). *The renewal of generosity: Illness, medicine, and how to live.* Chicago: University of Chicago Press.

Frankel, B. G., Speechley, M., & Wade, T. J. (1996). *The sociology of health and health care: A Canadian perspective.* Toronto: Copp Clark.

Freddolino, P. (1990). Mental health rights: Protection and advocacy. In Greenley, J. R. (Ed.), *Research in community and mental health* (Mental disorders in social context series, Vol 6, pp. 379–407). Greenwich, CT: JAI Press.

Freiden, T. R. (2010). A framework for public health action: The health impact pyramid. *American Journal of Public Health, 100*(4), 590–595.

Freidson, E. (1970a). *Profession of medicine.* New York: Dodd, Mead and Company.

Freidson, E. (1970b). *Professional dominance.* Chicago: Aldine.

Freud, S. (1905). *Three essays on sexuality.* London: Hogarth.

Frideres, J. S. (1994). Racism and health: The case of the Native people. In Bolaria, B. S., & Dickinson, H. (Eds.), *Health, illness and health care in Canada* (2nd ed.) (pp. 202–220). Toronto: Harcourt Brace.

Fritschi, L., Benke, G., Hughes, A. M., Kricker, A., Turner, J., Vajdic, C. M., . . ., & Armstrong, B. K. (2005). Occupational exposure to pesticides and risk of non-Hodgkin's lymphoma. *American Journal of Epidemiology, 162*(9), 849–857.

Fuller, C. (1998). Profit or non-profit: Are hospitals selling out? *Canadian Women's Health Network, 1*(4).

Gagan, D. (1989). For 'patients of moderate means': The transformation of Ontario's public general hospitals, 1880–1950. *Canadian Historical Review, 70*(2), 151–179.

Gaskell, J. (1987). Conceptions of skill and the work of women: Some historical and political issues. In Hamilton, R., & Barrett, M. (Eds.), *The politics of diversity* (pp. 361–80). London: Verso.

Gee, E. M. (2002). Misconceptions and misapprehensions about population aging. *International Journal of Epidemiology, 31*, 750–753.

General Accounting Office. (1992). *Hired farmworkers: Health and well-being at risk* (GAO publication No. GAO/HRD-92-46). Washington, DC: United States General Accounting Office. Retrieved from http://archive.gao.gov/t2pbat7/145941.pdf.

Gibson, D., & Fuller, C. (2006). *The bottom line: The truth behind private health insurance in Canada.* Newest Press: Edmonton, Alberta.

Giddens, A. (1991). *Modernity and self-identity. Self and society in the late modern age.* Cambridge: Polity Press.

Giddens, A. (1984). *The constitution of society: Outline of the theory of structuration.* Cambridge: Polity Press.

Gilland, B. (2002). World population and food supply: Can food production keep pace with population growth in the next half-century? *Food Policy, 27*, 47–63.

Gilliom, R. J., Barbash, J. E., Crawford, C. G., Hamilton, P. A., Martin, J. D., Nakagaki, N., . . ., & Wolock, D. M. (2006). *Pesticides in the nation's streams and ground water, 1992–2001.* Circular 1291; Washington, DC: USGS. Retrieved from http://ca.water.usgs.gov/pnsp/.

Glaser, B., & Strauss, A. (1967). *The discovery of grounded theory.* Chicago: Aldine.

Glass, G. V. (1976). Primary, secondary, and meta-analysis of research. *Educational Researcher*, 5, 3–8.

Glouberman, S., & Millar, J. (2003). Evolution of the determinants of health, health policy, and health information systems in Canada. *American Journal of Public Health*, 93(3), 388–392.

Goering, P., Wasylenki, D., & Durbin, J. (2000). Canada's mental health system. *International Journal of Law and Psychiatry*, 23, 345–59.

Goffman, E. (1959). *The presentation of self in everyday life*. Garden City, NY. Anchor Books.

Goffman, E. (1961). *Asylums*. Garden City, NY: Anchor Books.

Goffman, E. (1963). *Stigma: Notes on the management of spoiled identity*. Engelwood Cliffs, NJ: Prentice Hall.

Goldstein, M. S. (2000). The growing acceptance of complementary and alternative medicine. In Bird, C. E., Conrad, P., & Fremont, A. M. (Eds.), *Handbook of medical sociology* (pp. 284–297). Upper Saddle River, NJ: Prentice Hall.

Goode, W. J. (1969). The theoretical limits of professionalization. In Etzioni, A. (Ed.), *The semi-professions and their organization* (pp. 266–313). New York: Free Press.

Gorbach, S. L. (2001). Antimicrobial use in animal feed—time to stop. *New England Journal of Medicine*, 345(16), 1202–1203.

Gort, E., & Coburn, D. (1988). Naturopathy in Canada: Changing relationship to medicine, chiropractic and the state. *Social Science & Medicine*, 26, 1061–1072.

Goss, M. (1963). Patterns of bureaucracy among hospital staff physicians. In Freidson, E. (Ed.), *The hospital in modern society* (pp. 170–194). New York: Free Press.

Gove, W. (1982). *Deviance and mental illness*. Beverly Hills, CA: Sage.

Graham, D. J., Campen, D., Hui, R., Spence, M., Cheetham, C., Levy, G., . . ., & Ray, W. A. (2005). Risk of acute myocardial infarction and sudden cardiac death in patients treated with cyclo-oxygenase 2 selective and non-selective non-steroidal anti-inflammatory drugs: nested case-control study. *The Lancet*, 365(9458), 475–481.

Graham, H. (2004). Social determinants and their unequal distribution. *Milbank Quarterly*, 82(1), 101–124.

Gravel, R., & Beland, Y. (2005). The Canadian community health survey: Mental health and well-being. *Canadian Journal of Psychiatry*, 50, 573–579.

Greenberg, A., Angus, H., Sullivan, T., & Brown, A. D. (2005). Development of a set of strategy-based system-level cancer care performance indicators in Ontario, Canada. *International Journal for Quality in Health Care*, 17(2), 107–114.

Greenland, C., Griffin, J., & Hoffman, B. (2001). Psychiatry in Canada from 1951–2001. In Rae-Grant, Q. (Ed.), *Psychiatry in Canada: 50 Years, 1951–2000* (pp. 1–16). Ottawa: Canadian Psychiatric Association.

Greenwood, E. (1957). Attributes of a profession. *Social Work*, 2(July), 44–55.

Griffiths, L. (1997). Accomplishing team: Teamwork and categorization in two community mental health teams. *The Sociological Review*, 45, 59–78.

Grignon, M., & Bernier, N. F. (2012). *Financing Long-Term Care in Canada* (Vol. 33). Montreal: Institute for Research on Public Policy.

Grotto, D., & Zied, E. (2010). The standard American diet and its relationship to the health status of Americans. *Nutrition in Clinical Practice*, 25(6), 603–612.

Gunnell, D., Eddleston, M., Phillips, M. R., & Konradsen, F. (2007). The global distribution of fatal pesticide self-poisoning: Systematic review. *BMC Public Health*, 7, 357–371.

Gushulak, B. D., Pottie, K., Roberts, J. H., Torres, S., & DesMeules, M. (2011). Migration and health in Canada: Health in the global village. *Canadian Medical Association Journal*, 183(12), E952-E958.

Haas, J., & Shaffir, W. (1987). *Becoming doctors: The adoption of a cloak of competence*. Greenwich, Connecticut: JAI Press.

Haines, V. A., & Hurlbert, J. S. (1992). Network range and health. *Journal of Health and Social Behavior*, 33(3), 254–266.

Hall, E. M. (1980). *Canada's national-provincial health program for the 1980s: A commitment for renewal*. Ottawa: Department of National Health and Welfare.

Hall, O. (1948). The stages of a medical career. *American Journal of Sociology*, 53, 327–336.

Halpin, M., Phillips, M., & Oliffe, J. L. (2009). Prostate cancer stories in the Canadian print media: representations of illness, disease and masculinities. *Sociology of Health & Illness*, 31(2), 155–169.

Hankivsky, O., de Leeuw, S., Lee, J. A., Vissandjée, B., & Khanlou, N. (2011). Introduction: Purpose, overview, and contribution. In Hankivsky, O. (Ed.), *Health inequities in Canada: Intersectional frameworks and practices* (pp. 1–15). Vancouver: UBC Press.

Hanna, A. (2007). OMA Policy Paper: Interprofessional Care. Ontario Medical Association. Retrieved from https://www.oma.org/Resources/Documents/2007IPCPaper.pdf.

Harris, K. C., Kuramoto, L. K., Schulzer, M., & Retallack, J. E. (2009). Effect of school-based physical activity interventions on body mass index in children: A meta-analysis. *Canadian Medical Association Journal*, 180(7), 719–726.

Hart, K., & Pimental, D. (2002). Public Health and Costs of Pesticide. In Pimental, D. (Ed.), *Encyclopedia of pest management* (pp. 677–679). New York: Marcl Dekker.

Hartley, H. (2003). "Big Pharma" in our bedrooms: An analysis of the medicalization of women's sexual problems. *Advances in Gender Research*, 7, 89–129.

Hatch, L. R. (2000). *Beyond gender differences: Adaptation to aging in life course perspective*. Amityville, NY, Baywood Publishing.

Haug, M. R. (1973). Deprofessionalization: An alternate hypothesis for the future. *Sociological Review Monographs*, 20, 195–211.

Haug, M. (1979). Doctor patient relationships and the older patient. *Journal of Gerontology*, 34(6), 852–860.

Haug, M. R. (1988). A re-examination of the hypothesis of physician deprofessionalization. *The Milbank Quarterly*, 66, 48–56.

Haug, M. R., & Lavin, B. (1983). *Consumerism in medicine: Challenging physician authority*. Beverly Hills, CA: Sage.

Haydt, S. (2012). The forms of interdisciplinary primary care teams in Ontario: Implications for health equity. Paper presented at the Canadian Society for the Sociology of Health conference, Ottawa.

Health Canada. (n.d.). *Canada's health care system*. Ottawa: Author. Retrieved from www.hc-sc.gc.ca/hcs-sss/pubs/system-regime/2011-hcs-sss/index-eng.php#a13.

Health Canada. (2004). First Ministers' meeting on the future of health care 2004: A 10-year plan to strengthen health care. Ottawa: Author. Retrieved from www. hc-sc.gc.ca/hcs-sss/delivery-prestation/fptcollab/2004-fmm-rpm/index-eng.php.

Health Canada. (2009). *A statistical profile on the health of First Nations in Canada: Self-rated health and selected conditions, 2002 to 2005*. Ottawa: Author. Retrieved from www.hc-sc.gc.ca/fniah-spnia/pubs/aborig-autoch/index-eng.php.

Health Canada. (2010, December). Migration health: Embracing a determinants of health approach. *Health Policy Research Bulletin*. Ottawa: Author. Retrieved from www.hc-sc.gc.ca/sr-sr/alt_formats/pdf/pubs/hpr-rpms/bull/2010-health-sante-migr-eng.pdf.

Health Canada. (2011). *Cost and benefit analysis: Natural health products (Unprocessed product license applications) regulations*. Ottawa: Author. Retrieved from www.hc-sc.gc.ca/dhp-mps/prodnatur/legislation/acts-lois/gazette1/regul-regle_cba-aca-eng.php

Health Link BC. (2013). *BC health service locator App*. Retrieved from www.healthlinkbc.ca/app/.

Health Products and Food Branch. (2002, November 19). Recommended Canadian code of practice for food irradiation, Section 8. Health Canada and the Canadian Food Inspection Agency. Retrieved from www.hc-sc.gc.ca/fn-an/securit/irridation/code_of_practice-code_de_pratique01-eng.php#a5.2.

Helm Pharmaceuticals. (2007, Dec). Vibrel [Advertisement]. *En Route*, Air Canada inflight magazine.

Hempel, S. (2006). *The medical detective: John Snow and the mystery of cholera*. London: Granta.

Heritage, J., & Maynard, D. W. (2006). Problems and prospects in the study of physician-patient interaction: 30 years of research. *Annual Review of Sociology, 32*, 351–374.

Hertzman, C. (2000). The case for an early childhood development strategy. Isuma: *Canadian Journal of Policy Research, 1*(2), 11–18.

Herzlich, C. (2004). The individual, the way of life and the genesis of illness. In Bury, M., & Gabe, J. (Eds.), *The Sociology of Health and Illness: A Reader* (pp. 27–35). London and New York: Routledge.

Hevesi, D. (2007, June 9). Edwin Traisman, 91, dies; helped create iconic foods. *The New York Times*. Retrieved from www.nytimes.com/2007/06/09/us/09traisman.html?_r=1&oref=slogin.

Higginbottom, G. M. A. (2006). 'Pressure of life': Ethnicity as a mediating factor in mid-life and older peoples' experience of high blood pressure. *Sociology of Health & Illness, 28*(5), 583–610.

Hindhede, M. (1920). The effect of food restriction during war on mortality in Copenhagen. *Journal of the American Medical Association, 74*(6), 381–382.

Hindmarsh, J., & Pilnick, A. (2002). The tacit order of teamwork: collaboration and embodied conduct in anesthesia. *Sociological Quarterly, 43*(2), 139–164.

Hirshbein, L. D. (1998). Disciplining old age: The formation of gerontological knowledge. *Bulletin of the History of Medicine, 72*, 3, 594–5. Retrieved from http://muse.jhu.edu/login?auth=0&type=summary&url=/journals/bulletin_of_the_history_of_medicine/v072/72.3br_katz.html

Hirschkorn, K. A., Andersen, R., & Bourgeault, I. L. (2009). Canadian family physicians and complementary/alternative medicine: The role of practice setting, medical training, and province of practice. *The Free Library* (May, 1). Retrieved from www.thefreelibrary.com/Canadian family physicians and complementary/alternative medicine: . . .-a0201711471

Hirschkorn, K. A., & Bourgeault, I. L. (2005). Conceptualizing mainstream health care providers behaviours in relation to complementary and alternative medicine. *Social Science & Medicine, 61*(1), 157–70.

Hirschkorn, K. A., & Bourgeault, I. L. (2007). Actions speak louder than words: Mainstream health providers' definitions and behaviour regarding complementary and alternative medicine. *Complementary Therapies in Clinical Practice, 13*, 29–37.

Hites, R. A., Foran, J. A., Carpenter, D. O., Hamilton, M. C., Knuth, B. A., & Schwager, S. J. (2004). Global assessment of organic contaminants in farmed salmon. *Science, 303*(5655), 226–229.

Hiza, H. A. B., & Bente, L. (2007). *Nutrient Content of the U.S. Food Supply, 1909–2004: A Summary Report* (Home Economics Research Report No. 57). Washington, DC: Center for Nutrition Policy and Promotion, U.S. Department of Agriculture.

Hogg, W. (n.d.). *Comparison of primary care models in Ontario*. Ottawa: C. T. Lamont Primary Health Care Research Centre, Elisabeth Bruyère Research Centre.

Home Care Sector Study Corporation. (2003a). *Canadian Home Care Human Resources Study: Synthesis Report*. Ottawa: Human Resources Development Canada. Retrieved from www.cdnhomecare.ca/media.php?mid=1030

Home Care Sector Study Corporation. (2003b). *Canadian Home Care Human Resources Study: Technical Report*. Human Resources Development Canada (Ed.). Ottawa: Human Resources Development Canada. Retrieved from www.cdnhomecare.ca/media.php?mid=1035

Hopkins, L., Labonté, R., Runnel, V., & Packer, C. (2010). Medical tourism today: What is the state of existing knowledge? *Journal of Public Health Policy, 31*, 185–198.

Horowitz, M. D., Rosensweig, J. A., & Jones, C. A. (2007). Medical tourism: Globalization of the healthcare marketplace. *Medscape General Medicine, 9*(4), 33.

Horowitz, S. M. (2003). Applying the transtheoretical model to pregnancy and STD prevention: A review of the literature. *American Journal of Health Promotion, 17*(5), 304–328.

Houston, C. S. (2002). *Steps on the road to Medicare: Why Saskatchewan led the way.* Montreal & Kingston: McGill-Queen's University Press.

Hughes, D. (1988). When nurse knows best: Some aspects of nurse–doctor interaction in a casualty department. *Sociology of Health & Illness, 10*, 1–22.

Hughes, E. C. (1958). *Men and their work.* London: Free Press.

Hughes, E. C. (1962). Good people and dirty work. *Social Problems, 10*(1), 3–11.

Hum, D., & Simpson, W. (2001). A guaranteed annual income? From Mincome to the millenium. *Policy Options,* January/February, 78–82.

Iglehart, J. K. (1986). Canada's health care system (1). *New England Journal of Medicine, 315*(3), 202.

Illich, I. (1976). *Medical nemesis: The limits of medicine.* London: Penguin.

Inkster, D. (Writer and Director). (2007). 24 Days in Brooks [Video]. Thompson, B. (Producer). Ottawa: National Film Board of Canada.

International Dairy Foods Association v. Boggs 622 F. 3d 628 [2010] United States Court of Appeals, Sixth Circuit, Ohio.

International Federation of Organic Agriculture Movements. (2005). *The IFOAM basic standards for organic production and processing version.* Germany: International Federation of Organic Agriculture Movements.

Irvine, R., Kerridge, I., McPhee, J., & Freeman, S. (2002). Interprofessionalism and ethics: Consensus or clash of cultures?. *Journal of Interprofessional Care, 16*(3), 199–210.

Iyer, A., Sen, G., & Ostlin, P. (2008). The intersections of gender and class in health status and health care. *Global Public Health, 3*(S1), 13–24.

Jablonski, J. (2012). *Employment status and professional integration outcomes of IMGs in Ontario.* Unpublished undergraduate thesis. University of Ottawa, Ottawa, Ontario, Canada.

Jacoby, A., Snape, D., & Baker, G. A. (2005). Epilepsy and social identity: The stigma of a chronic neurological disorder. *The Lancet Neurology, 4*(3), 171–178.

James, W. P. T. (2008). WHO recognition of the global obesity epidemic. *International Journal of Obesity, 32,* S120–S126.

Janssen, P. A., Saxell, L., Page, L. A., Klein, M. C., Liston, R. M., & Lee, S. K. (2009). Outcomes of planned home birth with registered midwife versus planned hospital birth with midwife or physician. *Canadian Medical Association Journal, 181*(6-7), 377–383.

Jarvis, G. E. (2007). The social causes of psychosis in North American psychiatry: A review of a disappearing literature. *Canadian Journal of Psychiatry, 52*(5), 287–294.

Jaye, C., & Fitzgerald, R. (2010). The lived political economy of occupational overuse syndrome among New Zealand workers. *Sociology of Health & Illness, 32*(7), 1010–1025.

Jewson, N. D. (1976). The disappearance of the sick-man from medical cosmology, 1770–1870. *Sociology, 10,* 225–243.

Jeyaratnam, J. (1990). Acute pesticide poisoning: A major global health problem. *World Health Statistics Quarterly, 43*(3), 139–144.

Johnson, T. J. (1972). *Professions and power.* London: The Macmillan Press.

Johnson, T. J. (1977). The professions in the class structure. In Scase, R. (Ed.), *Industrial society, class cleavage and control* (pp. 93–110). London: George Allen & Unwin.

Jones, E., Farina, A., Hastorf, A., Markus, H., Miller, D., & Scott, R. (1984). *Social stigma: The psychology of marked relationships.* New York: Freeman. As cited in Jacoby, A., Snape D, & Baker G. A. (2005). Epilepsy and social identity: The stigma of a chronic neurological disorder. *The Lancet Neurology 4*(3), 171–178.

Jones, O. A., Maguire, M. L., & Griffin, J. L. (2008). Environmental pollution and diabetes: A neglected association. *The Lancet, 371*(9609), 287–288.

Joyce, K., & Loe, M. (2010). A sociological approach to ageing, technology and health. *Sociology of Health & Illness, 32*(2) 171–180.

Kanner, A. D., Coyne, J. C., Schaefer C., & Lazarus, R. S. (1981). Comparison of two modes of stress measurement: Daily hassles and uplifts verses major life events. *Journal of Behavioral Medicine, 4,* 1–39.

Kaplan, G. A., Everson, S. A., & Lynch, J. W. (2000). The contribution of social and behavioral research to an understanding of the distribution of disease: A multilevel approach. In Smedley, B. D. & Syme, S. L. (Eds.), *Promoting health: Intervention strategies from social and behavioral research* (37–80). Washington, DC: Institute of Medicine, Division of Health Promotion and Disease Prevention, National Academies Press.

Kaplan, G. A., Seeman, T. E., Cohen, R. D., Knudsen, L. P., & Guralnik, J. (1987). Mortality among the elderly in the alameda county study: Behavioral and demographic risk factors. *American Journal of Public Health, 77*(3), 307–312.

Katz, S. (1996). *Disciplining old age: The formation of gerontological knowledge.* Charlottesville: University Press of Virginia.

Kawachi, I., & Kennedy, B. (1997). Socioeconomic determinants of health: Health and social cohesion. *British Medical Journal, 314*(7086), 1037–1040.

Kazanjian, A. (1993). Health-manpower planning or gender relations? In Riska, E., & Wegar, K. (Eds.), *Gender, work and medicine* (pp. 147–171). Thousand Oaks, CA: Sage Publications.

Kelner, M. J., & Bourgeault, I. L. (1993). Patient control over dying: Responses of health care professionals. *Social Science & Medicine, 36*(6), 757–765.

Kelner, M., Bourgeault, I. L., Hébert, P. C., & Dunn, E. V. (1993). Advance directives: The views of health care professionals. *Canadian Medical Association Journal, 148*(8), 1331–1338.

Kelner, M., & Wellman, B. (2000). Introduction: Complementary and alternative medicine: challenge and change. In Kelner, M., Wellman, B., Pescosolido, B., & Saks, M. (Eds). *Complementary and alternative medicine: Challenge and change* (pp. 1–24). Melbourne: Harwood Academic Publishers.

Kelner, M., Wellman, B., Welsh, S., & Boon, H. (2006). How far can complementary and alternative medicine go? The case of chiropractic and homeopathy. *Social Science & Medicine, 63*, 2617–2627.

Kelsey, J. L., Whittemore, A. S., Evans, A. S., & Thompson, W. D. (1996). *Methods in observational epidemiology* (2nd ed.). New York: Oxford University Press.

Kendall, O., Lipskie, T., & MacEachern, S. (1997). Canadian health surveys, 1959–1997. *Chronic Diseases in Canada, 18*(2), 70.

Kessler, R. C., McGonagle, K. A., Zhao, S., Nelson, C. B., Hughes, M., Eshleman, S., . . ., & Kendler, K. S. (1994). Lifetime and 12-month prevalence of DSM-III-R psychiatric disorders in the United States: Results from the National Comorbidity Survey. *Archives of General Psychiatry, 51*(1), 8.

Key, T. J., Appleby, P. N., Spencer, E. A., Travis, R. C., Allen, N. E., Thorogood, M., & Mann, J. I. (2009). Cancer incidence in British vegetarians. *British Journal of Cancer, 101*(1), 192–197.

Kingsolver, B. (2008). *Animal, vegetable, miracle: A year of food life.* Toronto: Harper Perennial Canada.

Kirby, M. J. (2002, Oct.). *The health of Canadians—the federal role, volume six: Recommendations for reform.* The Standing Senate Committee on Social Affairs, Science and Technology. Final report on the state of the health care system in Canada. Ottawa: Author.

Kirby, M. J., & Keon, W. J. (2004). *Mental health, mental illness and addiction: Overview of policies and programs in Canada: Report 1.* Ottawa, ON: Standing Senate Committee on Social Affairs, Science and Technology.

Klawiter, M. (2004). Breast cancer in two regimes: the impact of social movements on illness experience. *Sociology of Health & Illness, 26*(6), 845–874.

Klegon, D. (1978). The sociology of professions: An emerging perspective. *Work and Occupations, 5*, 259–283.

Klein, R. (2010). What is health and how do you get it? In Metz, J. M., & Kirkland, A. (Eds.), *Against health: How health became the new morality* (pp. 15–25). New York: New York University Press.

Kobayashi, K. M., & Prus, S. G. (2005). Explaining the health gap between Canadian- and foreign-born older adults: Findings from the 2000/2001 Canadian Community Health Survey. *Journal of International Research Promotion Council, 63*(3), 269–273.

Kohler-Riessman, C. (1983/2003). Women and medicalization. In Weitz, R. (Ed.), *The politics of women's bodies: Sexuality, appearance & behavior* (2nd ed.) (pp. 46–63). New York: Oxford University Press.

Kopun, F. (2010, Sept 8). Genetically modified salmon is ready for dinner. *Toronto Star.* Retrieved from www.thestar.com/life/food_wine/2010/09/08/genetically_modified_salmon_is_ready_for_dinner.html.

Kosowan, G. (2001, July). Population aging prof breaks down myths. *Express News.* Edmonton: University of Alberta. Retrieved from www.archives.expressnews.ualberta.ca/article/2001/07/234.html.

Krause, N. M., & Jay, G. M. (1994). What do global self-rated health items measure? *Medical Care, 32*(9), 930–942.

Krever, H. (1997). *Commission of inquiry on the blood system in Canada.* Ottawa: Canadian Government Publishing.

Kristensen, P., Irgens, L. M., Andersen, A., Bye, A. S., & Sundheim, L. (1997). Birth defects among offspring of Norwegian farmers, 1967–1991. *Epidemiology, 8*, 537–544.

Lachmann, R. (1991). *Encyclopedic dictionary of sociology* (4th ed.). Guilford, CT: Dushkin.

Laforce, H. (1990). The different stages of the elimination of the midwife in Quebec. In Arnup, K., Levesque, E., & Roach Pierson, R. (Eds.), *Delivering motherhood* (pp. 36–50). New York, Routledge.

Lalonde, M. (1974). *A new perspective on the health of Canadians.* Ottawa: Ministry of Supply and Services Canada.

Lane, S., & Cibula, D. (2000). Gender and health. In Albrecht, G. L., Fitzpatrick, R., & Scrimshaw, S. (Eds.), *The handbook of social studies in health and medicine* (pp. 136–153). London: Sage.

Larkin, G. (1983). *Occupational monopoly and modern medicine.* London: Tavistock.

Larkin, M. (2011). The 'medicalization' of aging: what it is, how it harms, and what to do about it. *Journal on Active Aging* (Jan/Feb), 28–36.

Larsen, K., & Gilliland, J. (2008). Mapping the evolution of 'food deserts' in a Canadian city: Supermarket accessibility in London, Ontario, 1961–2005. *International Journal of Health Geographics, 7*(1), 16–31.

Larson, M. S. (1977). *The rise of professionalism: A sociological analysis.* Berkeley, CA: University of California Press.

Laumann, E. O., Paik, A., & Rosen, R. C. (1999). Sexual dysfunction in the United States. *Journal of the American Medical Association, 281*(6), 537–544. [Published erratum appears in JAMA (1999). *281*, 1174.]

Leicht, K., & Fennell, M. L. (2001). *Professional work: A sociological approach.* Malden, MA: Blackwell Publishers.

Lévesque, L. E., Brophy, J. M., & Zhang, B. (2006). Time variations in the risk of myocardial infarction among elderly users of COX-2 inhibitors. *Canadian Medical Association Journal, 174*(11), 1563–1569.

Lexchin, J. (2001). Pharmaceuticals: Politics and policy. In Coburn, D., Armstrong, H., & Armstrong, P. (Eds.), *Unhealthy times: Political economy perspectives on health care* (pp. 31–44). Toronto: Oxford University Press.

Lexchin, J. (2010). Pharmaceutical policy: The dance between industry, government, and the medical profession. In Bryant, T., Raphael, D., & Rioux, M. (Eds.), *Staying alive: Critical perspectives on health, illness, and health care* (2nd ed.) (pp. 371–394). Toronto: CSPI.

Li, P. S. (2008). The market value and social value of race. In Wallis, M. A., & Kwok, S. (Eds.), *Daily struggles: The deepening racialization and feminization of poverty in Canada* (pp. 21–34). Toronto: Canadian Scholar's Press.

Light, D. W. (1979). Uncertainty and control in professional training. *Journal of Health and Social Behavior, 20,* 310–322.

Light, D. W. (2000). The medical profession and organization change: From professional dominance to countervailing power. In Bird, C., Conrad, P., & Fremont, A. M. (Eds.), *Handbook of medical sociology* (5th ed.) (pp. 201–216). New Jersey: Prentice Hall.

Lincoln, Y. S., & Guba, E. G. (1985). *Naturalistic Inquiry.* Newbury Park, CA: Sage Publications.

Link, B. G., Dohrenwend, B. P., & Skodal, A. E. (1986). Socio-economic status and schizophrenia: Noisome occupational characteristics as a risk factor. *American Sociological Review, 51,* 242–258.

Link, B. G., & Phelan, J. (1995). Social conditions as fundamental causes of disease. *Journal of Health and Social Behavior, 35*(Extra Issue), 80–94.

Link, B. G., & Phelan, J. (1996). Review: Why are some people healthy and others not? The determinants of health of populations. *American Journal of Public Health, 86*(4), 598–599.

Lock, M. (1993). *Encounters with aging: Mythologies of menopause in Japan and North America.* Berkley: University of California Press.

Lock, M., & Kaufert, P. A. (Eds.). (1998). *Pragmatic women and body politics.* Cambridge: Cambridge University Press.

Loe, M. (2004). *The rise of Viagra: How the little blue pill changed sex in America.* New York and London: New York University Press.

Lorber, J. (1997). *Gender and the social construction of illness.* Thousand Oaks, CA: Sage.

Lorber, J. (2001). The night to his day: The social construction of gender. In Cohen, T. F. (Ed.), *Men and masculinity* (pp. 19–28). Toronto: Wadsworth.

Lorber, J., & Moore, L. J. (2002). *Gender and the social construction of illness.* Walnut Creek, CA: Altamira.

Lupton, D. (2000). The social construction of medicine and the body. In Albrecht, G. L., Fitzpatrick, R., & Scrimshaw, S. (Eds.), *The handbook of social studies in health and medicine* (pp. 50–63). London: Sage.

Lupton, D. (2001). Risk as moral danger: The social and political functions of risk discourse in public health. In Conrad, P. (Ed.), *The sociology of health and illness: Critical perspectives* (6th ed.) (pp. 394–401). New York: Worth Publishers.

Lupton, D. (2003). Power relations and the medical encounter. In Lupton, D. (Ed.), *Medicine as culture: Illness, disease and the body in western societies* (pp. 113–141). London: Sage.

MacAdam, M. (2004). Examining home care in other countries: The policy issues. *Home Health Care Management & Practice, 16*(5), 393–404.

MacDonald, K. M. (1985). Social closure and occupational registration. *Sociology, 19*(4), 541–556.

MacDonald, K. M., & Ritzer, G. (1988). The sociology of the professions: Dead or alive? *Work and Occupations, 15*(3), 251–272.

Macionis, J. J., Clarke, J. N., & Gerber, L. M. (1994). *Sociology: Canadian edition.* Toronto: Pearson.

Macionis, J. J., & Gerber, L. (2010). *Sociology* (6th ed.). Don Mills, ON: Pearson.

MacLachlan, I. (2001). *Kill and chill: Restructuring Canada's beef commodity chain.* Toronto: University of Toronto Press.

Maher, L. (1992). Punishment and welfare: Crack cocaine and the regulation of mothering. In Feinman, C. (Ed.), *The criminalization of a woman's body* (pp. 157–192). New York, London: The Haworth Press.

Markle, G. E., & McCrea, F. B. (2008). *What if medicine disappeared?* New York: State University of New York Press.

Marmot, M. G., Kogevinas, M., & Elston, M. A. (1987). Social/economic status and disease. *Annual Review of Public Health, 8*(1), 111–135.

Marmot, M. G., Rose, G., Shipley, M., & Hamilton, P. J. (1978). Employment grade and coronary heart disease in British civil servants. *Journal of Epidemiology and Community Health, 32*(4), 244–249.

Marmot, M. G., Shipley, M. J., & Rose, G. (1984). Inequalities in death—specific explanations of a general pattern? *The Lancet, 323*(8384), 1003–1006.

Marmot, M. G., Stansfeld, S., Patel, C., North, F., Head, J., White, I., . . ., & Smith, G. D. (1991). Health inequalities among British civil servants: The Whitehall II Study. *The Lancet, 337*(8754), 1387–1393.

Marshall, B. (2010). Science, medicine and virility surveillance: 'Sexy seniors' in the pharmaceutical imagination *Sociology of Health & Illness, 32*(2), 211–224.

Martel, L., Bélanger, A., Berthelot, J. M., & Carrière, Y. (2005). Healthy aging. In *Healthy today, healthy tomorrow? Findings from the National Population Health Survey.* Ottawa: Statistics Canada, Catalogue no. 82-618-MWE2005004.

Martin, E. (2001). *The woman in the body: A cultural analysis of reproduction.* Boston: Beacon Press.

Mason, J. (1988). Midwifery in Canada. In Kitzinger, K. (Ed.), *The midwife challenge* (pp. 99–133) London: Pandora.

Mathers C. D., Lopez, A. D., & Murray, C. J. L. (2006). The burden of disease and mortality by condition: Data, methods, and results for 2001. In Lopez, A. D., Mathers, C. D., Ezzati, M., et al. (Eds.), *Global burden of disease and risk factors.* Washington (DC): World Bank. Retrieved from www.ncbi.nlm.nih.gov/books/NBK11808/.

McAmmond, D. (2000). Food and nutrition surveillance in Canada: An environmental scan. Ottawa: Health Canada.

McBane, M. (2002, October 28). Senator Kirby's conflict. *The Hill Times,* Letter-to-the-Editor. Retrieved from http://healthcoalition.ca/wp-content/uploads/2010/02/kirby-conflict.pdf.

McCrea, F. B. (1983). The politics of menopause: The "discovery" of a deficiency disease. *Social Problems, 31*(1), 111–123.

McElroy, A., & Jezewski, M. A. (2000). Cultural variation in the experience of health and illness. In *The handbook of social studies in health and medicine* (191–209). London: Sage.

McFarland, B., Bigelow, D., Zani, B., Newsom, J., & Kaplan, M. (2002). Complementary and alternative medicine use in Canada and the United States. *American Journal of Public Health, 92*(10), 1616–1618.

McIntosh, C. N., Fines, P., Wilkins, R., & Wolfson, M. C. (2009). Income disparities in health-adjusted life expectancy for Canadian adults, 1991 to 2001. *Health Reports, 20*(4), 55–64. 82-003-X.

McKay, L. (2000). *Health beyond health care: Twenty-five years of federal health policy development.* Ottawa, Ontario, Canada: Canadian Policy Research Networks.

McKeown, T. (1972). An interpretation of the modern rise in population in Europe. *Population Studies, 26,* 345–382.

McKeown, T. (1979). *The role of medicine: Dream, mirage or nemesis?* Oxford, England: Basil Blackwell.

McKinlay, J. B. (1982). Toward the proletarianization of physicians. In Derber, C. (Ed.), *Professionals as workers: Mental labor in advanced capitalism* (pp. 37–62). Boston: G. K. Hall.

McKinlay, J. B. (1986). A case for refocusing upstream: The political economy of illness. In Conrad, P., & Kern, R. (Eds.), *The sociology of health and illness: Critical perspectives* (2nd ed.) (pp. 484–498). MacMillan.

McKinlay, J. B. (1996). Some contributions from the social system to gender inequalities in heart disease. *Journal of Health and Social Behavior, 38,* 1–26.

McMullin, J. A. (2000). Diversity and the state of sociological aging theory. *The Gerontologist, 40,* 517–530.

McNair, R., Stone, N., Sims, J., & Curtis, C. (2005). Australian evidence for interprofessional education contributing to effective teamwork preparation and interest in rural practice. *Journal of Interprofessional Care, 19*(6), 579–594.

Mead, G. H. (1934). Mind, self, and society. *Chicago: University of Chicago.*

Mechanic, D. (1961). The concept of illness behavior. *Journal of Chronic Disease, 15,* 189–194.

Mechanic, D. (1978). *Medical sociology* (2nd ed.). New York: The Free Press.

Mechanic, D. (1992). Health and illness behavior and patient-practitioner relationships. *Social Science & Medicine, 34*(12), 1345–1350.

Mechanic, D., & Volkart, E. H. (1960). Illness behavior and medical diagnosis. *Journal of Health and Human Behavior, 1*(2), 86–93.

Meltzer, B. N., Petras, J. W., & Reynolds, L. T. (1975). *Symbolic interactionism: Genesis, varieties, criticisms.* London: Routledge and Kegan Paul.

Mental Health Commission of Canada. (2009). Toward recovery and well-being: A framework for a mental health strategy for Canada. Ottawa: Author. Retrieved from www.mentalhealthcommission.ca/English/document/241/toward-recovery-and-well-being.

Mental Health Commission of Canada. (2012). Changing directions, changing lives: The mental health strategy of Canada. Ottawa: Author. Retrieved from www.mentalhealthcommission.ca/English/Pages/default.aspx.

Merleau-Ponty, M. (1962). *The phenomenology of perception.* London: Routledge.

Merriam-Webster Online (www.Merriam-Webster.com) copyright © 2014 by Merriam-Webster, Incorporated.

Merton, R. K., Reader, G. G., & Kendall, P. L. (Eds.), (1957). *The student physician: Introductory studies in the sociology of medical education.* Boston: Harvard University Press.

Metzel, J. M. (2010). Why "against health"? In Metzl, J. M., & Kirkland, A. (Eds.), *Against health: How health became the new morality* (pp. 1–11). New York: New York University Press.

Midwifery Act, 1991, S. O. 1991, c. 31. Government of Ontario. Retrieved from www.e-laws.gov.on.ca/Download/elaws_statutes_91m31_e.doc.

Mills, C. W. (1959). *The sociological imagination.* New York: Oxford University Press.

Mills, D. (2013). Menopause and perimenopause. Women to Women Health Clinic, Maine. Retrieved from www.womentowomen.com/category/menopause-perimenopause/.

Minkler, M., & Estes, C. L. (Eds.). (1991). *Critical perspectives on aging: The political and moral economy of growing old.* Amityville, NY: Baywood.

Mirowsky, J., & Ross, C. E. (1992). Age and depression. *Journal of Health and Social Behavior, 33,* 187–281.

Mishler, E. G., AmaraSingham, L. R., Hauser, S. T., Liem, R., & Osherson, S. D. (1981). *Social contexts of health, illness, and patient care.* Cambridge University Press.

Mitchell, A. E., Hong, Y. J., Koh, E., Barrett, D. M., Bryant, D. E., Denison, R. F., & Kaffka, S. (2007). Ten-year comparison of the influence of organic and conventional crop management practices on the content of flavonoids in tomatoes. *Journal of Agricultural and Food Chemistry, 55*(15), 6154–6159.

Mizrachi, N., Shuval, J. T., & Gross, S. (2005). Boundary at work: Alternative medicine in biomedical settings. *Sociology of Health & Illness, 27*(1), 20–43.

Monsanto. (n.d.). Company history. Retrieved from www.monsanto.com/whoweare/Pages/monsanto-history.aspx.

Monsanto. (n.d.). Genuity Roundup Ready 2 yield soybeans with acceleron performance: More beans per pod, more bushels per acre. Retrieved from www.monsanto.com/products/Pages/genuity-roundup-ready-2-yield-soybeans.aspx.

Monsanto. (n.d.). Is Monsanto going to develop or sell "terminator" seeds? Retrieved from www.monsanto.com/newsviews/Pages/terminator-seeds.aspx.

Monsanto. (2004). Monsantos Roundup Ready Corn 2 technology completes European Union food approval process. Retrieved from www.monsanto.com/products/Pages/genuity-roundup-ready-2-yield-soybeans.aspx.

Monsanto. (2005). Monsanto completes acquisition of Seminis. Retrieved from http://monsanto.mediaroom.com/index.php?s=43&item=158.

Moreau, D. T., Conway, C., & Fleming, I. A. (2011). Reproductive performance of alternative male phenotypes of growth hormone transgenic Atlantic salmon (Salmo salar). *Evolutionary Applications, 4*(6), 736–748.

Mosby, I. (2013). Administering colonial science: Nutrition research and human biomedical experimentation in Aboriginal communities and residential schools, 1942–1952. *Social History*, XLVI(91), 145–172.

Moseley, J. B., O'Malley, K., Petersen, N. J., Menke, T. J., Brody, B. A., Kuykendall, D. H., . . ., & Wray, N. P. (2002). A controlled trial of arthroscopic surgery for osteoarthritis of the knee. *New England Journal of Medicine, 347*(2), 81–88.

Moynihan, R. (2003). The making of a disease: female sexual dysfunction. *BMJ: British Medical Journal, 326*(7379), 45–47.

Moynihan, R., Heath, I., & Henry, D. (2002). Selling sickness: the pharmaceutical industry and disease mongering. *BMJ: British Medical Journal, 324*(7342), 886.

Moynihan, R., & Smith, R. (2002). Too much medicine? Almost certainly. *BMJ: British Medical Journal, 324*(7342), 859–860.

Mukherjee, D., Nissen, S. E., & Topol, E. J. (2001). Risk of cardiovascular events associated with selective COX-2 inhibitors. *Journal of the American Medical Association, 286*(8), 954–959.

Mulvale, G., Abelson, J., & Goering, P. (2007). Mental health service delivery in Ontario, Canada: How do policy legacies shape prospects for reform? *Health Economics, Policy and Law, 2*(4), 363–389.

Munro, S., Lewin, S., Swart, T., & Volmink, J. (2007). A review of health behaviour theories: how useful are these for developing interventions to promote long-term medication adherence for TB and HIV/AIDS? *BMC Public Health, 7*, 104.

Murphy, R. (1986). Weberian closure theory: A contribution to the ongoing assessment. *British Journal of Sociology, 37*, 21–41.

Mussell, A., Oginskyy A., & Hedley, G. (2008). The troubled corn economy of Ontario's livestock sector: A strategic policy analysis. Guelph, ON: George Morris Centre.

Muzzin, L., Brown, G. P., & Hornosty, R. W. (1994). Consequences of feminisation of a profession: The case of Canadian pharmacy. *Women & Health, 21*, 39–56.

Muzzin, L., Brown, G., & Hornosty, R. (1995). Gender, educational credentials, contributions and career advancement: A follow-up study in hospital pharmacy. *Canadian Review of Sociology and Anthropology, 32*(2), 151–168.

Navarro, V. (1976). *Medicine under capitalism.* New York: Prodist.

Navarro, V. (1986). *Crisis, health, and medicine: A social critique.* London: Tavistock.

Navarro, V. (1988). Professional dominance or proletarization? Neither. *The Milbank Quarterly, 66*(Suppl. 2), 57–75.

Navarro, V. (2009). What we mean by social determinants of health. *International Union for Health Promotion and Education [IUHPE] Global Health Promotion, 16*(1), 1–13.

Naylor, D. (1986). *Private practice, public payment.* Montreal: McGill University Press.

Naylor, R. L., Goldburg, R. J., Primavera, J. H., Kautsky, N., Beveridge, M. C., Clay, J., . . ., & Troell, M. (2000). Effect of aquaculture on world fish supplies. *Nature, 405*(6790), 1017–1024.

Neiterman, E. (2010). *The embodied experiences of pregnancy: Learning, doing and attaching meaning to pregnant body in different social contexts.* Unpublished doctoral dissertation. McMaster University, Hamilton, Ontario, Canada.

Nestel, S. (1996/1996). A new profession to the white population in Canada: Ontario midwifery and the politics of race. *Health and Canadian society, 4*(2), 315.

Nestle, M. (2000). Soft drink "pouring rights": marketing empty calories to children. *Public Health Reports, 115*(4), 308.

Nestle, M. (2003). *Safe food: Bacteria, biotechnology, and bioterrorism.* Berkeley, CA: University of California Press.

Nettleton, S. (1995). *The sociology of health & illness.* Cambridge, UK: Polity Press.

Norris, S. (2008). *Canada's blood supply ten years after the Krever Commission.* Ottawa: Parliamentary Information and Research Service, Library of Parliament.

North East LHIN. (2011). *Home first shifts care of seniors to home.* Retrieved from www.nelhin.on.ca/WorkArea/showcontent.aspx?id=11258.

Novek, J., Yassi, A., & Spiegel, J. (1990). Mechanization, the labor process, and injury risks in the Canadian meat packing industry. *International Journal of Health Services, 20*(2), 281–296.

Nurse Practitioner Association of Alberta. (2013). Nurse Practitioner Association of Alberta – Home page. Retrieved from www.albertanps.com/whatisnp.htm.

Oakley, A. (1980). *Women confined: Towards a sociology of childbirth.* Oxford: Martin Robertson.

O'Brien, M. (1989). *Reproducing the world.* Boulder, San Francisco, & London: Westview Press.

O'Brien-Pallas, L. L., Tomblin Murphy, G., Laschinger, H. K. S., White, S., & Milburn, B. (2004). *Survey of employers: Health care organizations' senior nurse managers.* Ottawa: Nursing Sector Study Corporation.

O'Connor, D. (2002). *Part one: A summary report of the Walkerton Inquiry: The events of May 2000 and related issues.* Toronto: Ontario Ministry of the Attorney General, Queen's Printer for Ontario.

OECD 2012. (2012, Aug 10). *Health data.* Paris: Author. Retrieved from www.oecd.org/health/healthpoliciesanddata/oecdhealthdata2012.htm.

Office of the Auditor General. (2010, Spring). *Report of the Auditor General of Canada to the House of Commons.* Ottawa: Minister of Public Works and Government Services Canada.

Offord, D. R., Boyle, M. H., Campbell, D., & Goering, P. (1996). One-year prevalence of psychiatric disorder in Ontarians 15 to 64 years of age. *Canadian Journal of Psychiatry/La Revue canadienne de psychiatrie, 41*, 559–563

Offord, D. R., Boyle, M. H., Szatmari, P., Rae-Grant, N. I., Links, P. S., Cadman, D. T., . . ., & Woodward, C. A.

(1987). Ontario Child Health Study: II. Six-month prevalence of disorder and rates of service utilization. *Archives of General Psychiatry, 44*(9), 832.

Omran, A. R. (1971). The epidemiologic transition: a theory of the epidemiology of population change. *The Milbank Memorial Fund Quarterly, 49*(4), 509–538.

Ontario Medical Association. (2009). New nurse practitioner clinics. Press Release. Retrieved from www.oma.org/Mediaroom/PressReleases/Pages/NewNursePractitionerClinics.aspx.

Ontario Ministry of Health and Long-Term Care. (2012). Community health centres. Toronto: Author. Retrieved from www.health.gov.on.ca/english/public/contact/chc/chc_mn.html.

Organic Monitor. (2010). *The global market for organic food & drink: Business opportunities & future outlook* (3rd ed.). London: Organic Monitor. Retrieved from www.organicmonitor.com/700340.htm.

Orton, F., Rosivatz, E., Scholze, M., & Kortenkamp, A. (2011). Widely used pesticides with previously unknown endocrine activity revealed as in vitro antiandrogens. *Environmental Health Perspectives, 119*(6), 794.

Papanikolaou, P. (2008). Book review. Aging and caring at the intersection of work and home life blurring the boundaries. *Quality in Ageing, 9*, 4, 44.

Park, J. (2005). Use of alternative health care. *Health Reports, 16*(2), 39–42.

Parkin, F. (1979). *Marxism and class theory: A bourgeois critique.* London: Tavistock.

Parry, N., & Parry, J. (1976). *The rise of the medical profession.* London: Croom Helm.

Parsons, T. (1951). *The social system.* Glencoe, Ill.: Free Press.

Pearlin, L. I. (1989). The sociological study of stress. *Journal of Health and Social Behavior, 30*(3), 241–256.

Pearlin, L. I., Menaghan, E. G., Lieberman, M. A., & Mullan, J. T. (1981). The stress process. *Journal of Health and Social Behavior, 22*(4) 337–356.

Pearlin, L. I., Schieman, S., Fazio, E. M., & Meersman, S. C. (2005). Stress, health, and the life course: Some conceptual perspectives. *Journal of Health and Social Behavior, 46*(2), 205–219.

Peden, A. H., Head, M. W., Ritchie, D. L., Bell, J. E., & Ironside, J. W. (2004). Preclinical vCJD after blood transfusion in a PRNP codon 129 heterozygous patient. *The Lancet, 364*(9433), 527–529.

Pederson, A., & Raphael, D. (2006). Gender, race and health disparities. In Raphael, D., Bryant, T., & Rioux, M. (Eds.), *Staying alive: Critical perspectives on health, illness, and health care* (pp. 159–191). Toronto: Canadian Scholar's Press.

Pehanich, M. (2003). Hail to the innovators: The food engineering hall of fame. *Food Engineering, 75* (9), 65–78.

Petrini, C. (2005). *Slow food nation.* New York: Rizzoli Ex Libris.

Pharmacy Act, 1991, S. O. 1991, CHAPTER 36. Toronto: Government of Ontario. Retrieved from www.e-laws.gov.on.ca/html/statutes/english/elaws_statutes_91p36_e.htm.

Phelan, J. C., Link, B. G., & Tehranifar, P. (2010). Social conditions as fundamental causes of health inequalities theory, evidence, and policy implications. *Journal of Health and Social Behavior, 51*(1 suppl), S28–S40.

Phillips, T. (2010). Debating the legitimacy of a contested environmental illness: A case study of multiple chemical sensitivities. *Sociology of Health & Illness, 32*(7), 1026–1040.

Piaget, J. (1932). *The moral judgment of the child.* London: Kegan Paul, Trench, Trubner and Co.

Piaget, J. (1952). *The origins of intelligence in children.* New York: International University Press.

Picot, G., Hou, F., & Coulombe, S. 2007. *Chronic low income and low-income dynamics among recent immigrants.* Ottawa: Statistics Canada. Catalogue no. 11F0019MIE—No. 294.

Pimentel, D., Houser, J., Preiss, E., White, O., Fang, H., Mesnick, L., . . ., & Alpert, S. (1997). Water resources: agriculture, the environment, and society. *BioScience, 47*(2), 97–106.

Pimentel, D., & Pimentel, M. (2003). Sustainability of meat-based and plant-based diets and the environment. *The American Journal of Clinical Nutrition, 78*(3), 660S–663S.

Pirog, R., & Benjamin, A. (2004). Food miles: A simple metaphor to contrast local and global food systems. Newsletter. Chicago: Hunger and Environmental Nutrition (HEN) Dietetic Practice Group of the American Dietetic Association.

Plamondon, J. (1985). Deinstitutionalization: Its implications and requirements. In *Deinstitutionalization: Costs and effects* (pp. 19–26). Ottawa: Canadian Council on Social Development.

Pollan, M. (2006). *The ominvore's dilemma: A natural history of four meals.* New York: Penguin.

Ponting, J. R. (Ed.). (1997). *First Nations in Canada: Perspectives on opportunity, empowerment, and self-determination.* Toronto: McGraw-Hill Ryerson.

Population Division of the Department of Economic and Social Affairs of the United Nations Secretariat. (2010). *World population prospects: The 2010 revision.* Geneva, Switzerland: United Nations.

Prakash S., & Valentine, V. (2006, June 8). Timeline: The rise and fall of Vioxx. *National Public Radio.* Retrieved from www.NPR.org.

Preibisch, K. L. (2007). Local produce, foreign labor: labor mobility programs and global trade competitiveness in Canada. *Rural Sociology, 72*(3), 418–449.

Prochaska, J. O., & DiClemente, C. C. (1983). Stages and processes of self-change of smoking: toward an integrative model of change. *Journal of Consulting and Clinical Psychology, 51*(3), 390.

Public Health Agency of Canada. (2008). Fact sheet—Methicillin-resistant staphylococcus aureus. Retrieved from www.phac-aspc.gc.ca/id-mi/mrsa-eng.php.

Public Health Agency of Canada. (2010). *The Chief Public Health Officer's report on the state of public health in Canada, 2010.* Ottawa: Author. Retrieved from www.phac-aspc.gc.ca/cphorsphc-respcacsp/2010/fr-rc/cphorsphc-respcacsp-06-eng.php.

Public Health Agency of Canada. (2011). Fact sheet—Clostridium difficile (C. difficile). Ottawa: Author. Retrieved from www.phac-aspc.gc.ca/id-mi/cdiff-eng.php.

Putney, N. M., & Bengtson, V. L. (2005). Family relations in changing times: A longitudinal study of five cohorts of women. *International Journal of Sociology and Social Policy, 25*(3), 92–119.

Puxley, C. (2013, Dec 25). Attempt to get nurse to check on Brian Sinclair was 'just passed off', inquest told. *CTV News.* Retrieved from www.ctvnews.ca/canada/attempt-to-get-nurse-to-check-on-brian-sinclair-was-just-passed-off-inquest-told-1.1511604#ixzz2oW3o9XEO.

Rachlis, M. (2005). *Prescription for excellence: How innovation in saving Canada's health care system.* Toronto, Ontario: HarperPerennialCanada, HarperCollins Publishers.

Rachlis, M., & Kushner, C. (1989). *Second opinion: What's wrong with Canada's health-care system and how to fix it.* Toronto: Collins Publishers.

Radley, A. (1994). *Making sense of illness: The social psychology of health and disease.* London: Sage.

Raj, A. (2011, December 7). Beyond the border: Harper, Obama announce deal to bolster security, reduce trade barriers. *Huffington Post.* Retrieved from www.huffingtonpost.ca/2011/12/07/beyond-the-border-perimeter-security-canada_n_1134463.html.

Raphael, D. (2009). Social determinants of health: An overview of key issues and themes. In Raphael, D. (Ed.), *Social determinants of health: Canadian perspectives, (2nd ed.)* (pp. 2–19). Toronto: Canadian Scholars' Press.

Raphael, D. (2010). Social determinants of health: an overview of concepts and issues. In Bryant, T., Raphael, D., & Rioux, M. (Eds.), *Staying alive: Critical perspectives on health, illness and health care.* Toronto: Canadian Scholars' Press.

Ratcliffe-Brown, A. R. (1940). On social structure. *The Journal of the Royal Anthropological Institute of Great Britain and Ireland, 70*(1), 1–12.

Ratnasingham, S., Cairney, J., Rehm, J., Manson, H., & Kurdyak, P. A. (2012). *Opening eyes, opening minds: The Ontario burden of mental illness and additions report.* An ICES/PHO Report. Toronto: Institute for Clinical Evaluative Sciences and Public Health Ontario. Retrieved from www.oahpp.ca/opening-eyes-opening-minds.

Redding, C. A., Rossi, J. S., Rossi, S. R., Velicer, W. F., & Prochaska, J. O. (2000). Health behavior models. *The International Electronic Journal of Health Education, 3*(Special Issue), 180–193.

Regush, N. M. (1987). *Condition critical.* Toronto: Macmillan.

Reisig, V. M. T., & Hobbis, A. (2000). Food deserts and how to tackle them: A study of one city's approach. *Health Education Journal, 59*(2), 137–149.

Revenson, T. A., Schiaffino, K. M., Deborah Majerovitz, S., & Gibofsky, A. (1991). Social support as a double-edged sword: The relation of positive and problematic support to depression among rheumatoid arthritis patients. *Social Science & Medicine, 33*(7), 807–813.

Reverby, S. (1987). *Ordered to care.* Cambridge: Cambridge University Press.

Richardson, G., & Maynard, A. (1995). Fewer doctors? More nurses? Centre for Health Economics, Working Paper Series. York, UK: University of York. Retrieved from www.york.ac.uk/media/che/documents/papers/discussionpapers/CHE Discussion Paper 135.pdf.

Richter, E. D. (2002). Acute human pesticide poisonings. In Pimentel, D. (Ed.), *Encyclopedia of pest management* (pp. 3–6). New York: Dekker.

Riessman, C. K. (1983). Women and medicalization: A new perspective. *Social Policy, 14*, 3–18.

Roberge, R., Berthelot, J. M., & Wolfson, M. (1995). The Health Utility Index: Measuring health differences in Ontario by socioeconomic status. *Health Reports, 7*(2), 25–32.

Robins, L. N., Helzer, J. E., Croughan, J., & Ratcliff, K. S. (1981). National Institute of Mental Health diagnostic interview schedule: its history, characteristics, and validity. *Archives of General Psychiatry, 38*(4), 381.

Robins, L. N., Locke, B. Z., & Regier, D. A. (1991). An overview of psychiatric disorders in America. In Robins, L. N., & Regier, D. A. (Eds.), *Psychiatric disorders in America: The Epidemiologic Catchment Area Study* (pp. 328–366). New York: The Free Press.

Robins, L. N., & Reiger, D. A. (1991). *Psychiatric disorders in America: The Epidemiologic Catchment Area Study.* New York: Free Press.

Rockwell, J. (2010). Deconstructing housework: Cuts to home support services and the implications for hospital discharge planning. *Journal of Women & Aging, 22*(1), 47–60.

Romanow, R. (2002). *Building on values: The future of health care in Canada.* (Final Report). Commission on the Future of Health Care in Canada. Ottawa: National Library of Canada.

Romanow, R. (2012, January 8). Stephen Harper's hands-off stance could signal end to national healthcare system. *The National Post.* Retrieved from http://news.nationalpost.com/2012/01/08/stephen-harpers-hands-off-stance-could-signal-end-to-national-health-care-system-romanow/.

Rootman, I., & Raeburn, J. (1994). The concept of health. In Pederson A, O'Neill, M., & Rootman, I. (Eds.). Health promotion in Canada: Provincial, national and international perspectives (pp. 56–71). Toronto: Saunders WB.

Rosenhan, D. L. (1973). On being sane in insane places. *Science, 179*(4070), 250–258.

Rosenhan, D. L. (1975). On being sane in insane places. In Scheff, T. (Ed.), *Labeling madness* (pp. 54–74). New Jersey: Prentice Hall.

Rosenstock, I. M. (1974). Historical origins of the health belief model. *Health Education Monographs, 2*, 1–8.

Rosser, W., Colwill, J., Kasperski, J., & Wilson, L. (2011). Progress of Ontario's family health team model: A patient-centred medical home. *Annals of Family Medicine, 9*(2), 165–171.

Rothman, B. Katz. (1993). *The tentative pregnancy: How amniocentesis changes the experience of motherhood.* New York: Norton Press.

Royal College of Physicians and Surgeons of Canada. (1993). *Expert panel on human safety of RBST.* Report of the Royal College of Physicians and Surgeons of Canada. Ottawa: Health Canada.

Rule, D. C., Broughton, K. S., Shellito, S. M., & Maiorano, G. (2002). Comparison of muscle fatty acid profiles and cholesterol concentrations of bison, beef cattle, elk, and chicken. *Journal of Animal Science, 80*(5), 1202–1211.

Rushing, B. (1991). Market explanations for occupational power: The decline of midwifery in Canada. *American Review of Canadian Studies, 21*(1), 7–27.

Saks, M. (1983). Removing the blinkers? A critique of recent contributions to the sociology of professions. *Sociology Review, 31,* 1–21.

Sampson, R. J., & Laub, J. H. (1993). *Crime in the making: Pathways and turning points through life.* Harvard University Press, Cambridge Massachusetts.

Scallan, E., Hoekstra, R. M., Angulo, F. J., Tauxe, R. V., Widdowson, M. A., Roy, S. L., . . ., & Griffin, P. M. (2011). Foodborne illness acquired in the United States—major pathogens. *Emerging infectious diseases, 17*(1), 7.

Scheff, T. (1966). *Being mentally ill: A sociological theory.* Chicago: Aldine.

Scheff, T. (1984). *Being mentally ill: A sociological theory* (2nd ed.). Chicago: Aldine.

Schlosser, E. (2005). *Fast food nation: The dark side of the all-American meal.* New York: Harper Perennial.

Schneider, J. W., & Conrad, P. (1980). In the closet with illness: Epilepsy, stigma potential and information control. *Social Problems, 28*(1), 32–44.

Schuurman, H. J., & Pierson 3rd, R. N. (2008). Progress towards clinical xenotransplantation. *Frontiers in Bioscience: A Journal and Virtual Library, 13,* 204.

Seale, C., & Charteris-Black, J. (2008). The interaction of class and gender in illness narratives. *Sociology, 42*(3), 453–469.

Segall, A. (1976). The sick role concept: Understanding illness behavior. *Journal of Health and Social Behavior, 17,* 162–169.

Segall, A. (1997). Sick role concepts and health behavior. In Gochman, D. S. (Ed.), *Handbook of health behaviour research* (pp. 289–300). New York: Plenum Press.

Segall, A., & Chappell, N. (2000). *Health and health care in Canada.* Toronto: Prentice Hall.

Seierstad, S. L., Seljeflot, I., Johansen, O., Hansen, R., Haugen, M., Rosenlund, G., . . ., & Arnesen, H. (2005). Dietary intake of differently fed salmon; the influence on markers of human atherosclerosis. *European Journal of Clinical Investigation, 35*(1), 52–59.

Selye, H. (1956). *The stress of life.* New York: McGraw-Hill.

Semeniuk, I. (2013, Jan 25). How poverty influences a child's brain development. *The Globe and Mail.* Retrieved from www.theglobeandmail.com/technology/science/brain/how-poverty-influences-a-childs-brain-development/article7882957/.

Seminis. (n.d.). About Seminis. Retrieved from http://us.seminis.com/about/default.asp.

Senate of Canada. (2005). The evidence on rBST. 1999; 38th Parliament 1st Session Standing Committee on Health. Ottawa: Parliament of Canada.

Sered, S., & Agigan, A. (2008). Holistic sickening: Breast cancer and the discursive worlds of complementary and alternative practitioners. *Sociology of Health & Illness, 30*(4), 616–631.

Shandel, T., & Johnson, G. (Writers). (1983). *Bitter medicine* [documentary]. Montreal: National Film Board of Canada.

Shapiro, M. (1978). *Getting doctored: Critical reflections on becoming a physician.* Kitchener, ON: Between the Lines.

Sharkey, S., Larsen, L., & Mildon, B. (2003). An overview of home care in Canada: Its past, present, and potential. *Home Health Care Management & Practice, 15*(5), 382–390.

Shaw, G. M., Wasserman, C. R., O'Malley, C. D., Nelson, V., & Jackson, R. J. (1999). Maternal pesticide exposure from multiple sources and selected congenital anomalies. *Epidemiology, 10*(1), 60–66.

Shenk, D., Kuwahara, K., & Zablotsky, D. (2004). Older women's attachments to their home and possessions. *Journal of Aging Studies, 18*(2), 157–169.

Shenton, A. K. (2004). Strategies for ensuring trustworthiness in qualitative research projects. *Education for Information, 22*(2), 63–75.

Shields, M. (2006). Overweight and obesity among children and youth. *Health Reports, 17*(3), 27–42.

Shrout, P. E., Dohrenwend, B. P., & Levav, I. (1986). A discriminate rule for screening cases of diverse diagnostic types: Preliminary results. *Journal of Consulting Clinical Psychology, 54,* 314–319.

Siegel, K., Lune, H., & Meyer, I. H. (1998). Stigma management among gay/bisexual men with HIV/AIDS. *Qualitative Sociology, 21*(1), 3–24.

Sinclair, U. (2004). *The jungle.* New York: Pocket Books.

Singer, P. (2002). *Animal liberation: A new ethics for our treatment of animals.* New York: Ecco.

Singh, G. K., Miller, B. A., & Hankey, B. F. (2002). Changing area socioeconomic patterns in US cancer mortality, 1950–1998: Part II—Lung and colorectal cancers. *Journal of the National Cancer Institute, 94*(12), 916–925.

Sivapalasingam, S., Friedman, C. R., Cohen, L., & Tauxe, R. V. (2004). Fresh produce: A growing cause of outbreaks of foodborne illness in the United States, 1973 through 1997. *Journal of Food Protection, 67*(10), 2342–2353.

Smith, A., & Fiddler, J. (2009). Making the gift of life safety: The Canadian tainted blood scandal and its regulatory consequences. In Bolaria, S. (Ed.), *Health, illness, and health care in Canada* (pp. 491–506). Toronto: Nelson.

Smith, A., & MacKinnon, J. B. (2007). *The 100-mile diet: A year of local eating.* Toronto: Vintage.

Smith, B. E. (1981). Black lung: The social production of disease. *International Journal of Health Services, 11*(3), 343–359.

Smith, D. E. (1993). The standard North American family SNAF as an ideological code. *Journal of Family Issues, 14*(1), 50–65.

Smith, K. E., Besser, J. M., Hedberg, C. W., Leano, F. T., Bender, J. B., Wicklund, J. H., . . ., & Osterholm, M. T. (1999). Quinolone-resistant Campylobacter jejuni infections in Minnesota, 1992–1998. *New England Journal of Medicine, 340*(20), 1525–1532.

Smoyer-Tomic, K. E., Spence, J. C., & Amrhein, C. (2006). Food deserts in the Prairies? Supermarket accessibility and neighborhood need in Edmonton, Canada. *The Professional Geographer, 58*(3), 307–326.

Smylie, J., Fell, D., & Ohlsson, A. (2010). The Joint Working Group on First Nations, Indian, Inuit, and Métis infant mortality of the Canadian Perinatal Surveillance System. A review of Aboriginal infant mortality rates in Canada–striking and persistent Aboriginal/non-Aboriginal inequities. *Canadian Journal of Public Health, 101*(2), 143–48.

Sontag, S. (1978). *Illness as metaphor.* New York: Random House.

Spitzer, R. L., Endicott, J., Fleiss, J. L., & Cohen, J. (1970). The psychiatric status schedule: A technique for evaluating psychopathology and impairment in role functioning. *Archives of General Psychiatry, 23*(1), 41.

Spoel, P. (2004). The meaning and ethics of informed choice in Canadian midwifery. Paper prepared for Laurentian University. Sudbury: Laurentian University, pp. 1–11.

Standing Committee on Social Affairs, Science and Technology. (2006). *Out of the shadows at last: Transforming mental health, mental illness and addiction services in Canada.* Final report on Mental Health, Mental Illness and Addiction. Ottawa: Author.

Standing Senate Committee on Agriculture and Forestry. (1999). *rBST and the drug approval process.* (Interim report). Ottawa: Author. Retrieved from www.parl.gc.ca/Content/SEN/Committee/361/agri/rep/repintermar99-e.htm

Stanton, B. F. (1993). Changes in farm size and structure in American agriculture in the twentieth century. In Hallam, A. (Ed.), *Size, structure and the changing face of American agriculture* (pp. 587–627) Boulder, CO: Westview Press.

Starr, P. (1982). *Social transformation of American medicine: The rise of a sovereign profession and the making of a vast industry.* New York: Basic Books.

Starzl, T. E., Fung, J., Tzakis, A., Todo, S., Demetris, A. J., Marino, I. R., . . ., & Michaels, M. (1993). Baboon-to-human liver transplantation. *The Lancet, 341*(8837), 65–71.

Statistics Canada. (1980). *Income distributions by size in Canada.* Ottawa: Author, Supply and Services Canada.

Statistics Canada. (1983). *Historical statistics of Canada* (2nd ed.). (Catalogue no. 11-516-XIE). Ottawa: Author.

Statistics Canada. (1995). *Births and deaths, 1995.* (Catalogue no. 84-210-XIB). Ottawa: Author.

Statistics Canada, Special Surveys Division. (1997). *National Longitudinal Survey of Children and Youth: Users handbook and microdata guide* (Cycle 1, Release 2). Ottawa: Author.

Statistics Canada. (2001). *Perspectives on labour and income,* the online edition. December(2), 12. Ottawa: Author. Retrieved from www.statcan.gc.ca/pub/75-001-x/01201/6036-eng.html.

Statistics Canada. (2002). Life tables—Canada, provinces and territories, 1995–1997. (Catalogue no. 84-537). Ottawa: Author.

Statistics Canada. (2006a). Census of Agriculture, Farm Data and Farm Operator Data. (Catalogue no. 95-629-XWE). Ottawa: Author.

Statistics Canada. (2006b). Health-adjusted life expectancy, at birth and at age 65, by sex and income group, Canada and provinces, occasional (years) (CANSIM Table 102-0121). Ottawa: Author.

Statistics Canada. (2006c). *Report on the demographic situation in Canada.* (Catalogue no. 91-209-XIE). Ottawa: Author.

Statistics Canada. (2007a). *Aboriginal health and well-being.* Ottawa: Author. Retrieved from www41.statcan.gc.ca/2007/10000/ceb10000_004-eng.htm.

Statistics Canada. (2007b). *A portrait of seniors in Canada.* Ottawa: Ministry of Industry.

Statistics Canada. (2007c). *Residential care facilities 2005/06.* (Catalogue no. 8-237-X). Ottawa: Author.

Statistics Canada. (2008a). *Canada at a glance, 2008.* (Catalogue no. 12-581-XPE). Ottawa: Author.

Statistics Canada. (2008b). Life expectancy, abridged life table, at birth and at age 65, by sex, Canada, provinces and territories, annual (years) (CANSIM Table 102-0511). Ottawa: Author.

Statistics Canada. (2008c). Report on the demographic situation in Canada, 2005 and 2006. (Catalogue no. 91-209-X). Ottawa: Author.

Statistics Canada. (2010a). *Canadian Health Measures Survey (CHMS) data user guide: Cycle 1.* Ottawa: Author.

Statistics Canada. (2010b). *Population projections for Canada, provinces, and territories, 2009 to 2036.* Ottawa: Author.

Statistics Canada. (2010c). *Residential care facilities survey guide: Instructions and definitions.* Ottawa: Author. Retrieved from www23.statcan.gc.ca/imdb-bmdi/document/3210_D1_T1_V15-eng.pdf.

Statistics Canada. (2011). Population unemployment rates among those aged 25–54 by education and immigrant status in 2010 (CANSIM table 282-0106). Ottawa: Author.

Statistics Canada. (2011, December). Canadian business patterns database. Ottawa: Author. Retrieved from www.ic.gc.ca/cis-sic/cis-sic.nsf/IDE/cis-sic622etbe.html.

Statistics Canada. (2012, May 31). Deaths, 2009. Statistics Canada, *The Daily.* Ottawa: Author. Retrieved from www.statcan.gc.ca/daily-quotidien/120531/dq120531e-eng.pdf.

Statistics Canada (2012a). *Canada year book, 2012*. (Catalogue no. 11-402-X). Ottawa: Author. Retrieved from www.statcan.gc.ca/pub/11-402-x/11-402-x2012000-eng.htm.

Statistics Canada. (2012b). Leading causes of deaths in Canada, 2009. (CANSIM Table 102-0561). Ottawa: Author.

Statistics Canada. (2012c). The Canadian population in 2011: Age and sex. (Catalogue no. 98-311-X2011001). Ottawa: Author. Retrieved from www12.statcan.gc.ca/census-recensement/2011/as-sa/98-311-x/98-311-x2011001-eng.pdf.

Statistics Canada. (2012d). Health adjusted life expectancy by sex, 2005/2007. (CANSIM, table 102-0122 and Catalogue no. 82-221-X). Ottawa: Author. Retrieved from www.statcan.gc.ca/tables-tableaux/sum-som/l01/cst01/hlth67-eng.htm.

Statistics Canada. (2012, October 5). Employment by class of worker and industry (based on NAICS1)—Seasonally adjusted. (Catalogue 11-001-X). *The Daily*, Table 2. Ottawa: Author.

Straus, R. (1957). The nature and status of medical sociology. *American Sociological Review, 22*(2), 200–204.

Streiner, D. L., Cairney, J., & Lesage, A. (2005). Psychiatric epidemiology in Canada and the CCHS Study. *Canadian Journal of Psychiatry, 50*(10), 571–572.

Stone, D. (1999). Learning lessons and transferring policy across time, space and disciplines. *Politics, 19*(1), 51–59.

Storch, J. L. (2010). Ethics in nursing practice. In Kuhse, H., & Singer, P. (Eds.), *A companion to bioethics* (2nd ed.) (pp. 551–562). Oxford, UK: Wiley-Blackwell.

Strong-Boag, V. (1979). The girl of the new day: Canadian working women in the 1920s. *Labour/Le Travail, 4*, 131–164.

Sutherland, R. W., & Fulton, M. J. (1990). *Health care in Canada*. Ottawa: The Health Group.

Sutherns, R. (2005). So close yet so far: Rurality as a determinant of women's health. *Canadian Woman Studies, 24*(4), 117–122.

Suzuki, D. (2000). Experimenting with life. *Yes!, 1*(14), 1–4.

Swartz, D. (1977). The politics of reform: Conflict and accommodation in Canadian health policy." In Panitch, L. (Ed.), *The Canadian state: Political economy and political power* (pp. 311–343). Toronto: University of Toronto Press.

Szasz, T. S. (1961). *The myth of mental illness: Foundations of a theory of personal conduct*. New York: Harper.

Szasz, T. S. (1967). *The myth of mental illness: Foundations of a theory of personal conduct*. New York: Harper & Row.

Szasz, T. S., & Hollender, M. H. (1956). A contribution to the philosophy of medicine: the basic models of the doctor-patient relationship. *Archives of Internal Medicine, 97*(5), 585.

Szreter, S. (2002). Rethinking McKeown: The relationship between public health and social change. *American Journal of Public Health, 92*(5), 722–725.

Tacon, A. G., & Metian, M. (2008). Global overview on the use of fish meal and fish oil in industrially compounded aquafeeds: Trends and future prospects. *Aquaculture, 285*(1), 146–158.

Tanner, C. M., Kamel, F., Ross, G. W., Hoppin, J. A., Goldman, S. M., Korell, M., . . ., & Langston, J. W. (2011). Rotenone, paraquat, and Parkinson's disease. *Environmental health perspectives, 119*(6), 866.

Task Force Two. (2006). *Canada's physician workforce: Occupational human resources data assessment and trends analysis* (Final Report). *A physician human resource strategy for Canada: Final report*. Ottawa: Canadian Labour and Business Centre, Canadian Policy Research Networks Retrieved from www.physicianhr.ca/reports/TF2FinalStrategicReport-e.pdf.

Tavernise, S. (2013, December 11). F.D.A. restricts antibiotics use for livestock. *The New York Times*. Retrieved from www.nytimes.com/2013/12/12/health/fda-to-phase-out-use-of-some-antibiotics-in-animals-raised-for-meat.html?nl=todaysheadlines&emc=edit_th_20131212.

Thoits, P. A. (1995). Stress, coping, and social support processes: Where are we? What next? *Journal of Health and Social Behavior, 35*(Extra issue), 53–79.

Tholl, W. G. (1994). Health care spending in Canada: Skating faster on thinner ice. In Blomqvist, A., & Brown, D. M. (Eds.), *Limits to care: Reforming Canada's health system in an age of restraint* (pp. 53–89). Toronto: C. D. Howe Institute.

Thorslund, M., & Norström, T. (1993). The relationship between different survey measures of health in an elderly population. *Journal of Applied Gerontology, 12*(1), 61–70.

Timmermans, S., & Haas, S. (2008). Towards a sociology of disease. *Sociology of Health & Illness, 30*(5), 659–676.

Tjepkema, M. (2006). Adult obesity. *Health Reports, 17*(3), 9–25.

Todd, E. C. (1989). Costs of acute bacterial foodborne disease in Canada and the United States. *International Journal of Food Microbiology, 9*(4), 313–326.

Torrance, G. M. (1998). Socio-historical overview: The development of the Canadian health care system. In Coburn, D., D'Arcy, C., Torrance, G. M., & New, P. (Eds.), *Health and Canadian society: Sociological perspectives* (3rd ed.) (pp. 3–22). Toronto: University of Toronto Press.

Toscano, V. (2005). Misguided retribution: Criminalization of pregnant women who take drugs. *Social & Legal Studies, 14*(3), 359–386.

Tremblay, M. S., & Willms, J. D. (2003). Is the Canadian childhood obesity epidemic related to physical inactivity? *International Journal of Obesity, 27*(9), 1100–1105.

Trottier, H., Martel, L., Houle, C., Berthelot, J. M., & Légaré, J. (2000). Living at home or in an institution: What makes the difference for seniors? *Health Reports, 11*(4), 49–59.

Turner, B. (1992). *Regulating bodies: Essays in medical sociology*. London: Routledge.

Turner, B. (1995). *Medical power and social knowledge* (2nd ed.). Beverly Hills, CA: Sage.

Turner, B. (1996). *The body and society: Explorations in social theory*. Thousand Oaks, CA: Sage.

Turner, B. (2004). *The new medical sociology: Social forms of health and illness*. New York: W. W. Norton and Co.

Turner, B. (2010). *Vulnerability and human rights*. University Park, PA: Penn State Press.

Turner, L. (2002). Bioethical and end-of-life care in multi-ethnic settings: Cultural diversity in Canada and the USA. *Morality, 7*(3), 285–301.

Turner, R. J., & Avison, W. R. (1992). Innovations in the measurement of life stress: Crisis theory and the significance of event resolution. *Journal of Health and Social Behavior, 33*, 36–50.

Turner, R. J., & Noh, S. (1988). Physical disability and depression: A longitudinal analysis. *Journal of Health and Social Behavior, 29*, 23–37.

Twaddle, A. C. (1969). Health decisions and sick role variations: An exploration. *Journal of Health and Social Behavior, 10*(2), 105–114.

United Nations Food and Agriculture Organization. (n.d.). Global capture production 1950–2009. Rome, Italy: Author. Retrieved from www.fao.org/fishery/statistics/global-capture-production/query/en.

United States Department of Agriculture, Economic Research Service.(n.d.). Food CPI and expenditures. Washington, DC: Author. Retrieved from www.ers.usda.gov/Briefing/CPIFoodAndExpenditures/Data/Expenditures_tables/table1.htm.

Vaillant, G. (2002). *Aging well*. Boston, MA: Little, Brown and Company.

Valverde, M. (1985). *Sex, power and pleasure*. Toronto: Women's Press.

van Balen, E., Font, R., Cavallé, N., Font, L., Garcia-Villanueva, M., Benavente, Y., . . ., & de Sanjose, S. (2006). Exposure to non-arsenic pesticides is associated with lymphoma among farmers in Spain. *Occupational and Environmental Medicine, 63*(10), 663–668.

Varcoe, C., & Rodney, P. (2009). Constrained agency: The social structure of nurses' work. In Bolaria, B. S., & Dickinson H. (Eds.), *Health, illness, and health care in Canada* (4th ed.) (pp. 122–151). Toronto: Nelson Education.

Varul, M. Z. (2010). Talcott Parsons, the sick role and chronic illness. *Body & Society, 16*(2), 72–94.

Veenstra, G. (2007). Social space, social class and Bourdieu: Health inequalities in British Columbia, Canada. *Health and Place, 13*, 14–31.

Veenstra, G. (2009). Racialized identity and health in Canada: results from a nationally representative survey. *Social Science & Medicine, 69*(4), 538–542.

Verbrugge, L. M., & Wingard, D. L. (1987). Sex differentials in health and mortality. *Women & Health, 12*(2), 103–145.

Vinten-Johansen, P., Brody, H., Paneth, N., Rachman, S., & Rip, M. (2003). *Cholera, chloroform and the science of medicine: A life of John Snow*. London, Oxford: University Press.

Vioxx, Celebrex (2004, December 17). Concerns over popular arthritis drugs. *CBC News Online*. Retreived from www.cbc.ca/news/background/drugs/cox-2.html.

Virchow, R. (1848/2006). Report on the typhus outbreak of Upper Silesia. *American Journal of Public Health, 96*(12), 2102–2105.

Wade, T. J. (2001). Delinquency and health among adolescents: Multiple outcomes of a similar social and structural process. *International Journal of Law and Psychiatry, 24*(4-5), 447–467.

Wade, T. J., & Brannigan, A. (2010). Estimating population trends through secondary data: Attractions and limitations of national surveys. In Cairney, J., & Streiner, D. (Eds.), *Mental disorder in Canada: An epidemiologic perspective* (pp. 73–91). Toronto: University of Toronto Press.

Wade, T. J., & Cairney, J. (1997). Age and depression in a nationally representative sample of Canadians: A preliminary look at the National Population Health Survey. *Canadian Journal of Public Health, 88*(5), 297–304.

Wade, T. J., & Cairney, J. (2000a). The effect of sociodemographics, social stressors, health status and psychosocial resources on the age-depression relationship. *Canadian Journal of Public Health, 91*(4), 307–312.

Wade, T. J., & Cairney, J. (2000b). Major depressive disorder and marital transition among mothers: Results from a national panel study. *Journal of Nervous and Mental Disease, 188*(11), 741–750.

Wade, T. J., & Pevalin, D. J (2004). Marital transitions and mental health. *Journal of Health and Social Behavior, 45*(June), 155–170.

Wade, T. J., Pevalin, D. J., & Brannigan, A. (1999). The clustering of severe behavioural, health and educational deficits in Canadian children: Preliminary evidence from the National Longitudinal Survey of Children and Youth. *Canadian Journal of Public Health, 90*(4), 253–259.

Wade, T. J., Veldhuizen, S., & Cairney, J. (2011). Prevalence of psychiatric disorder in lone fathers and mothers: Examining the intersection of gender and family structure on mental health. *Canadian Journal of Psychiatry, 56*(9), 567–573.

Waitzkin, H. (1989). A critical theory of medical discourse: Ideology, social control, and the processing of social context in medical encounters. *Journal of Health and Social Behavior, 30*, 220–239.

Waitzkin, H. (1983). *The second sickness: Contradictions of capitalist health care*. New York: Free Press.

Wajcman, J. (1991). Patriarchy, technology, and conceptions of skill. *Work and Occupations, 18*(1), 29–45.

Waldron, I. (1995). Contributions of biological and behavioral factors to changing sex differences in ischaemic heart disease mortality. In Lopez A., Caselli G., & Valkonen T. (Eds.), *Adult mortality in developed countries: From description to explanation.* (pp. 161–178). Oxford: Clarendon Press.

Walters, V. (1982). State, capital and labour: The introduction of federal-provincial insurance for physician care in Canada. *Canadian Review of Sociology and Anthropology, 19*, 157–172.

Wardwell, W. I. (1992). The future of chiropractic. In Brown, P. (Ed.) *Perspectives in medical sociology* (2nd ed.), (pp. 485–506). Long Grove, IL: Waveland Press.

Wardwell, W. I. (1994). Alternative medicine in the United States. *Social Science & Medicine, 38*(8), 1061–1068.

Wasylenik, D. (2001). The paradigm shift from institution to community. In Rae-Grant, Q. (Ed.), *Psychiatry in Canada: 50 years*. Ottawa: Canadian Psychiatric Association.

Watts, R. (2010, March 11). Part nurse, part doctor, no job. Victoria *Times Colonist*. Retrieved from www2.canada.com/victoriatimes-colonist/news/capital_van_isl/story.html?id=0ee01466-887c-4e9d-bf86-e750bcdce3be.

Weber, M. (1958). *The protestant ethic and the spirit of capitalism.* (Talcott Parsons trans.) New York, Charles Scribner's Sons.

Wegener, H. C. (1999). The consequences for food safety of the use of fluoroquinolones in food animals. *New England Journal of Medicine, 340*(20), 1581.

Wegner, E. (1990). Deinstitutionalization and community-based care for the chronic mentally ill. In Greenley, J. R. (Ed.), *Research in community and mental health, volume 6: Mental disorders in social context* (pp 295–323). Greenwich, CT: JAI Press.

Weinstein, R. M. (1990). Mental hospitals and the institutionalization of patients. In Greenley, J. R. (Ed.), *Research in community and mental health, volume 6: Mental disorders in social context* (pp. 273–294). Greenwich CT: JAI Press.

Weinstein, R. M. (1982). The mental hospital from the patient's point of view. In Gove, W. (Ed.), *Deviance and mental illness* (pp. 121–146). Beverly Hills: Sage.

Weitz, R. (1996). *The sociology of health, illness, and health care: A critical approach*. New York: Wadsworth Publishing Co.

West, C. (1984). *Routine complications: Troubles with talk between doctors and patients*. Bloomington: Indiana University Press.

West, C., & Zimmerman, G. L. (1987). Doing gender. *Gender & Society, 1*(2), 125–151.

Wheaton, B. (1994). Sampling the stress universe. In Avison, W. R., & Gotlib, I. H. (Eds.), *Stress and mental health: Contemporary issues and prospects for the future* (pp. 77–114). New York: Plenum.

Wilensky, H. (1964). The professionalization of everyone? *American Journal of Sociology, 70*(September), 137–158.

Wilkinson, R. G. (1996). *Unhealthy societies: The afflictions of inequality*. London, England: Routledge.

Williams, G. (1984). The genesis of chronic illness: narrative reconstruction. *Sociology of Health & Illness, 6,* 175–200.

Williams, S. J. (2005). Parsons revisited: From the sick role to . . .? *Health, 9*(2), 123–144.

Willis, E. (1989). *Medical dominance: The division of labour in the Australian health care system* (2nd ed.). Sydney: George Allen and Unwin.

Winson, A. (2004). Bringing political economy into the debate on the obesity epidemic. *Agriculture and Human Values, 21*(4), 299–312.

Witz, A. (1992). *Professions and patriarchy*. London: Routledge.

Woodruff, T. J., Zota, A. R., & Schwartz, J. M. (2011). Environmental chemicals in pregnant women in the United States: NHANES 2003–2004. *Environmental Health Perspectives, 119*(6), 878.

World Economic Forum. (2013). *Global risks 2013* (8th ed.). Geneva: Author.

World Health Organization. (1948). Preamble to the Constitution of the World Health Organization as adopted by the International Health Conference, New York, 19–22 June, 1946; signed on 22 July 1946 by the representatives of 61 States (Official Records of the World Health Organization, no. 2, p. 100) and entered into force on 7 April 1948. New York: Author.

World Health Organization. (1978, Sept 6–12). International Conference on Primary Health Care, Alma-Ata, USSR. Retrieved from www.who.int/publications/almaata_declaration_en.pdf.

World Health Organization. (1986). *Ottawa charter for health promotion*. Geneva, Switzerland: World Health Organization European Office.

World Health Organization. (1992). *ICD-10 classifications of mental and behavioural disorder: Clinical descriptions and diagnostic guidelines*. Geneva: Author.

World Health Organization. (2003). *The world health report, 2003*. Geneva: Author.

World Health Organization. (2008). Closing the gap in a generation: Health equity through action on the social determinants of health. Commission on Social Determinants of Health. Geneva, Switzerland: World Health Organization European Office.

Wotherspoon, T. (1994). Colonization, self-determination, and the health of Canada's first nations peoples. In Bolaria, B. S., & Bolaria, R. (Eds.), *Racial minorities, medicine and health* (pp. 247–268). Halifax: Fernwood.

Wotherspoon, T. (2009). Transformation in Canadian nursing and nurse education. In Bolaria, B. S., & Dickinson, H. (Eds.), *Health, illness, and health care in Canada* (pp. 99–121). Toronto: Nelson Education.

Wright, D., Moran, J., & Gouglas, S. (2003). The confinement of the insane in Victorian Canada. In Porter R., & Wright, D. (Eds). *The confinement of the insane: International perspectives, 1800–1985* (pp. 100–128). New York: Cambridge University Press.

Wu, Z., Noh, S., Kaspar, V., & Schimmele, C. M. (2003). Race, ethnicity, and depression in Canadian society. *Journal of Health and Social Behavior, 44*(3), 426–41.

Yiridoe, E. K., Bonti-Ankomah, S., & Martin, R. C. (2005). Comparison of consumer perceptions and preference toward organic versus conventionally produced foods:

A review and update of the literature. *Renewable Agriculture and Food Systems, 20*(4), 193–205.

Yoshida, K. K. (1993). Reshaping of self: A pendular reconstruction of self and identity among adults with traumatic spinal cord injury. *Sociology of Health & Illness, 15*(2), 217–245.

Young, J. T. (2004). Illness behaviour: A selective review and synthesis. *Sociology of Health & Illness, 26*(1), 1–31.

Zborowski, M. (1969). *People in pain.* San Francisco: Jossey-Bass.

Zeytinoglu, I. U., Denton, M., Davies, S., & Plenderleith, J. M. (2009). Casualized employment and turnover intention: Home care workers in Ontario, Canada. *Health Policy, 91*(3), 258–268.

Zimmerman, G. L., Olsen, C. G., & Bosworth, M. F. (2000). A "stages of change" approach to helping patients with change behavior. *American Family Physician, 61,* 1409–1416.

Zola, I. K. (1972). Medicine as an institution of social control. In Conrad, P. (Ed.), *The sociology of health and illness: Critical perspectives* (pp. 404–414). New York: Worth.

Zola, I. K. (1994). Medicine as an institution of social control. In Conrad, P., & Kern, R. (Eds.), *The sociology of health and illness: Critical perspectives* (6th ed.) (pp. 392–402). New York: St. Martin's Press.

Index

Page numbers followed by "*f*" indicate figures, and those followed by "*t*" indicate tables.

cognitive development, theories of, 195–196
cohort study, 116
cold pasteurization, 281
collaborative practice, 79
community clinics, 97
community connectedness, 18
community health care
    primary care, in, 95
    primary care models, 95–96t
    private, fee-for-service (FFS) medical practice, 95
    social organization of health care, 95–99
Community Health Centres (CHCs), 79, 95, 97–98
community psychiatric services, 184–185
community shared agriculture (CSA), 296
Community Treatment Orders, 186
comorbidity, 168
complementary and alternative medicine (CAM), 66
    acupuncture, 71, 228
    and cancer, 245
    chiropractic medicine, 229
    defined, 70–71, 228–229
    and globalization, 229
    health care division of labour, 70–72
    holistic sickening, 245
    homeopathy, 71, 72, 228
    Interdisciplinary Network on Complementary and Alternative Medicine (IN-CAM), 230
    naturopathy, 70–72
    Traditional Chinese Medicine (TCM), 71, 228
    use of, 229–230
Composite International Diagnostic Interview (CIDI), 167
comprehensiveness, 41
concealable dimension of stigma, 243
concentrated animal feeding operations (CAFOs), 299
conceptual level, of medicalization, 258
concrete operations stage, 195
concurrent validity, 19
The Condition of the Working Class in England (Engels), 134
conflict theory, 6. See also materialism
constant comparison, 25
constellation of multiple characteristics, 122–124

construct validity, 19, 167
consumerism, 216, 225
consumers. See patients
contemplation stage, 219
content analysis, 25
continuing care, 203
continuity theory of aging, 192–193
control, 6
    components of, 59–60
    experimental control, 20
    and health inequalities, 144
    and medical dominance, 60
    statistical control, 21
control group, 20
convalescent homes, 85
Cooley, Charles, 9
cost-sharing, with governments, 37–38, 41
cottage hospitals, 87
course dimension of stigma, 243
credat emptor, 61
criterion validity, 167
critical gerontology, 193
critical perspectives on aging, 193
Critical Public Health (Labonté), 160
Critical to Care: The Invisible Women in Health (Armstrong), 92
critical voices, 184
cross-sectional survey, 21
cultural/behavioural argument, 146
cultural gerontophobia, 191–192
culture. See also ethnicity
    and illness, 249–250
cumulative effects, 140

D

daily hassles, 180
Danish natural experiment, 298
data
    comparison of quantitative and qualitative methods, 17t
    primary data, 18
    secondary data, 18
    sources of, 18
    tertiary data, 18
death. See mortality
death-ways, 210
decision-making power, 144
definition of the situation, 9
deinstitutionalization
    community psychiatric services, 184–185
    patient rights and critical voices, 184
    phases of, 186
demedicalization, 261–262
dementia, 198

Denton, Margaret, 209
dependence of society on care symptom, 266
dependence of society on drugs symptom, 266
dependent variable, 17
depersonalization, 89–90, 256
depression
    and ethnicity, 173
    and marital status, 177
    and race, 173
    and social causation, 176–177
    and stress process, 177
    and women, 181
deprofessionalization, 65, 226
deskilling, 67
despair task, 198
detail men, 270
diabetes, 109, 293
Diagnostic and Statistical Manual of Mental Disorders (DSM), 11, 165, 166, 261, 272
diagnostic imperialism, 257
diagnostic interviews, 167
Diagnostic Interview Schedule, 167
Diagnostic Interview Schedule for Children (DISC), 169
diagnostic services, 47
dilution, 278
direct measures of health, 110–111
direct-to-consumer marketing, 271
Discipling Old Age: The Formation of Gerontological Knowledge (Katz), 200
disciplining old age, 200
discreditable stigma, 242
discredited stigma, 242
discrimination, 8, 193, 263
disease
    causes of, 141, 143
    defined, 3
    etiology of, 255
    postmodernism, 11
    and socio-economic status, 141–143
    validation of, 3
disengagement theory of aging, 192
dispensing vs. prescribing medicine, 69
disruptiveness dimension of stigma, 243
distal risk factors, 141, 158, 160, 161
distribution, problem with HHR, 75, 76–78f
doctors. See also medical socialization
    American, 54
    and clinical iatrogenesis, 265–266

ownership of, 205
utilization of, 205
workers in, 205–206
low income cut-offs (LICO), 144

M

MacKinnon, J. B., 296
macro level
of aging, 194
described, x
of feminism, 7
of materialism, 6
measurement of, 18
by neo-Marxist theories, 62
of postmodernism, 11
sex and gender differences, 150
of theoretical frameworks, 4, 4f
Walkerton Inquiry, 292
mad cow disease, 283–284
maintenance stage, 219
males. *See* men
mandate, 61
Manitoba *Mincome* experiment,
147–148
marginal practitioners, 71
marital status
and depression, 177
and mental disorder, 173–174
and mental illness, 170, 172t,
173–174
marketing
direct-to-consumer
marketing, 271
food, 277
by pharmaceutical industry,
269–271
market model, 51, 228
Marmot, Michael, 144, 159
Marshall, Barbara, 199
Marx, Karl, 6, 9
Marxism, 143
massage, 71
mastery, 181
matched-group design, 20–21
materialism, 9
assumptions of, 4, 4f
class differences, 146–147
described, 6–7
health and sickness, 12
and quantitative methods, 16
Matthews, Anne Martin, 211
McKeown, Thomas, 126, 134, 138
McKeown thesis, 126, 134, 138
Mead, George Herbert, 9, 195
mean age, 119

meaning, 25–26
means of production, 6
measurement, and quantitative
methods, 17–18
measurement artifact, 146
Mechanic, David, 223–224
Mechanic's four dimensions for
assessing illness, 223–224
mechanistic-based perspective, 2, ix
Medical Care Act (1966), 40–41, 135
medical dominance
defined, 60
diagnostic imperialism, 257
rise and fall of, 64–66
medical encounter. *See* provider-
patient interaction
medical equipment companies, 268
medical gaze, 84, 256, 262
medical-industrial complex, 83
medical information, 65, 226
medicalization
of ADHD, 257, 258–259
of aging, 191
of alcoholism, 259
of childbirth, 259–261
defined, 255
demedicalization, 261–262
and healthism, 262–264
levels of, 257–258
and medical equipment
companies, 268
and pharmaceutical industry,
268–273
of pregnancy, 259–261
remedicalization, 261–262
and social constructionism, 258
of society, 257–264
of women's bodies, 12, 259–261
medicalization of expectation
symptom, 267
medicalization of prevention and early
diagnosis of illness symptom, 267
medicalization of the human lifespan
symptom, 266–267
medical knowledge
government and regulation, 257
medical model, 256–257
social construction of, 255–257
medical model, development of,
256–257
medical socialization, 9, 63, 64
medical sociology. *See also* sociology
of health
and antiracism, 9
described, x–xiii

and Parson's sick role, 238
and postcolonialism, 8–9
medical technologies,
103–105
medical tourism, 102
countries of destination for, by
world region, 231t
defined, 231
and globalization, 231–232
and transplant tourism, 232
Medicare. *See also* Canadian health
care system
before, 31–34
and CAM, 230
and class, 42
extended health services, 203
future of, 50–52
insured services, 203
national, start of, 37–39
National Forum on Health
(NFH), 47
public health care, sustainability
of, 53
reforms, 50–52
term used in United States, 41
Medicare in Saskatchewan, 34
medicine. *See also* complementary
and alternative medicine
(CAM)
anthroposophical medicine, 71
botanical medicine, 71
clinical iatrogenesis,
265–266
dispensing *vs.* prescribing, 69
history of, 256–257
telemedicine, 104
Western, allopathic
medicine, 84
membership, as social closure, 60
men. *See also* gender
and cancer, 247–248
and heart disease, 246–247
leading cause of death, 126, 127t,
149–150
life expectancy of, 126–129,
149–150
risky behaviour of, 152
seeking medical help, 151, 226
and treatment imperative, 247
Men and Their Work (Hughes), 61
menopause, 249
mental disorder, 165, 172t. *See also*
mental illness
Mental Health Commission of Canada
(MHCC), 46, 187